T0073261

ENDING EPIDEMICS

A History of Escape from Contagion

RICHARD CONNIFF

The MIT Press
Cambridge, Massachusetts
London, England

The MIT Press would like to thank the anonymous peer reviewers who provided comments on drafts of this book. The generous work of academic experts is essential for establishing the authority and quality of our publications. We acknowledge with gratitude the contributions of these otherwise uncredited readers.

This book was set in Adobe Garamond and Berthold Akzidenz Grotesk by Westchester Publishing Services. Printed and bound in the United States of America.

Library of Congress Cataloging-in-Publication Data

Names: Conniff, Richard, 1951– author.
Title: Ending epidemics : a history of escape from contagion / Richard Conniff.
Description: Cambridge, Massachusetts : The MIT Press, [2023] |
    Includes bibliographical references and index.
Identifiers: LCCN 2022016588 (print) | LCCN 2022016589 (ebook) |
    ISBN 9780262047968 (hardcover) | ISBN 9780262373852 (epub) |
    ISBN 9780262373869 (pdf)
Subjects: LCSH: Epidemics—History.
Classification: LCC RA649 .C67 2023 (print) | LCC RA649 (ebook) |
    DDC 614.4—dc23/eng/20220715
LC record available at https://lccn.loc.gov/2022016588
LC ebook record available at https://lccn.loc.gov/2022016589

10 9 8 7 6 5 4 3 2 1

For those who have given their lives
to the cause of ending epidemics

Contents

Preface: The Healing

In our hearts, none of us believed the pandemic would come next year, or even within our lifetimes. We may have wallowed in the eye-bleeding horrors of *The Hot Zone* or the rampant infectiousness of the movie *Contagion*, but it was voyeuristic: we were thrilled and yet managed to keep these viral horrors separate from our own lives.

The turning point for me came just after midnight one day in my first month of COVID-19 lockdown, on reading a news report of deaths in a pandemic hotspot. "Some crematories in New York City are incinerating bodies at four times the normal rate," it said. "Hospitals have run out of body bags or turned to forklifts to transfer piles of corpses into makeshift mobile morgues." This wasn't London in a plague year. It was now, in neighborhoods that I knew. And it suddenly seemed strange that we could ever have felt safe, or would ever do so again.[1]

Why was it so shocking? Where had we come by the implausible sense of our safety? It's based on how those of us born since World War II have spent our lives, without quite recognizing just how fortunate we have been. This is mainly true in the developed world. But low-income nations have also shared in the benefits, especially in this century. Thanks to modern medical discoveries, a swarm of diseases that were once our ancestors' familiar lot have faded away, in many cases within living memory. That's the subject of this book: It's the story of humanity's long and, until now, extraordinarily successful struggle against infectious diseases.

If this were another time in our history, we would be accustomed to sickness and death from diseases including malaria, diphtheria, yellow fever, scarlet fever, plague, polio, cholera, tetanus, tuberculosis, typhus, typhoid fever, and smallpox. Quaint-seeming terms like *blood poisoning*, from causes as trivial as a splinter, or *lockjaw*, from a rusty nail, would still be on every mother's tongue. We would expect children to spend long weeks laid up with whooping cough, mumps, chicken pox, and measles. One child in three would die before reaching school age.

Depending on how old you are, you can count off these diseases according to how close an escape you have made. Polio, for instance, caused permanent paralysis in 21,300 Americans and killed 3,150 in 1952, shortly before the Salk vaccine arrived. Measles was infecting more than 530,000 American children in an average year and killing 440 before the arrival of a vaccine in 1963. And in 1974, on the brink of eradication, smallpox still infected 218,000 people worldwide and killed about a third of them.[2]

I can count off this history of escape from infectious disease in my own family, and it's a measure of how recent, dramatic, and personal this change has been: Growing up in the Bronx in the 1920s, my uncle had polio, and it left him on crutches for life. But "polio season" became summer again for me, after my grade school class reluctantly lined up in 1956 to receive Jonas Salk's new polio vaccine. I came down with measles, on the other hand, in the prevaccine peak epidemic of 1958 and was laid out for a week, with voices whispering outside my bedroom door and the curtains drawn tight to block out the sun. In the United States, measles killed 552 children that year. I also had most of the other childhood diseases, as did my classmates. My children had just one, chicken pox, for which a vaccine became available only in 1995.

To say this happened in living memory may, however, overstate the case. It is the catch-22 of vaccines and, in truth, of all infectious disease discoveries: they save us from diseases, then cause us to forget the diseases from which they have saved us. You get a sense of how clueless we were about epidemics before COVID-19 by the casual way we used the word, with our anxious talk about the obesity epidemic, the autism epidemic, even the tanning epidemic, and of course the epidemic of anxiety.

Once a disease like measles appears to be gone from our lives, we become lax, or worse. Well-meaning parents increasingly avoid vaccinating their children, particularly when it comes to the measles-mumps-rubella (MMR)

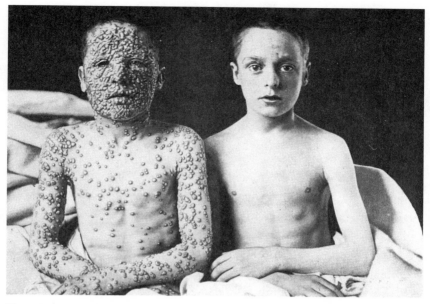

Figure 0.1

During an earlier era in vaccine hesitancy, Dr. Allan Warner, a physician in Leicester, England, took this photo to remind people what they were risking. Both boys were exposed to smallpox on the same day. Only one had been vaccinated.

vaccine. As a result, a major measles outbreak in 2019 sickened children in Europe, the United States, and other areas that vaccination had once made measles-free. Parents had forgotten that children with measles can die or suffer permanent intellectual disability. They forgot that an outbreak of rubella in the 1960s resulted in twenty thousand American children being born with brain damage, including autism and other abnormalities. Much as our forebears were fatalistically accepting of epidemic diseases, we had become naively oblivious to them.

Even the HIV/AIDS epidemic did not change this overall picture, despite the suffering and death it continues to cause. When antiretroviral therapy became available in the 1990s, people who tested positive accepted it and found they could lead normal lives again. Worldwide life expectancy, having more than doubled in the twentieth century, continued to edge upward—until COVID-19.

THE STRUGGLE TO REMEMBER

This book started out as a conscious effort to remember. One day I was checking my yellow international immunization card, which I keep with my passport, and found myself puzzling over the entry for Tdap. I recognized the *t* for *tetanus* and the *p* for *pertussis*, or whooping cough. But I was ignorant about the *d*. Even pediatricians now tend to know diphtheria only from textbooks. But before the development of serum therapy in the 1890s and effective vaccines in the twentieth century, diphtheria was among the great terrors of childhood. It killed more than three thousand young Americans one year in the mid-1930s, when my parents were in high school. It is once again killing children today in Venezuela, Yemen, and other areas where political upheaval has disrupted the delivery of vaccine.

Among other symptoms, diphtheria clots a child's throat with a gray membrane of dead cells, which can cause death by strangulation. In past epidemics, it was sufficiently contagious to take down whole families of children—whole streets of them—leaving only the shattered parents behind in the sudden quiet. (I write about it in chapter 22.) From diphtheria, I soon found myself digging back into the story of the people who came to understand such terrible diseases and consign them to history.

My interest is specifically in how researchers found ways to save us from some of the deadliest infectious diseases and how their stories can help us continue to escape such diseases well into the future. Past accounts of medical discovery tended to hagiography, perhaps because the grateful writers still had personal experience of the diseases being overcome. Winston Churchill, who saw a friend die of typhoid in South Africa and whose father is said to have died from tertiary syphilis, once wrote that the beatific choir should make room for Saint Anesthesia, Saint Antiseptic, and Saint Penicillin, each with a suitable feast day. He wasn't entirely joking.[3]

For today's readers, though, that note of veneration feels misplaced. Maybe that's another symptom of our having forgotten the diseases medical discoverers cured or prevented. But we have also come to recognize that heroes too often turn out, on closer examination, to be problematic. As a group, until the mid-twentieth century, medical discoverers were almost exclusively white and male. They frequently came from families that were relatively wealthy or of the "right" social class. Most lived in nations subsidized by empire, able to extract wealth, knowledge, and products from colonized countries and with a financial system capable of supporting education and scientific research. They accomplished great things. But like athletes caught using performance-enhancing drugs, it can seem as if they should go into the history books with an asterisk.

Marginalized groups were often vehemently denied any credit, even when their contribution to a medical advance was public knowledge. During a 1721 smallpox epidemic in Boston, for instance, African-born residents of the city revealed a method to prevent this deadly disease. It worked, but their role was minimized and ridiculed from the start. And when a woman introduced the same method in England, based on first-hand experience in Turkey, her recompense included a heaping bowlful of misogynist bile. (I write about these cases in chapter 6.)

As I worked on this book, I tried where possible to position individuals we think of as lone geniuses within the network of people on whom they depended. Louis Pasteur, for instance, was always known to be an ambitious and enthusiastic self-promoter, but he depended on largely unacknowledged contributions by physician Émile Roux, among others (I write about them in chapters 17 and 21). It's possible to say this while still recognizing Pasteur as a master of experimental science and brilliant at choosing the right path from one experiment to the next. Likewise, Joseph Lister, who introduced antiseptics to the operating room, depended throughout his career on research performed in their home laboratory by Agnes Syme, his wife—and yet Lister excluded her from any credit for their work. (I write about them in chapter 15.) Jonas Salk acknowledged that his polio vaccine benefited from a key contribution by John Enders, but he overlooked Isabel Morgan, who developed a crucial forerunner of the vaccine (see chapter 30).

Legend to the contrary, no great medical discovery was ever the unaided work of a lone genius or wholly original. New ideas don't just appear out of nowhere and instantly change everything. Instead, they rise up over and over like waves and mostly beat themselves out against the sand, unnoticed. It takes special circumstances, lucky timing, the subtle influence of previous waves, before an idea gathers strength and becomes a tsunami. Beta versions of a discovery may appear repeatedly before taking hold. The work we end up labeling *genius* was rarely just a matter of making a discovery. It was also about making the discovery *known* well enough to break through the wall of tradition-bound indifference. It was about building a case to make the discovery *believed* beyond reasonable doubt.

Nor has any great discovery ever resulted from the special blessing of the gods. Everything resulted first from favorable circumstances, and then from long preparation, followed by endlessly patient watching and thinking about the problem at hand (with a certain amount of discreet eavesdropping on what others were doing and thinking), followed by experimentation, repeated over and over, with small variations, frequent failures, no guarantee of eventual success, and frustration leading at times to the brink of madness.

The idea that great scientists come with abundant flaws and that medical discovery has always depended on collaboration may at first seem less inspiring. But I have found medical discoverers much easier to understand as leading figures in a network of collaborators than as heroic demigods. Their quirks and missteps remind us that people with ordinary failings can nonetheless achieve great and heroic things together. Knowing how they struggled with familiar human issues (and with one another) ought to make it easier for rising scientists, particularly those feeling marginalized by gender, race, or sexual orientation, to set aside imposter syndrome and walk more confidently in their own footsteps.

Among other characteristics, it seemed to me as I was working on this book that past medical discoverers were often adept not just at synthesizing existing lines of research, but also at imagining how to push them forward in surprising ways. They consistently displayed an urge to see things with their own eyes, rather than rely on what they learned in classrooms or textbooks. During an 1835 autopsy, for instance, medical student and amateur botanist James Paget looked more closely at gritty specks in muscle, which his instructors described as bits of bone. With the help of a microscope, Paget discovered that they were, in fact, cysts containing parasitic worms. "I believe," he explained, "that I alone 'looked-at' them and 'observed' them: no one trained in natural history could have failed to do so." (See chapter

10.) Paying close attention to the complex lives of plants and animals was good training for observing the symptoms of patients and the behaviors of microbes.[4]

It struck me, as I did my research, that the study of the diseases of humans and other animals is itself a branch of natural history. It's a story of coming to understand the human body as a habitat and many human diseases as a colonization of that habitat. Diseases also have their own evolutionary history, appearing or disappearing, becoming more virulent or less so, jumping from one species to another, with baffled humans struggling to figure it all out before it kills us. Medical discovery itself is not linear, one great idea emerging from another in a neat progression. It's more like evolution—branchy, confused, with lots of false starts and dead ends. We don't "conquer disease," the trope of past medical histories. More often, medical discoveries enable us to fend off diseases for a time as they emerge, evolve, and then reemerge.

In what follows, I have attempted to weave together all the threads of discovery into a single story of the struggle against disease across three centuries. It starts with the first description of bacteria on April 24, 1676 (chapter 1) and ends with the eradication of smallpox and the last known death from it on September 11, 1978 (chapter 31). Readers will object that HIV/AIDS, Ebola, COVID-19, and other emerging diseases have taught us too well that the story does not end there. But the eradication of smallpox was a turning point in human history and remains a powerful model for what humans can still achieve when we set aside differences and work together against disease.

In between these two events, I focus on a series of key developments that persuaded the medical world to stop seeking the causes of epidemic disease in noxious miasmas, bodily humors, or divine dyspepsia. Instead they learned to focus on pathogens—and also on dramatic improvements in sanitation, control of disease-carrying arthropods, the proliferation of antiseptics, the discovery of antibiotics and other antimicrobials, and the development of new vaccines and technologies.

If I sometimes dwell on the dreadful symptoms of past diseases, that's deliberate, a reminder of just how much we owe the researchers who enabled us to escape these symptoms. It's also a reminder of how important it is to muster public will for the inconvenient work of preventing or controlling these diseases.

As you read, it will help to set aside present knowledge. Forget what you know about bacteria, say, or mosquitoes, and instead try stepping back into the minds of our forebears. Imagine a time when all anyone really understood about infectious disease was death, often coming in a terrifying rush of symptoms that either drove away the victim's loved ones or kept them close to become victims themselves. Then imagine what it took to make sense of these unknown and unimaginable forces and somehow stop them. Putting ourselves in the minds of our predecessors and in the face of such diseases is a way to appreciate how hard it was to achieve the sense of safety we take for granted.

It may also turn out to be useful practice for other pandemics still to come.

1 WHAT THE DRAPER SAW

The life of one seventeenth-century Dutch merchant was more fortunate than most. Antoni van Leeuwenhoek (1632–1723) lived to be ninety, seemingly unscathed by infectious disease. But he saw death all around him. He lost two infant siblings while still a child, then his father when he was just five, and his stepfather when he was fifteen. Later, he lost four of his five children by his first wife, who died when she was just thirty-six. His second wife survived twenty-three years of marriage and produced one child, who also died.

Leeuwenhoek was not, however, driven by a compulsion to understand why this should be so. He was a draper, a cloth merchant, knowledgeable in matters of button loops and bombazine, not human physiology. And yet his work, or rather what he did in the hours before and after work, would begin the unraveling of the dark secrets of infectious disease.

Leeuwenhoek was born into a family of basket-makers and brewers in a spacious, three-story canal house in Delft, a coastal city of more than twenty thousand people. Delft merchants were among the founding partners in the Dutch East India Company, the world's first transnational corporation. The wealth it produced in the colonial trade for spices, sugar, and other commodities translated into opportunity at home, much as poverty elsewhere sent genius packing off unnoticed to an early grave. It's a measure of Delft's prosperity in the Dutch Golden Age that Leeuwenhoek's christening was entered into the baptismal registry of the city's Nieuwe Kerk on the same page as another newborn of 1632 named Johannes Vermeer, and each lived to fulfill his native genius.

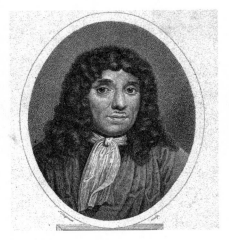

Figure 1.1
Leeuwenhoek in a 1686 portrait (Wellcome Collection).

In 1654, after a six-year internship with an Amsterdam merchant, Leeuwenhoek returned to Delft to establish his own fabric business. He married, purchased a home around the corner from the central market square, and began to play a part in civic affairs. To science, though, he was "merely an ordinary shopkeeper, holding a few minor municipal appointments," in the words of one biographer. Nor was he physically memorable. Contemporary portraits depict him in sumptuous robes and a periwig, but they also capture the shallow eyes, set slightly wide in a round face, above a substantial nose and an abbreviated pencil mustache.[1]

A NEW VISIBLE WORLD

People tend now to remember Leeuwenhoek as the inventor of the microscope. But that essential discovery in the history of medicine emerged in the late 1500s, a lifetime before his birth. His fascination with microscopes dates only from the 1660s, and it was a book that awakened him to the discoveries being made possible by magnification.

"By the means of Telescopes, there is nothing so far distant but may be represented to our view; and by the help of Microscopes, there is nothing so small, as to escape our inquiry," British polymath Robert Hooke wrote in *Micrographia*, published in 1665. "Hence there is a new visible World discovered to the understanding . . . and in every little particle of its matter, we now behold almost as great a variety of Creatures, as we were able before to reckon up in the whole Universe itself."[2]

Micrographia was the first true scientific picture book, with finely detailed illustrations in the author's own hand. London diarist Samuel Pepys bought an early copy that January, and he sat up until 2:00 a.m. on a Saturday night with what he pronounced "the most ingenious book that ever I read in my life." Hooke depicted a Gargantuan flea in extreme close-up, on a gatefold page wider than the book itself, so the flea seemed to leap cat-like into the reader's lap. He made "a small white spot of hairy mould" found on the leather cover of a book look like a flower garden on spindly stalks. These "Microscopical Mushroms" were actually the reproductive structures of a small fungus belonging to the genus *Mucor*. It was the first description by any human observer of a microbial life form.[3]

Micrographia may initially have caught Leeuwenhoek's eye as a fabric merchant, an occupation that relied on the equivalent of a jeweler's loupe to make thread counts. The book's illustrations included a piece of fine linen

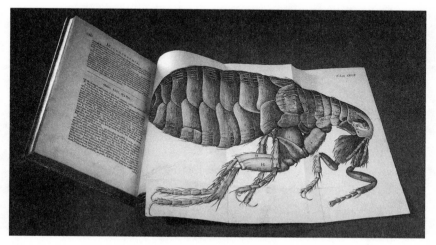

Figure 1.2
Robert Hooke's flea attempts an escape (Wellcome Collection).

magnified to look like "coarse Matting," as Hooke put it, and a bit of taffeta silk ribbon seeming "like a very convenient substance to make. . . . Door-matts." But Hooke urged readers "to proceed further, and to attempt greater things in the same and different wayes." Leeuwenhoek took heed, moving beyond fabrics into the biological world, where he would travel widely over the rest of his life.

Hooke preferred to work with a conventional compound microscope, a tube with lenses at each end, mounted on a stand, which he said was easier on the "weakness" of his eyes. But he also described a technique that seems to have become the basis for Leeuwenhoek's very different single-lens microscopes. It involved heating "a very clear piece of a broken Venice Glass" with a candle, drawing the glass out into threads, and then heating these threads in the flame till a small globule formed on the end. After the maker ground off the rough parts of this globule and polished it with Tripoli buffing compound, it could be mounted as a pinhole lens in what looked like a handheld magnifying glass, usually about three or four inches long. To examine a specimen, Leeuwenhoek generally glued it to a pin or sometimes placed it on a glass plate mounted in front of the lens. One screw, which doubled as a handle, allowed him to move the specimen up or down. Another screw moved it in or out. He could thus position the specimen in front of the lens for a precise focus as he held the instrument up to his eye.[4]

In the spring of 1673, eight years after publication of *Micrographia*, a letter arrived at the Royal Society in London from a Delft physician who was a fellow of the society. "I am writing to tell you," he began, "that a certain most ingenious person named Leewenhoeck has devised microscopes which far surpass those which we have hitherto seen." He enclosed a letter in which Leeuwenhoek described some of his first rudimentary findings. The physician urged the society to "test the skill of this most diligent man" by "proposing to him more difficult problems of the same kind." With this introduction, Leeuwenhoek began a lifelong correspondence with the Royal Society, where Robert Hooke himself was then curator of experiments. He had moved on from microbes to roam brilliantly across the scientific universe. Leeuwenhoek, by contrast, stuck with a shopkeeper's patience to his microscopes. The skill and curiosity with which he explored the microbial world over the next half century would transform the human body and the planet itself from the intimately familiar to something astonishingly strange and populous.

AN ABUNDANCE OF LITTLE ANIMALS

Almost from the start, Leeuwenhoek saw things no one ever had. He was apparently blessed with excellent vision and he was able to grind his lenses more finely than others could, enabling him to magnify his specimens by as much as three hundred times their actual size and resolve objects almost down to a micron. He worked in a room with a northeastern exposure lit by a bank of leaded-glass casement windows, of the sort familiar from numerous Vermeer paintings. Like Vermeer, Leeuwenhoek made himself a master of finding the best light for any given subject, by flinging open the shutters or drawing them tight, adjusting the curtains, working by candlelight, or other means he chose to keep secret.[5]

He was also a skilled craftsman at the precise metalwork needed to position and hold each lens, producing more than five hundred different magnifying devices over the course of his career, each suited to a different subject. His workroom was equipped with small smelting furnaces, metalworking machinery, a glassblowing table, lens-grinding materials, and other equipment. Then there were the specimens: "Van Leeuwenhoek made thin slices of optical nerves, brains, hair, tongue, spleen, muscle, eye, tendon, bone marrow, skin and fat, as well as all kinds of botanical materials," Lesley A. Robertson and her coauthors write in *Antoni van Leeuwenhoek: Master of the Minuscule*. "He boiled brains to make them easier to handle or reveal structures more clearly. Sometimes, he found it necessary to wash away soft tissue, or let it . . . rot away."[6]

Leeuwenhoek reported his observations in letters to the Royal Society. Henry Oldenburg, a German immigrant who was then secretary there, translated them into English, edited them, and deemed them remarkable enough to publish in issue after issue of the society's *Philosophical Transactions*. What Leeuwenhoek was seeing bordered on the fantastical. A sample of water from a nearby lake contained an "abundance of little animals, some of which were roundish," he wrote, others oval, some "whitish, others pellucid," still others with "green and very shining little scales." A few of these creatures were plodding, but "the motion of most of them in the water was so swift," Leeuwenhoek wrote, "and so various, upwards, downwards, and round about, that I confess I could not but wonder at it." Leeuwenhoek was peering for the first time into the unsuspected world of microorganisms that behaved like animals. He was describing protozoa, a group of single-celled microorganisms that includes both free-living and parasitic species.[7]

Leeuwenhoek sometimes called the microscopic creatures he was describing "little eels or worms," sometimes "exceedingly small insects or animals," and sometimes just "animalcules," a Latin diminutive. It would be another sixty years before Carolus Linnaeus would devise the system of naming living things by genus and species. Along with nonexistent nomenclature, Leeuwenhoek lacked anything remotely like standard units of measurement at the microscopic scale. He made do with homely comparisons. One sort of "little animals" was "a thousand times smaller than the eye of a louse." Another was as small relative to a cheese mite as a bee is to a horse. Leeuwenhoek intended none of these comparisons casually. He took the development of a system of measurements as seriously as he did the making of lenses and microscopes. Such comparisons led him to make the eye-widening estimate that a single drop of water could contain a million of these minute creatures.[8]

Apart from the seemingly outlandish observations, this relatively new correspondent often wrote in a conversational tone, interspersed with opinions and details of his personal life. "He sets down his views—frequently quite mistaken and even ridiculous views—with childish and charming simplicity," British microbiologist Clifford Dobell wrote, with obvious affection, in his 1932 biography of Leeuwenhoek, "and he has no feeling of embarrassment in telling the Royal Society the most intimate details about his blood, his sweat, or his urine; or about his sicknesses or his habits or his little vanities."[9]

This extreme candor was a product of unquenchable curiosity, not exhibitionism. Oldenburg had specifically asked Leeuwenhoek to focus on the secretions of the human body, and Leeuwenhoek duly examined his own semen, among other things. He obtained it not by "sinfully defiling" himself, he wrote in 1677, but "before six beats of the pulse had intervened" after ejaculation, presumably during intercourse with his very patient wife. He thus became the first person to describe spermatozoa.[10]

Leuwenhoek may have thought that omitting minor details could compromise what he correctly regarded as major scientific observations. He relied on Oldenburg to edit out what seemed irrelevant. But Leeuwenhoek's apparent naiveté and "ridiculous views" also cast a persistent shadow on the remarkable things he discovered. Visiting on behalf of the Royal Society in 1685, a student in nearby Leiden tut-tutted that Leeuwenhoek was "quite a stranger to letters, master neither of Latin French or English, or any other of the modern tongues besides his own." He was thus prone to "very odd accounts of things, nay sometimes sutch as are wholy irreconsilable with all truth." Even decades after Leeuwenhoek was firmly established as one of the geniuses of the day, a visitor could still remark, one eyebrow lifted, that he "has been accused of seeing more with his imagination than with his magnifying glasses."

Leeuwenhoek's foibles did not compromise his science: "Despite the imperfections of his language and his lack of scientific education," Dobell wrote, the letters are "a model for all other workers. He never confuses his facts with his speculations. When recording facts he invariably says 'I have observed . . . ,' but when giving his interpretations he prefaces them with 'but I imagine . . .' or 'I figure to myself . . .' Few scientific workers . . . have had so clear a conception of the boundary between observation and theory, fact and fancy, the concrete and the abstract."[11]

THIS SO WONDERFUL A SPECTACLE

Leeuwenhoek was adamant about what he was seeing, while acknowledging that it might seem unbelievable. Informed that "people of great knowledge in Paris" doubted another of his observations, he replied, "I do not mind this at all. What I wrote on this subject is perfectly true." They were welcome to come see for themselves.[12]

On October 9, 1676, Leeuwenhoek sent off his "Letter 18," now regarded as the founding document for the science of microbiology. It ran to seventeen-and-a-half folio pages of tightly written script. The letter represented a year's research into Leeuwenhoek's "little animals" and contained 145 observations, in water from well, river, sea, and rooftop, as well as in water infused with peppercorns, ginger, clove, and nutmeg. (The colonial spice trade was everywhere in Leeuwenhoek's research.)[13]

Letter 18 consisted mainly of things he saw on specific dates, without any unifying narrative thread. "I have couched my observations in the form of a journal," Leeuwenhoek explained to a colleague, "merely that they be better credited in England" and among those disbelievers in Paris. He was emphatic about the care with which he made his observations. "*Note*," he advised the Royal Society, "that when I say, I have view'd the water, I mean, that . . . in scrutinizing 3 or 4 drops I may do such a lot of work that it keeps me in a sweat." That care and diligence enabled him to see a host of protozoa and other microorganisms, many of them described accurately enough, despite the lack of proper nomenclature, for modern scientists to recognize them by genus or species.[14]

The most momentous of these sightings took place on April 24, 1676. While examining a sample he had prepared earlier that month of water with whole peppercorns mixed in, Leeuwenhoek "discern'd in it, to [his] great wonder, an incredible number of [very] little animals of divers kinds." Three of them were of types he had seen before, but "the 4th sort of creatures" were so small he thought "ten hundred thousand of them could not equal the dimensions" of a grain of coarse sand. Microbiologists now regard this as the first unmistakable description of bacteria, the organisms responsible for so many of our infectious diseases.

Leeuwenhoek could scarcely contain his excitement at the sheer number of these organisms. "For me this was among all the marvels that I have discovered in nature the most marvellous of all," he wrote, "and I must say that, for my part, no more pleasant sight has yet met my eye than this of so many thousands of living creatures in one small drop of water, all huddling and moving, but each creature having its own motion."

The reaction at the Royal Society was more like consternation. The learned gentlemen there temporized for five months. When they finally published Letter 18 in March, they inserted a cautionary note at the idea of hundreds of thousands of organisms in a single drop of water: "This Phaenomenon and some of the following ones seeming to be very extraordinary, the Author hath been desired to acquaint us with his method of observing, that others may confirm such Observations as these."[15]

For all his candor about his personal life, Leeuwenhoek could be secretive about his methods. But he now followed through on his offer to have other scholars look on as he worked, so they could see what he saw. Their testimonials revealed that Leeuwenhoek studied his water samples in a capillary glass tube the thickness of a horse hair, divided into measured parts. Leeuwenhoek also explained the homely comparisons he used to estimate microbial populations. He started with a drop of water the size of a green pea, and the number of millet seeds that would fit in a pea. With a bookkeeper's attention to detail, he worked his way downward from there to smaller and smaller units of measure. He also upped his count for the number of organisms seen in a single drop of water to more than eight million.[16]

Seeking to replicate Leeuwenhoek's work, the Royal Society turned to Robert Hooke, who was already beginning to develop a reputation for quarrelsome rivalries. Called on now to deal with this microscopic newcomer, Hooke sounded like an old gunslinger reluctantly retrieving his weapons. "I put in order," he wrote "such remainders as I had of my former Microscopes (having by reason of a weakness in my sight omitted the use of them for many years.)" Then he prepared an infusion of peppercorns in water and set to work certain he "would discover things much smaller than such as the aforesaid Mr. Leeuwenhoeck had affirmed these creatures to be."

At first, he found nothing at all. He gave up for most of a week, until "finding it a warm day, I examined again the said water; and then much to wonder I discovered vast multitudes of those exceeding small creatures, which Mr. Leeuwenhoeck had described." After trying out other microscopes and other lighting arrangements, "I discovered many other sorts very much smaller than those I first saw, and some of these so exceeding small, that millions of millions might be contained in one drop of water. I was very much surprized at this so wonderful a spectacle." He could hardly have imagined that nature could contain "so exceedingly minute animal productions. But nature is not to be limited by our narrow apprehensions."[17]

Instead of quarrelling with Leeuwenhoek, Hooke then became his great advocate. He published "*a letter of the Ingenious and Inquisitive* Mr. Leeuwenhoeck of Delft," together with his own findings. "The prospect of those small animals" was so pleasing to all who saw them, Hooke wrote to Leeuwenhoek, that King Charles II "was desirous to see them and very well pleasd with the Observation and mentiond your Name at the same time."[18]

In 1680, a vellum diploma, embossed with the Royal Society's red seal and shipped in a silver box, announced to the shopkeeper from Delft that he was henceforth a Fellow of the Royal Society. It was the great honor of Leeuwenhoek's life. He had his portrait painted with the diploma prominently displayed in the foreground. And an envious Dutch colleague sneered that this new "great man of the century" had inquired, on receiving his fellowship, if he would still be obliged to "take a back seat in the presence of a doctor of medicine!" But beyond its significance for Antoni van Leeuwenhoek, his discovery of microorganisms meant that thoughtful researchers could begin to explore the link between microorganisms and infectious diseases. Deliverance from epidemic disease was now possible.[19]

2 DEADLY PRECONCEPTIONS

It was possible—but it didn't happen. Leeuwenhoek himself came so tantalizingly close to the link between microorganisms and disease that the reader possessed of modern knowledge at times wants to shout, "Wait, Antoni! Go back!" One anonymous reader did just that, writing to *Philosophical Transactions* soon after it published Letter 18 to suggest that Leeuwenhoek's work "may prompt us to suspect that our Air is also vermiculated"—that is, alive with "worms"—particularly "in seasons of general Infections of Men or Animals."[1]

Leeuwenhoek hadn't found microorganisms in the air, as the editors noted in an aside to that reader's letter. But he found them in other places that might have suggested their role in disease. In 1681, for instance, he advised the Royal Society, with his customary candor, that "I . . . ordinarily have a fairly thick stool in the morning." But a bout of diarrhea had led him to apply his microscope to a sample, in which he found "animalcules moving very prettily," with bodies "a little longer than broad," and bellies "flattish and furnished with several legs, with which they moved through the clear matter" like "a wood-louse running up against a wall." It was a protozoan parasite now called *Giardia*, which causes one of the more debilitating forms of diarrhea. Leeuwenhoek recognized that these animalcules did not normally turn up in his stool samples, but it seems not to have occurred to him that they might have been the cause of his discomfort.[2]

Likewise, in 1683, Leeuwenhoek applied his microscope to his own dental plaque and sent a letter, with such clear illustrations of microorganisms living there that a modern microbiologist could recognize some of the same bacterial species that inhabit our mouths today. Leeuwenhoek also sampled plaque from a man who claimed never to have cleaned his mouth and found the animalcules "so excessively numerous that all the water seemed to live." But he made no attempt to connect these bacterial communities with tooth decay or other health problems, except perhaps "a stinking mouth." Leeuwenhoek was caught up instead, understandably, in the wonderment that there could be "more animals in the unclean matter on the teeth in one's mouth than there are men in a whole Kingdom." His genius lay in seeing well and describing what he saw, not in saying what it meant.[3]

HUMORAL THINKING

To understand why Leeuwenhoek's discoveries did not immediately revolutionize medical thinking, it's necessary to backtrack a little and understand the world contemporary physicians inhabited. Humoral theory dominated medicine then, and it must have seemed like a beautifully complete paradigm for understanding the human body and its many malfunctions. Health consisted of a balance among four bodily fluids—blood, black bile, yellow bile, and phlegm. Sickness had to do with something in the individual's makeup that threw these fluids out of their natural equilibrium, in response to miasmas (noxious air or atmosphere), effluvia (emanations from the decay of bodily matter), telluric forces (movements within the earth), or the alignment of the heavens (*influenza* at first meant "influenced by the stars"), among other factors. Infectious diseases did not exist as we now think of them, caused by distinct pathogens originating outside the human body, nor was there much medical consideration of diseases being passed contagiously from one person to another.

Hippocrates (ca. 460–370 BC), the "father of medicine," had promulgated humoral theory in an effort to shift medical thinking about disease toward natural causes. He meant it as a move away from demonic theory, the tendency to attribute disease to the wrath of the gods. Galen (129–200 AD), a Greek physician in the Roman Empire, expanded on the humoral idea and made it the foundation of Western medicine. Middle Eastern thinkers—notably, Persian polymath Avicenna (Ibn Sīnā, ca. 980–1037)—preserved the idea through the middle ages in Europe and also spread it across the Islamic world and east to China.

Humoral theory *seemed* logical. Each of the four humors (blood, black bile, yellow bile, and phlegm) corresponded to one of four temperaments (sanguine, melancholic, choleric, phlegmatic), four seasons (spring, autumn, summer, winter), and the four supposed elements (air, earth, fire, water). It made it possible to link changes in health to weather or season in ways that seemed plausible and at times contained hints of truth. A physician might have attributed the sicknesses of people living in a marshy neighborhood, for instance, to a humoral imbalance brought on by swampy miasmas, while a modern epidemiologist would focus instead on the danger of mosquito-borne diseases. And where a humoral doctor might have attributed a diarrhea outbreak in an urban neighborhood to putrid vapors, the epidemiologist might instead suspect a contaminated water supply. The humoral system also seemed to explain the role of human behaviors in disease. When eating or drinking too much produced a bellyache or throbbing head, for instance, it could seem as if these behaviors had disrupted the humoral equilibrium.

Not least, humoral theory seemed believable to patients. It provided highly active measures that physicians and patients necessarily performed together, to purge out-of-balance humors. "These interventions were supposed to be painful—it was the smart that they produced which drew the humours or cajoled Nature into action," medical historian Hannah Newton has written. The humoral physician was no mere servant of nature, "he was goading nature into doing what he thought was necessary."

Human physiology was arranged conveniently for this purpose. "God that made the body of man hath not in vain created so many wayes and passages to purge forth the humours," a sixteenth-century Dutch physician exulted. They could be cast out via the nostrils by blowing or bleeding, the palate by sneezing and spitting, the lungs by coughing, the stomach by vomiting, and the skin by sweating, all in addition to the exuberant productions of bowel, bladder, and genitals. First, though, a Scottish physician of the same era wrote, the body "must be prepared and the humors must be made fluxible," to bring the disease to a crisis and allow the humors to flow. "Imagery of food preparation and cookery was used in this context,"

Newton writes. "Nature 'chopped' and 'melted' the thick humours, so that they could be more easily evacuated." Bloodletting was the most common humoral remedy, a pint at a time, more than a tenth of the total blood supply for an average adult, often repeated at intervals of days or even hours. Practitioners and patients alike appear to have been equally impressed with the results, except presumably in cases of death.[4]

Understanding how humoral theory could have dominated medicine for more than two thousand years is a struggle for modern readers, beginning with the vocabulary, which continues to shape how we speak even now, though in confusing ways. Hippocrates did not of course use the word *humor*. He used *chymos*, meaning "juice" or "sap." That got translated into *humor* based on the Latin *umor*, meaning "moisture," as in the word *humidity*. The language becomes especially tangled because the association between bodily humors and temperaments has stayed with us. Among his more than one hundred uses of the word, Shakespeare has both a "black oppressing humour" (*Love's Labour's Lost*) and a "merry humour" (*Comedy of Errors*). The merrier meaning has prevailed, and a word that started out with bodily fluids now refers to stuff that makes us laugh. (But maybe that's not such a stretch, after all). Even stranger, the word *phlegm*, from Ancient Greek *phlegein*, meaning "to burn," has evolved into *phlegmatic*, a word we now use for people who are cold and unemotional. Our word *melancholy* comes directly from humoral theory's black bile (Greek *melankholia*)—but that's hardly what we think about when we hear Frank Sinatra singing "My Melancholy Baby." Humoral theory, one historian writes, is "embedded as a sort of verbal fossil in our language."[5]

The real difficulty in understanding the persistence of humoral medicine isn't the language, though. It's the divergence from our idea of reality. Hippocrates, Galen, and all their followers, the French immunologist Charles Richet complained in a 1910 talk, "describe humours which they had never seen, and which no one will ever see, for they do not exist." The human body contains blood and bile, of course, but the terms *black* or *yellow bile* are meaningless for us, and the phlegm of humoral theory was not the stuff we clear from our throats but some unknown product of the pituitary gland. "What can we say," Richet went on, "of this fanciful classification of humours into four groups, of which two are absolutely imaginary?" One thing we can say is that people are prone to the conventional wisdom of their times. Richet, for example, was a proponent of European racial superiority and a spiritualist who coined the word *ectoplasm*.[6]

A more surprising explanation for the persistence of humoral theory is that physicians did not just imagine the humors they described, but actually saw them in the blood they drew. In the early 1920s, a Swedish pathologist named Robin Fåhraeus helped popularize the erythrocyte sedimentation rate, a test that requires leaving a blood sample to coagulate for an hour in a glass tube. In a healthy patient, the sedimentation rate is slow and the result is a uniform red. You could say it's balanced. But in certain inflammatory conditions, sedimentation occurs so rapidly that the sample breaks down into four distinct layers. That seemed useful to Fåhraeus for recognizing conditions that produce systemic inflammation, like colitis or rheumatoid arthritis.

Beyond that, he saw a correspondence between the layered blood sample and humoral theory, with the bottom layer of densely packed red blood cells corresponding to black bile, the translucent red layer just above that to blood, the thin layer above that to yellow bile, and the white layer on top to what the ancients called *phlegm*. In blood samples from sick patients, the phlegm—what we now call *plasma*—can make up more than half the sample. That's why the Ancient Greeks believed, Fåhraeus wrote, that phlegm was "by far the most important cause of almost all diseases."

Fåhraeus did not cite evidence in humoral writings to back up this theory. But when doctors bled their patients, which they did alarmingly often, they noted whether the blood was, as one of them put it, "well coloured, and in such proportion as is usual in healthful persons." Subsequent researchers have, however, generally reverted to the idea that the four humors originated in speculative natural philosophy.[7]

CONTAGION

This brings us back to the question on which hundreds of millions of human lives hung—or rather, would be lost: Why didn't Leeuwenhoek's detailed descriptions of protozoa and bacteria, or the work of scientists and physicians before and long after, lead to new insights into contagion, or perhaps even to recognition that pathogens cause disease?

The idea that certain diseases, particularly plague and leprosy, could be contagious had ancient roots. Quarantines were a familiar tool in epidemics, to keep out people from areas believed to be infected. So was isolation of infected individuals within a community. But these practices existed apart from conventional medicine. For centuries, medical thinkers seem not to have asked just what a quarantine was keeping out or what mysterious factor was getting through when a seemingly contagious disease began to spread. And when these questions became gradually more common from the mid-seventeenth century on, anticontagionist thinkers fended them off, often with good reason: questions and suppositions did not add up to evidence.

A contagionism proponent might suspect some seed or other unknown disease factor could pass from a sick person to a new victim by various means. But patients sometimes fell sick when no direct source of contagion was apparent, or they remained inexplicably healthy even as beloved family members fell sick and died all around them. Epidemics broke out in areas where no sick person was known to have visited. Or they sometimes raged through a particular village or neighborhood—and then stopped there without spreading to nearby areas.[8]

Concepts we now take for granted were entirely unknown then. Physicians didn't realize that some people could be hidden carriers of disease, suffering no symptoms even as they infected those around them. They recognized that people sometimes acquired resistance through prior exposure to certain diseases, but they had no idea at all about the role of genetic variation, or inheritance, in shaping individual susceptibility to different diseases. They didn't understand that disease could arrive in their drinking water or their food, or be transmitted by animals, including the livestock that shared their land and even their homes. Above all, doctors didn't understand that the tightly interwoven infectious illnesses of humans and other animals were the product of yet other living things, or that these living things—what we call *microbes*—each had its own peculiar ecology.

Unfamiliar diseases and their microbes were meanwhile teaching terrifying new lessons about the deadly price of ignorance almost everywhere.

3 FOREIGN BODIES

Two related events in the era before Leeuwenhoek might have led to new ways of thinking about the nature of contagion. The first began almost the moment European explorers stepped ashore in the New World in 1492. Native Americans were soon slipping away before an invading army of unfamiliar infectious diseases, from measles to smallpox. Just in the first century of colonization, according to one recent estimate, these diseases took the lives of fifty-six million people.[1]

The modern understanding is that New World people and their immune systems had been separated from Old World diseases since the collapse of the land bridge across the Bering Strait more than ten thousand years earlier. Thus they had no acquired immunity to infectious diseases that had meantime become common, particularly the zoonotic diseases routinely encountered by Old World people in their close dealings with domesticated livestock herds. The newcomers also tended to arrive from crowded Old World communities, where they and their forebears had survived a long list of infectious diseases, with population-wide effects on immune resistance. So smallpox, for instance, might kill between 15 and 30 percent of European victims, but 90 percent of some Native American tribes.[2]

European colonizers didn't understand at first that they were giving diseases to the people they encountered. But they rejoiced once they recognized that the great dying was underway. King James I of England celebrated "the utter Destruction, Devastation, and Depopulation of that whole Territorye" after a mysterious plague annihilated Native American populations in Massachusetts in about 1617. This was in the official Charter of New England, sending the Puritans off in the *Mayflower*. God had brought Europeans "to a Country wonderfully prepared for their Entertainment" by a "prodigious Pestilence," Puritan minister Cotton Mather (1663–1728) explained in a 1702 history of the settlement, "so that the *Woods* were almost cleared of those pernicious Creatures, to make Room for a *better growth*." This pestilence not only killed "vast Multitudes" but also conveniently left "those Tawny Pagans" who survived "smitten into awful and humble Regards of the *English*."[3]

The colonists exploited their sense of physiological, social, and moral superiority to justify the taking of land—and even souls—by a kind of religious eminent domain. An early missionary who proselytized among American tribes won praise in a contemporary Jesuit history for exerting "the greatest care . . . to let no infant miss baptism." That way, when smallpox "opportunely" intervened, he gathered in "a rich harvest of these innocent souls." The sense of European superiority, together with a strong dose of humoralism, led to a theory of "American degeneracy," proposed by an eighteenth-century French naturalist: humans and animals in "these melancholy regions" were supposedly weaker because of the hostile climate and the dense forests, "overloaded with humid and noxious vapours."[4]

A MOST PRESUMPTUOUS POX

The grand experiment that was killing tens of millions of people across the Americas made almost no difference, however, to people trying to understand the nature of infectious diseases. Medical thinkers focused instead on a disease much closer to the heart of European life. Physicians at first "cared not even to behold" this new disease, much less "to touch the infected," Ulrich von Hutten wrote in his *De Morbo Gallico* (The French Disease), published in 1519. It was unlike anything they had ever encountered. The earliest victims "had *Boils* that stood out like Acorns, from whence issued such filthy stinking Matter," he wrote, "that whosoever came within the Scent, believed himself infected . . . the very Aspect [was] as shocking as the Pain itself, which yet was as if the Sick had lain upon a Fire."[5]

Patients in the first wave of the outbreak suffered pustules on the skin, which "mutate into ulcers" and "spread to the nervous parts and attack the bones," Italian physician Girolamo Fracastoro (1478–1553) reported. Some victims suffered "the complete destruction of the lips, others of the nose, and others of all their genitals." Death was quick and agonizing at first. But within a few decades, the disease shifted form, and the agony, though less obvious, was drawn out over years or even decades.[6]

It had no name at first, except for a sort of geographical finger-pointing. To the Russians, it was "the Polish disease," and the Poles deemed it a product of Germany. In India, where colonizers carried it in 1498, it became "the Portuguese evil," and in Japan in 1515, it was "the Chinese ulcer." In truth, no one knew where it came from. But it traveled faster than any disease before it, by way of colonization and commerce. Fracastoro later gave the disease a lasting name minus the geographical slurs. Sometime between 1510 and 1530, he turned the pandemic into the unlikely subject of an epic poem. It featured a shepherd tending the many flocks of his king. In despair, when a summer drought begins killing his sheep, the shepherd blasphemes the god in charge of such phenomena. The god then curses shepherd, king, and nation with "a hideous leprosy," on which he also bestows the shepherd's name—*Syphilus*. It would in time displace the uglier common name, "the pox."[7]

The European outbreak probably began with the first voyage of Christopher Columbus to the New World. On returning to Spain in 1493, Columbus went to Barcelona, with some of his crew and captives—women taken as sex slaves—to report to his royal sponsors, King Ferdinand and Queen Isabella. There, a physician wrote that he treated members of the expedition for a disease "never seen or recognized or found in medical books." From Barcelona, syphilis skipped across the Mediterranean to Italy, probably by way of sailors, mercenaries, or prostitutes attached to the army sent out to defend Ferdinand and Isabella's hereditary claim to Naples. In 1495, all the elements of a superspreading event momentarily came together when an invading French army marched into Naples unopposed. They seem to have remained only long enough for soldiers to consort with prostitutes and to court, or rape, local women. When the French king subsequently disbanded his troops, they scattered back to every corner of Europe, bearing to their wives and lovers the gift of the spiral-shaped bacteria known today as *Treponema pallidum*.[8]

The willingness of many victims to describe their experiences with syphilis in print represented a dramatic change in medicine. "The advent of syphilis marks the beginning of a new approach to disease itself, leading physicians out of their traditional dependence upon medieval and classical texts," according to historian Bruce Thomas Boerher, "and instead forcing them to interact with each other, and with their patients and patrons, to an unprecedented degree." Publishing was a key element in this transformation. Commercial printing had become commonplace since Johannes Gutenberg's invention of the movable-type printing press a half-century earlier.

By one count, a dozen medical tracts about the new disease appeared just between 1497 and 1501, including some of the first narratives of a disease written by the patient. People may have been willing to discuss their symptoms frankly because syphilis was still a mysterious calamity afflicting much of the adult population. Victims did not at first understand that they were dealing with a sexually transmitted disease, given how little anyone understood about the causes of any medical condition, and also given the dormancy period of as much as six weeks between infection and the onset of symptoms.[9]

The search for remedies was the driving topic. Surgeons, sensing a business opportunity, applied hot irons to the scourge of swellings, knobs, and sores. This unthinkable cruelty proving useless, they moved on to ointments made of bayberry, burnt salt, turpentine, and almost anything else they could lay their hands on. Mercury became the dominant syphilis treatment in about 1500, as an ointment to be slathered onto the skin, an elixir to be drunk, or fumes to be inhaled. Some patients submitted three or four times a day to treatment in a heated chamber, with a pan over a fire releasing mercury and other substances into the air.

Symptoms of syphilis and mercury poisoning overlapped and became confused. Hutten and his contemporaries took the excess flow of saliva produced by mercury for a draining out of corrupted humors. When sores afflicted the mouth, throat, and lungs, he wrote, "a stinking Matter continually was voided from these Places . . . which sort of Cure was indeed so terrible, that many chose rather to die than to be eased thus of their Sickness." The treatment itself could be fatal. In a single day, one practitioner killed three patients "through such excessive Heat their Hearts failed them."[10]

Hutten, infected in the second wave of syphilis, submitted repeatedly to this treatment while still in his twenties. His physicians sweated and bled him. They fed him an assortment of elixirs. But no remedy brought lasting relief, and he wrote that a close friend, seeing "me so bitterly vexed with Pain, that I could neither rest by Night, nor take my Food by Day, advised me to kill my self." Some fellow sufferers ran like madmen, "not only their Hands and Feet, but their whole Bodies trembling: Some also were forced to mumble and stammer in their Speech as long as they lived, without any Remedy." Some victims—of the disease or its remedies—hanged themselves or slit their own throats.[11]

LITTLE STEEMY BODIES

The idea that a disease could be something carried in the bodies of people aboard ships, or on horseback, and thus spread from one end of the earth to the other, was only dimly beginning to take shape. In the first printed medical book in English, 1547's *Breviary of Helthe*, the author, a physician, warned that the disease could be acquired from lying in bedsheets, or sitting on a toilet or saddle, lately used by "a pocky person." But "specially it is taken" when a pocky person "doth synne in lechery the one with another." Hutten acknowledged that syphilis rarely occurred in those "not given to Fornication or bodily Lust" and that "the more a Man is addicted to these Pleasures, the sooner he catcheth it." But he preferred to attribute his own disease to the dire circumstances of his life as a wandering writer.[12]

One practical remedy that soon appeared was an early version of the condom, introduced by a Catholic priest named Gabriele Falloppio (1523–1562). Having taken his vows primarily for financial support, he went on to become a brilliant anatomist at the University of Padua. He was the first person to describe numerous anatomical features, including the tubes leading from the ovaries to the uterus, which now bear his name. He also introduced the term *vagina* and was one of the first medical authorities to describe the function of the clitoris. The condom he devised was, however, meant solely to protect the male. Out of concern for "the frame of mind of the prostitutes," he wrote, one could hardly show up for an assignation carrying prophylactic ointments. Instead, he recommended carefully cleaning the penis after sex, and then placing it in the linen sheath he had invented, soaked with medications, and tied up with a ribbon, for a period of recovery.[13]

The cavalier attitude to the fate of women was characteristic of the time. Hutten, for instance, advised men recovering from the new disease to abstain from "the fleshly act" mainly to avoid aggravating their own sickness, not out of concern that they might infect their partners. Eustachio Rudio, a medical professor at Padua, put it more plainly: "Paid women . . . are worth preserving not for their own health, but primarily for the sake of their male customers." When a British physician advanced a vaguely animalcular explanation of syphilis in 1670, women were still of interest only as a cause of disease, not as victims in need of treatment. He thought syphilis had arisen in the heat of intercourse between a diseased Frenchman and a "fretted Neapolitan Whore" creating "little steemy bodies, or atoms." These proliferated in her body, as only living things could do, to infect other men who slept with her.[14]

TAKING THE WOOD

Hope came finally from a shade tree. Sometime between 1506 and 1516, wood from the guaiacum tree began to be imported into Europe from the Caribbean. There, Hutten wrote, all the inhabitants are "at some times diseased with this Sickness, as we are with the *Measles* and *Small-Pox*; nor have they any surer Remedy therefore than this." In Hutten's minutely detailed recipe, one pound of wood chips or sawdust slowly simmered in eight pounds of water yielded a faintly muddy, sour-tasting liquid, to be chugged down twice a day, and a powder to be applied to the sores. The treatment regimen entailed sitting under a heap of blankets in a heated room while being slowly starved and purged. The patient consumed about a quarter pound of guaiacum a day for thirty days, on a diet otherwise sufficient only "to keep off Fainting."

"The principal and chief Effect of this Wood," Hutten promised his readers (and himself), "is to heal the *French Pox*, which it does effectually eradicate even though of long standing." He offered caveats. The treatment worked only "gradually to cleanse and purify" the corrupted blood and "to expel the hurtful Humours nourishing the Distemper." It could also be painful. In some patients, "it maketh the Bones bare, in some the Sinews and Veins" in the course of searching and destroying "the putrid Flesh infected with the Sickness." But he added, as if preaching a sermon, "it then I say healeth up the same."[15]

Readers looked up from their despair and sang "Alleluia," or at least the ones who could afford guaiacum did. "Soon Hutten's book had a popularity and distribution such as had few medical works of any period," physician Robert S. Munger wrote, in a 1949 history of guaiacum. "Reprinted, paraphrased, and translated into several languages, it quickly became established as the guide to the treatment of syphilis." Demand for guaiacum soared, and so did the price.[16]

Being freed from mercury poisoning might have been enough to make guaiacum feel like a miraculous cure, for a little while. It also "allowed the patient's disease a chance to abate on its own, a characteristic of syphilis not then understood," Munger wrote. Wishful patients mistook the temporary relief for an effect of the treatment. And when some patients showed no benefit from the supposed panacea, then the patient was to blame, not the medicine. Guaiacum would remain popular until the twentieth century, when science finally demonstrated that it was completely useless against syphilis. Hutten was among the many syphilitics who found this out on their own. In a July 1523 letter to a friend, he wondered if "the unhappy fate . . . that pursues us so bitterly" would ever be checked. A few weeks later, at the end of summer, he died, age thirty-four.[17]

Syphilis had driven home the frightening reality of contagion. But the answer to one key question was still missing: Contagion how? Learned men would go on seeking the answer in the corruption of the air, in decomposing organic matter, in the weather, and in the stars. But a few early medical thinkers began to speculate about the actual mechanism by which sickness might pass from one person to another.

4 PRECURSORS

In his 1546 tract *Contagion, Contagious Diseases and Their Treatment*, Girolamo Fracastoro largely set aside the idea that diseases arose from miasmas, or from some predisposing humoral imbalance in the victim. Instead, he argued that *seminaria*—that is, germs or seeds—were to blame and that a given germ was specific to a particular disease, causing a "certain precisely similar corruption" in anyone those germs infected. Moreover, germs could "generate and propagate other germs precisely like themselves, and these in turn propagate others," as an infection became epidemic.

Germs could spread by direct contact, Fracastoro wrote, or by means of *fomites*—that is, clothes, bedding, or other objects that had been in contact with a sick person. A third means of transmission, at a distance through the air, might be "hard to explain," he admitted, and yet it was familiar to physicians from the way "pestiferous fevers" or phthisis (tuberculosis) commonly infected other members of the household who had not been in direct contact with a known victim.[1]

Fracastoro had trained at the University of Padua, then Europe's leading center of medical learning. He set up practice in his hometown of Verona and became known as a thinker on matters from astronomy to marine fossils, as well as medicine. He looked the part. In his portrait by Titian from about 1528, Fracastoro is about fifty years old, brow slightly knit as in mid-thought, deep-set eyes peering inquisitively to the side, above a thin, pointed nose and a full beard. Draped across his broad shoulders, he wore the pelt of a lynx, a species said to be so keen-sighted it could see through walls. (Italy's leading scientists, Galileo among them, would later join together in the *Accademia dei Lincei*, the Academy of the Lynx-Eyed.)

Unfortunately, the idea that disease spread through invisible particles in the air—what another physician in Verona derided as "some absurd seedlets"—sounded close enough to "foul exhalations" for most physicians to skip past the original thinking and stick to their miasmas. In truth, even modern scholars with microbiological expertise have been confused about exactly what Fracastoro had in mind with his seminaria. But Fracastoro's ideas about contagion, and his vocabulary of *seminaria* and *fomites*, spread across Europe and became "part of the normal discourse of the learned physician," according to medical historian Vivian Nutton.[2]

An early twentieth-century medical historian marveled that Fracastoro seemed "by some remarkable power of divination or clairvoyance, to have seen morbid processes in terms of bacteriology" when bacteria were still unknown. Fracastoro wrote not only before Leeuwenhoek actually saw and described bacteria, but decades before the development of the microscope itself, or the scientific method for testing the validity of his ideas by experimentation. Fracastoro's "clairvoyance" depended only on his eyes, for observing his patients closely, and his mind, for thinking clearly, without regard for current dogma. Nobody would mistake his work for modern medical thinking. Like many contemporaries, Fracastoro allowed, for instance, for the malign influence of the stars in disease outbreaks. But readers should reflect, American microbiologist Thomas D. Brock suggested, on what we ourselves "would have invented to explain the observable facts of syphilis or tuberculosis in the year 1546."[3]

SEDUCED BY SPONTANEOUS GENERATION

Jesuit priest Athanasius Kircher (1602–1680) was another early thinker to propose that living organisms might be the agents of infectious diseases. This German-born polymath conducted research across such broad areas of interest, from music theory to Egyptology, that he was dubbed *Germanus Incredibilis*—but also just "a scholarly windbag." In 1656, when plague struck Rome, Kircher volunteered to help in overcrowded hospitals. There, with a rudimentary microscope, he examined blood from a plague victim and pronounced it "so crowded with worms as to well nigh dumbfound me."[4]

This was almost twenty years before Leeuwenhoek's description of microorganisms in the human body. Moreover, Kircher was not shy about directly connecting his "worms" to disease. He wrote that "all putrid matter swarms with a brood of worms without number which are invisible to the unaided eye." And once this poisonous corruption comes into existence, it "gives rise to an evil breath, which is exhaled into the air, carrying with it the poisonous corpuscles." These cling to the bedding, the garments and hands of bystanders, he wrote, "and even insinuate themselves into the very pores . . . and cause the commencement of an epidemic." Thus some modern scholars have credited Kircher as the first to attribute infectious disease to a *contagium animatum*, a living agent of disease.[5]

Kircher did not, however, bother to describe in any detail what he claimed to have seen. "Not one of his allusions to minute organisms carries with it the conviction of a serious primary interest in microscopical details as was characteristic of contemporary microscopists," American biologist Harry Beal Torrey wrote in a scathing 1938 critique. In stark contrast to Leeuwenhoek, "Kircher appears to have been concerned less with observations than arguments, more with the origin of living creatures from putrefying substances than the creatures themselves." Modern researchers have largely concluded that the "worms" Kircher saw in the blood of plague victims were ordinary red blood cells, clumped together in lines, or "rouleaux."[6]

Kircher also perpetuated the common belief that these "worms" could arise from nothing—or rather, from almost anything, if it became putrid, or if a body contained "corruption" hidden somewhere within. Among other experiments intended to demonstrate spontaneous generation, he urged readers to leave a piece of meat out at night "exposed to the lunar moisture" until "all the putridity drawn from the moon has been transformed into numberless little worms of different sizes." Spontaneous generation made almost any nonsense plausible, as Kircher amply demonstrated. And as long as certain lower organisms could come out of nowhere, as if by magic, it was impossible to think coherently about the true causes of disease.

Kircher's credulous approach had one beneficial result for the understanding of infectious disease: it led a contemporary to subject spontaneous generation to genuinely rigorous testing. Francesco Redi (1626–1697) was a physician and naturalist advising Cosimo de' Medici III, the sixth Grand Duke of Tuscany. He had been educated by Jesuits and normally held them "in deference," according to translator Mab Bigelow. But it's hard to miss the needle in Redi's recounting of his attempts to carry out some of Kircher's more fanciful experiments. "As Father Kircher had stated that scorpions are reborn from dead scorpions themselves, if exposed to the sun and sprinkled with sweet basil and water, I risked a second and a third experiment," Redi wrote, with muted glee, "only to be disappointed and to wait in vain the desired young scorpions, instead of which I always got flies."[7]

Redi then began to observe the arrival of flies around pieces of meat set out in boxes. When maggots inevitably followed, he put a lid on top to keep them from escaping. As they developed into flies of the same species, he recorded the details with a naturalist's attentiveness and occasional delight. The hind legs of one species were so red "they would put cinnabar to shame." These observations convinced Redi that the worms found on dead animals were "all generated by insemination and that the putrefied matter in which they are found" was merely a place "where animals deposit their eggs at the breeding season, and in which they also find nourishment." But belief, he wrote, "would be vain without the confirmation of experiment."

He set out samples of different meats in four open flasks, and also in four flasks "well closed and sealed" with strong paper to keep out flies. Maggots duly appeared in the open flasks and not in the sealed ones. But Redi worried, as modern scientists would, about a possible confounding effect: The stale air in the sealed flasks might somehow have prevented spontaneous generation of maggots. So he set out new meat samples in four open flasks and four flasks covered with "a fine Naples veil, that allowed the air to enter." Again, the maggots appeared only in the open flasks and not within the closed flasks, though flies attracted by the meat sometimes hovered above the closed flasks and their maggots soon appeared on top of the veil. "Hence as I have shown," Redi concluded, "no dead animal can breed worms." Spontaneous generation was a myth.[8]

Kircher responded huffily that Redi must not have properly followed the published directions: "Just because one or the other of [the experimenets] was unsuccessful when he tried it, he concludes that Kircher must be wrong." His new book asserted that insects need not have been brought aboard Noah's Ark with the other animals. They would simply reappear later by spontaneous generation.

Redi, now considered the founder of parasitology, went on to describe more than 180 parasites, including deer ticks, human roundworms, and sheep liver flukes. He continued to develop the fundamental method in scientific experimentation of keeping one group of a particular parasite untreated, as a control group, while testing a remedy against another group of that same species. He also provided further evidence against spontaneous generation in a medical context by demonstrating that parasites produce eggs, from which their young emerge.

Even Redi did not, however, entirely escape the seductive appeal of spontaneous generation when it came to the many worms found in and around plants. One way they got there was from eggs deposited by insects, much as he had demonstrated with meat. But "the other way," he wrote, "which I esteem worthy of credence," was that the "soul or principle which creates the flowers and fruits of living plants" also "produces the worms of these plants." Naturalists leapt to correct this error, and Redi regretted it in his correspondence. But his own susceptibility suggests why belief in spontaneous generation would persist unabated for more than two hundred years after Redi decisively proved that it didn't actually happen: spontaneous generation was like a magic trick that people could witness any day of the week with their own eyes, if they did not look too carefully. (And who wanted to look carefully at maggots on rotting meat?) Even for the great minds of the scientific revolution, including Rene Descartes and Francis Bacon, the powerful evidence of what they *seemed* to see, supported by ancient authorities, triumphed over experimental proof.[9]

It would take humble diseases and uncelebrated scientists to make progress toward the true causes of disease.

5 RIDICULOUS DISEASES, INCONCEIVABLE IDEAS

Scabies did not rank among the great scourges of the day, like syphilis or smallpox. It killed no one, and it was easy to ignore because it mainly afflicted the poor and unwashed. It is a skin condition, and its name derives from the Latin word for the chief response of victims, which is to scratch (*scabere*). It shows up first as a fierce itching almost anywhere on the body. Hence its other common name, "the itch." Scratching and a vigilant immune system soon produce a pimple-like rash. The itching becomes even more intense at night. If untreated, particularly in people with a compromised immune system, scabies can ultimately cover large portions of the body in a scabby layer resembling a crusted bread loaf.

Women everywhere, and seemingly from time immemorial, have connected these symptoms with the presence of tiny creatures in the skin, now known to be mites. Pricking them out with a sewing needle was the only effective treatment against scabies, which commonly afflicted their children. This remedy turns up, among many other places, on Tahiti, where women used bamboo splinters to pick mites out of two infected sailors when HMS *Endeavour* visited in 1769. It's also in *Romeo and Juliet*, where Shakespeare describes the fairy queen Mab's wagon being drawn by a gnat "not half so big as a little round worm, pricked from the finger of a lazy maid." The remarkable Benedictine Abbess Hildegard of Bingen (1098–1179) declared that *minutissimi vermiculi*, "the tiniest worms," were not just a corollary, but the cause of scabies. Medical men nonetheless stuck with the idea from Galen that scabies arose from "melancholic juices," or from Avicenna that it was a product of "corrupt blood."[1]

Then, in 1687, a young physician from Livorno, Italy, named Giovanni Cosimo Bonomo (1663–1696) wrote a letter to Francesco Redi, detailing the mite's role in causing scabies. Bonomo wrote that he had frequently "observed that the Poor Women, when their children are troubled with the *Itch*, do with the point of a Pin pull out of the Scabby Skin little Bladders of Water and crack them like Fleas upon their Nails." Under Bonomo's microscope, one of these bladders had turned out to be "a very minute Living Creature," he wrote, "in shape resembling a Tortoise, of whitish colour . . . of nimble motion with six Feet, a sharp Head, with two little Horns at the end of the Snout."[2]

This was an excellent description of an animal that is no more than a half-millimeter in size, except that the scabies mite, a tick-like arachnid, actually has eight legs, not six. "I have good reason to conclude," he wrote, "that the affliction is nothing but a continuous biting and chewing" by these mites. Redi edited the letter and published it. Giovanni Maria Lancisi (1654–1720), personal physician to the Pope, promptly intervened to dismiss the idea that human diseases might have zoological origins. Lancisi was a skilled anatomist who made important contributions in cardiology and other medical fields. But he was a resolute believer in humoral theory. He admonished Bonomo that scabies had an underlying humoral basis, which preceded the infestation by mites. Perhaps mindful of Galileo's encounter with papal authority, Bonomo backed away.[3]

Resistance to the idea that mites caused scabies was hardly limited to the Church. Even literal firsthand experience could prove unpersuasive. Joseph Adams (1756–1818), a British physician, was a careful observer of the inheritance of medical disorders. But in 1801, on a visit to Madeira, he turned his attention to smaller fry. When an old woman showed him how to extract scabies mites with a needle, Adams and a companion had the clever holiday idea of infecting themselves, in the interest of science. Live mites placed on the tender skin between the fingers soon produced the expected result, and Adams diligently recorded the progress of the disease. Weirdly, though, he went on to assert that what he had given himself wasn't actually scabies but some other itch.

The medical world's inability to accept the mite as the cause of scabies had to do partly with the difficulty of finding it. The common mistake was to prick with a needle at the pustule on the surface of the skin. But this served only to irritate the patient, as any number of mothers could have advised: the mite resides not in the pimple, but in a burrow off to the side. Doctors probably also dismissed the mite as the cause of the disease because it was easier to blame the victims for their poverty and filthy living conditions.

Bonomo's insight would nonetheless soon play a key part in explaining the nature of contagious diseases, in another context far removed from the great human epidemics of the age.

CATTLE AND CONTAGIONISM

In the summer of 1711, a shipment of oxen originating in Hungary made the trip across the Adriatic into northeastern Italy. Just outside Padua, a single ox went astray, according to contemporary accounts, and was given shelter in the stable of a farm belonging to the Borromeo family. Days later, the cattle there began to fall sick. Their eyes and noses ran and they suffered acute diarrhea, leading to rapid death. The new disease soon decimated herds across the region. Families dependent on cattle for milk, cheese, and meat, and on oxen to plow their fields, faced starvation.[4]

Rinderpest (German for "cattle plague") did not, however, cause any illness in humans, which helped to undercut conventional humoral theories about how people become sick. "Many of the explanations invoked for human diseases—excess indulgence, late nights, too much good/rich food, anxiety, evildoing (by the cattle), and divine wrath—could not be introduced to confuse the situation," medical historian Margaret DeLacy wrote in *The Germ of An Idea*, "although some did claim that the suffering of the cattle was divine retribution for human sin."

Instead, "rinderpest favored the development of contagionism," according to DeLacy, first because it was so clearly contagious. The appearance of symptoms within four or five days after exposure made it easy for farmers to recall contact with a sick animal. Cattle herds were "relatively discrete entities," and their infrequent meetings with other herds tended to stick in the memory. Accounts of pandemics rarely begin with a detail as precise as an ox in the stable at the Borromeo family farm.[5]

The new disease caught the attention of Bernardino Ramazzini (1633–1714), a professor of medicine at the University of Padua. Delivering his annual lecture to faculty and students that November, barely two months after the original shipment of oxen, he dismissed old ideas about astrological influences or atmospheric miasmas, which would presumably have sickened humans as much as their livestock. He also batted aside objections that it was inappropriate to discuss animal diseases in the context of human health. Instead, he likened rinderpest to smallpox, for the pustules that were one of its symptoms, and to syphilis, for the rapid and pervasive spread of infection. He focused on how inanimate "seeds of disease easily multiply and widely propagate themselves . . . in a suitable and susceptible subject." A sick animal's "virulently poisoned breath" could carry the infection into the body of a healthy one. The contagion also "spread through the secretions and the excreta of ailing and dead oxen," leaving stables and pastures "contaminated to the injury of other oxen subsequently using them." Fumigating contaminated stables and isolating the sick were his sensible remedies.[6]

Unfortunately, they proved insufficient. When the cattle plague reached Rome in the summer of 1713, Giovanni Maria Lancisi, the same papal physician who had bigfooted Bonomo on the question of scabies mites, once again intervened. He successfully advocated killing and burying all infected animals, along with strict limits on movement of cattle, and immediate jailing of merchants who violated the rules. Farmers raged against the loss of their herds, but culling stopped the spread of disease in Rome, and again the next year when others employed the technique in London.

The immediate success of culling sick animals may have inspired Lancisi to propose an even more remarkable preventive measure soon after, against an unrelated disease. In the low-lying regions around Rome, he had been studying the persistent problem of malaria. Lancisi concluded in 1717 that marshes were to blame not just for their noxious emanations, but also for their resident "evil insects," and he recommended draining swamps as a remedy. He also mentioned the possibility of living organisms in the blood of malaria victims. But he preferred to think mosquitoes were merely carrying some inanimate poison from the swamps to nearby residents.[7]

The idea that living creatures could routinely bring disease and death to humans clashed with the fundamental Western belief that God had made the world for the good of mankind. It was less threatening, according to DeLacy, "to attribute contagion to inanimate forces, to leave the nature of the agent unspecified," or to regard insects as external agents, "biting and gnawing the body, not as inimical vital entities growing and multiplying within their host."[8]

THE HUMAN BODY AS FOOD AND HABITAT

It fell to a young and unknown writer, without academic or papal credentials, to build the essential lesson of the rinderpest outbreak into a persuasive argument. Carlo Francesco Cogrossi (1682–1769) had graduated from the University of Padua and gone on to practice medicine in Crema, near Milan. He set down his observations on "this savage epidemic" in a letter to a former professor: naturalist and medical researcher Antonio Vallisneri (1661–1730). It was a good choice. In a careful study of flies that parasitize rosebushes, Vallisneri had demonstrated that spontaneous generation didn't happen in plants any more than it did in rotten meat. That made him a receptive audience for the idea that diseases didn't just appear out of nowhere either.[9]

In a letter dated September 3, 1713, Cogrossi asked for his old teacher's indulgence as he laid out a "bizarre hypothesis." Watching maggots on animals dying of rinderpest had led him to "philosophize on the itch"—that is, scabies: "a contagious disease, yes, but a ridiculous one." He noted Bonomo's demonstration a quarter century earlier that this disease is "due to very minute worms, or invisible mites, which gnaw the human skin and hollow out tiny dens for themselves in it." Anyone who doubted it could see the evidence with their own eyes through a microscope. He also described how easily scabies spread "whenever these very nimble animalcules cross from one body to another either by actual contact or on some article of clothing."

Cogrossi seemed reluctant to move too directly to his main argument about rinderpest. Instead, he laid out the character of scabies for several more paragraphs, as a sort of intellectual foundation. Quoting Vallisneri's own "indisputable principle" that "all insects are generated from their proper parents, feed on food proper to them, and dwell in surroundings proper to them," Cogrossi stated the logical implication: for scabies mites, the proper food and habitat was the human body.[10]

Differences in individual susceptibility to scabies reminded Cogrossi of differences in susceptibility to other contagious diseases, particularly rinderpest: while some people would contract scabies "at the slightest opportunity and will get rid of it only with difficulty," Cogrossi wrote, others seemed to enjoy such a natural immunity that they could sleep "freely in the most ragged sheets" of public inns "without having to carry their own along on the trip." Likewise, some cattle remained surprisingly resistant to rinderpest, even as the rest of the herd went down around them. But differences in susceptibility did not distract from his point. Noting the many tiny "worms" or "insects" described by "the famous Dutchman" Antoni van Leeuwenhoek, Cogrossi wrote: "There can be invisible insects from which the epidemic of oxen derives," much as scabies "derives from the grubs" found in human skin.

Two pages later, he restated this "bizarre hypothesis" more emphatically: "If therefore such tiny living creatures are so readily met everywhere, and they can penetrate into the most hidden recesses of animals, why is it not permissible to suspect that in the epidemic among oxen the poisonous insects can pass from one animal to another of similar kind and through the [mouth], the nose, and even the passages in the skin creep into the blood and introduce there irreparable and fatal disorders?"[11]

What was bizarre about the hypothesis, he acknowledged, was that something trivial enough to be exhaled on the breath "can demolish with such great vehemence and activity the huge living machine of an ox," while leaving people and other animals untouched. "This is not easy for me to understand." He knew that if he presented the idea to most of "our long-robed peripatetics," they would laugh at the inconceivable notion "that there could be in nature animalcules so tiny and so subtle." One argument in favor of his hypothesis, he thought, was that small creatures could proliferate rapidly, like "that enormous spread of locusts and grubs by which sometimes corn has been devoured and consumed over vast regions until whole peoples died of hunger." Thus one ox in the barn of the Borromeo family outside Padua could contain the start of an epizootic that would demolish herds across Italy.

Vallisneri replied that the same line of thought had occurred to him, adding, "I shall always find it easier to understand that a living thing, rather than an inanimate thing, can pass from a man or animal to another man or animal; and that it can multiply with the immense fertility which is natural for insects."[12]

THE ANIMALCULE HYPOTHESIS

The publication in 1714 of Cogrossi's letter and Vallisneri's reply was the culmination of an extraordinary period of collective insight into the true character of infectious disease. And all of it took place within the lifetime of one of the key participants, Antoni van Leeuwenhoek. Medical historian Lise Wilkinson traced what she called "a straight line of development," beginning with the argument put forward by British physician William Harvey (1578–1657) that all animals, even humans, emerge from the egg. The pace of this developing insight gathered speed with Leeuwenhoek's Letter 18 and its eye-opening description of vast numbers of animalcules even within the human body, soon followed by "Francesco Redi's elegant refutation of the theory of spontaneous generation and his definitive formulation of the concept of parasitism" in 1687. The line of thought then built to what Wilkinson called "the final, all-important link in the chain, the real turning-point to which Cogrossi refers at length," Bonomo's 1687 demonstration that mites cause scabies. But surely the real turning point was the one Cogrossi himself achieved by lifting Bonomo's work out of the realm of a "ridiculous" itch and instead using it to argue persuasively that mere animalcules could sweep across the countryside, killing animals as massive as an ox.[13]

Even Lancisi, the resolute humoralist, confessed to being "torn in mind" on reading Cogrossi and Vallisneri. He "would add [his] own vote" to their "plausible conjecture" if he could actually see the proposed animalcules in the blood of infected cattle, or in victims of malaria. Until then, though, he could say only that the developing theory of contagion was "very probable but not yet certain."

This was an entirely "realistic and comprehensive picture of the facts as known," according to Wilkinson. The experimental evidence Lancisi wanted could not in fact be produced "in an age which had neither sufficiently powerful microscopes nor the general experimental techniques needed to obtain unequivocal results." Medical researchers then had no way to grow bacteria in a culture or to isolate bacterial strains into pure cultures for detailed study, as later researchers would do. They lacked the tools even to *suspect* the existence of viruses. It would be another 150 years of itching and bleeding and puking and dying before those experimental means would arrive to save the day.

6 BUYING THE POX

At 3:00 a.m. on a Tuesday in mid-November 1721, someone stopped in front of a prosperous home in Boston's North End. He lit the fuse on a bomb and hurled it at the window of what had until recently been the bedroom of Rev. Cotton Mather, a preacher and powerful voice in colonial affairs. By chance, it hit a metal window mullion, knocking off the fuse, and it landed in the bedroom with a thud rather than a boom. The weight alone might have been enough to kill if it had hit someone, never mind the gunpowder in an upper chamber. The oil and turpentine in a lower chamber, Mather wrote, would "have laid the House in Ashes." A note tied to the fuse by a string said, "COTTON MATHER, *You Dog, Dam you: I'll inoculate you with this, with a Pox to you.*"[1]

It was easy enough to imagine Mather, that holy monster, as a target of local outrage. From about 1700 on, many Boston residents disdained him as a dark, insinuating force behind the hanging of nineteen people in the Salem witch trials of the early 1690s. According to one popular account, Mather had even addressed an uneasy crowd from horseback at the execution site, to ensure that the hangings proceeded. For that, and other offenses, one early antagonist had left a drawing of a hanged man at his front gate. Another, a drunken ship captain, showed up at his door, cutlass drawn, "content to lie a year in Hell" for the satisfaction of killing him, apparently to avenge some stern words from the pulpit. "Knotts of riotous Young Men," Mather complained, still later, gather "under my Window in the Middle of the Night, and sing profane and filthy Songs."[2]

In 1721, though, his would-be killer was an anti-vaxxer, before vaccines even existed. That spring, twenty-nine years after the witch trials, Mather had waded back into controversy, proposing to stop an epidemic with a daring medical technique that would become a precursor to vaccination. It was as odd as if "Tail Gunner" Joe McCarthy had put his 1950s red-baiting behind him and reemerged in the 1980s as an AIDS activist. The disease in question was smallpox. Back then, when it swept through at ten- or fifteen-year intervals, every child born in the aftermath of one epidemic grew up in the likelihood of being mowed down or mauled by the epidemic that inevitably followed. Surviving the disease conferred lifetime immunity. But for anyone without this acquired immunity, and especially for parents of unprotected children, smallpox was the great abiding terror.

The disease came on "with Sickness or Shiverings, flushing Heats," and miscellaneous pains, according to Zabdiel Boylston (1680–1766), a Boston physician and surgeon of that era. These symptoms might pass at first for some lesser illness, like chicken pox or measles. But after three or four days, red spots developed into bumps. They filled with fluid and rose up as irregular but sharply defined yellow pustules, volcanic islands on the skin, often indented in the middle, and with a reddened corona. Hundreds of them could cover the face, the limbs, the trunk. They could clot the eyelids shut, or constrict nostrils, mouth, and throat, and make breathing an agony. They sometimes gave off the stench of rotting flesh.[3]

In the best cases, the pustules gradually leaked and crusted over, beginning after five days, and fell off after ten, often leaving the underlying skin badly pitted. In the worst cases, the sick fell into "Ravings and Deliriums; Convulsions, and other Fits," Boylston wrote. The pustules could be so numerous that they blended together to become "confluent" smallpox. Swaths of skin could slough away, leaving patients "as if in the Fire, or scalded with boiling Water." In the worst cases, victims died horribly from failure of multiple organs, or pneumonia. But survival could seem worse: "Some who live are Cripples," wrote Boylston, "others Idiots, and many blind all their Days" or disfigured. When a strikingly attractive British woman of that era came down with smallpox, the instruction to her doctor from an unnamed relative was: "Preserve her beauty or take her life."[4]

A WONDERFUL PRACTICE

Smallpox found its way to Boston Harbor late that April. It had been nineteen years since the city's last epidemic, time enough to raise a generation of fresh victims. Cotton Mather had warned months earlier of "the speedy approach of the destroying Angel" and now felt the need to "ly in the Dust" before God lest he seem vain at "seeing [his] poor praediction accomplished." He had been preparing for this moment for years, as if in need of redemption.

Surprisingly, the moment also needed Mather. He was a proud, emotionally unstable figure, long-winded, prone to imperiousness, and quick to treat critics as agents of Satan. But from childhood, Mather had also been a keen student of science and medicine. He considered it his duty to consult knowledgeably with physicians about the health of his flock. When parishioners were too poor for physicians, he administered medical care himself. New England's tradition of clergymen doubling as physicians was "the angelical conjunction," Mather thought. Saving bodies and souls was the same holy work. Mather also had personal reason to be interested in medical progress. He had lost his first wife to cancer and his second to measles, and he would see thirteen of their fifteen children die.[5]

On June 6, Mather circulated a proposal among Boston's physicians about "a *Wonderful Practice* lately used in several Parts of the World" to defend against smallpox. At first glance, this preventive measure must have seemed almost as terrifying as the sickness itself: A physician would find a patient with a milder case of smallpox and puncture one of the ripe pustules to draw off "variolous matter"—that is, pus. (*Variola* was a Latin coinage meaning "varied pock marks." It survives today as the name of the smallpox virus.) The physician then stored this treasure and portioned it out to willing patients, via an incision in the skin. The promise of "variolation" was that it would produce immunity to future attacks, after a "kind" case of one of the deadliest diseases on Earth. Symptoms appeared within a week.

Variolation—sometimes called *engrafting* or *inoculation*—had ancient roots. According to one account, a Buddhist nun first introduced it in eleventh-century China, where the standard practice was to blow powdered smallpox scabs into a healthy patient's nostrils. Elsewhere, inoculation through the skin was the usual method. No one understood why variolation was any safer than getting smallpox by natural means. But with an epidemic bearing down, explanations mattered less than the evidence that it seemed to work.

Western science had only recently become aware of the practice. A brief description from a physician in Constantinople appeared in *Philosophical Transactions* in 1714, followed by a more detailed account from a Venetian physician on the coast of Turkey. Mather invoked these reports to bolster his argument: "Let it be considered," he declared, "That these Communications come from Great Men . . . and are address'd unto very Eminent Persons" and presented with "the Approbation of the Royal Society (as Illustrious a Body as are in the World)."[6]

In fact, Mather had first learned of the technique years earlier at the opposite end of the social spectrum. His source was "a *Guramantee*-Servant of my own," with *Guramantee* meaning someone who had passed through a notorious fort on the coast of Ghana and *servant* meaning slave. Mather had given this man the New Testament name Onesimus, from the Greek

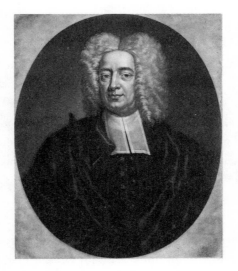

Figure 6.1
Cotton Mather had no portrait made of the African-born man, his "servant," who taught Boston how to stop smallpox (Metropolitan Museum of Art).

for "useful." No other name survives. He was "a pretty Intelligent Fellow," said Mather, who reported that the procedure "was often used among the *Guramantese*, & whoever had the Courage to use it was forever free from the fear of the Contagion."[7]

Mather found corroborating accounts, and scars from the procedure, among other African-born Bostonians. To minimize the perception that variolation might just be a scheme to kill white people, he devised clumsy dialect for what his informants told him. But he also wrote, "I don't know why 'tis more unlawful to learn of *Africans*, how to help against the *Poison* of the *Small Pox*, than it is to learn of our *Indians*, how to help against the *Poison* of a *Rattle-Snake*." In truth, African use of variolation was sophisticated. Another Boston clergyman learned that in Africa, "when Young men among them wanted to go a trading two or three hundred Miles off, but were afraid because they had not yet had the Small-Pox," they went to someplace where the disease was active. After being variolated there, they could "then go & trade anywhere without fear." They were practicing what we call *travel medicine*.[8]

Boston's medical community recoiled from Mather's proposal, with a single exception: Zabdiel Boylston knew how bad smallpox could be. As an apprentice, he had deliberately exposed himself to the disease in the expectation that a quick recovery would enable him to help treat patients. Instead, he became so sick he was given up for dead at one point, but survived with only pockmarks and a profound horror of the disease. Boylston had gone on to become a medical innovator, removing kidney stones and performing the first mastectomy in North America. As the new epidemic worsened, he recognized that his children "were daily in danger" of infection "from [his] visiting the Sick in the natural way." On June 26, despite "a Cloud of Opposers," he performed his first three variolations. The patients were Jack, the enslaved assistant in his medical practice; Jack's two-and-a-half-year-old son; and his own six-year-old son. Jack showed little response, having apparently been exposed to smallpox in his youth. But the two boys experienced "a kind and favourable Small-Pox," with about a hundred pustules apiece.

Word of this success only angered city residents as smallpox made its way among them. "They rave, they rail, they blaspheme," Mather wrote in his diary, "they talk not only like Ideots but also like *Franticks*, And not only the Physician who began the Experiment," he continued, now seeming to fob off responsibility onto Boylston, "but I also am an Object of . . . their furious Obloquies and Invectives." Boylston likewise was "put into a very great Fright" by the "Rage of the People against" what he had done. But he inoculated others who came to him seeking the new treatment.[9]

THE WORK OF "IGNORANT WOMEN"

The same high-pitched debate, full of slander and savagery, was playing out on both sides of the Atlantic. The great proponent of variolation in Britain was Lady Mary Wortley Montagu, a poet, wit, and celebrated beauty, who moved easily through aristocratic and literary circles. She had lost a beloved brother to smallpox in 1713 and survived the disease herself, somewhat scarred, in 1715. (In a poem thinly disguising her own experience, she wrote, "There let me live, in some deserted place / There hide in shades this lost Inglorious Face.") So when she encountered variolation in 1718, as the wife of the British consul in Turkey, she had their six-year-old son variolated by the consulate's British doctor and "an old *Greek* Woman" who showed him the method.[10]

Back in England in 1721, with smallpox killing friends and neighbors, Lady Montagu asked the same doctor, Charles Maitland, to variolate her daughter. Maitland called in medical backup for moral support and to witness the effectiveness of the method. Caroline, Princess of Wales, took notice as Montagu's daughter recovered. She persuaded her father-in-law, King George I, to authorize a test of the method on a half-dozen condemned inmates, with the test subjects to win their freedom if they lived. At Newgate Prison that August, Maitland administered variolation to three men and three women, witnessed by twenty-five other doctors and surgeons and accompanied by a great public baying and wailing both for and against the experiment. The inoculations went smoothly. One of the women subsequently slept in the same bed with a boy suffering from smallpox, to prove she had acquired immunity to the disease.

Other successful experiments followed, including one on a group of orphans. The Princess of Wales, no longer willing to risk smallpox "the natural way," had her two daughters variolated. This was effectively a royal warrant for the practice and helped overcome resistance in Britain. Contemporary accounts tended, however, to minimize the role of the two women, instead substituting their husbands' names. "This was not wilful inaccuracy, but sound public relations," wrote Isobel Grundy, in her biography *Lady Mary Wortley Montagu*. Failure "to suppress the heavy female involvement . . . would only give an opening for misogynist bile."[11]

Misogyny found an opening in any case. Strangers accosted Lady Montagu in the street "to hoot at her as an unnatural mother, who had risked the lives of her own children." William Wagstaffe, a British physician, swiped at her in print as "some *sanguine* traveler from *Turkey*." He raged that "an experiment practiced only by a few *Ignorant Women*, amongst an illiterate and unthinking People, shou'd on a sudden, and upon a slender Experience, so far obtain in one of the Politest Nations in the World as to be receiv'd into the *Royal Palace*." In Boston, the physician William Douglass likewise thought variolation needed to be managed "by abler hands than *Greek old women, madmen, and fools*."[12]

Opponents of variolation raised valid objections: People who had been variolated often went about their normal lives, even receiving visitors, instead of being isolated like other smallpox patients—but being less sick didn't mean they were less contagious. Use of a living donor also introduced the risk of secondary infections—for instance, if the donor was infected with syphilis. But reasonable objections tended to be stated in the most inflammatory language possible. William Douglass characterized variolation advocates as murderers. Of their reliance on African-born informants, he added: "There is not a Race of Men on Earth more False Lyars."[13]

Douglass had recently arrived from the mother country expecting to make his fortune as Boston's only physician with an actual medical degree. He took it as an affront to have a colonial minister like Mather intruding on his professional sphere, and Boylston was merely "a certain *cutter for the stone*." Why were religious leaders giving more trust to the "groundless *Machinations of Men*," he wondered, in a letter published July 24, 1721, "than to our Preserver in the ordinary course of nature?" It was inconsistent with devotion to "the *all-wise Providence* of GOD Almighty." A week later, a half-dozen clergymen took back the religious argument, asking "what hand or art of *Man* is there in this Operation more than in *bleeding, blistering* and a Score more things in Medical use? Which are all consistent with a *humble Trust in our Great Preserver.*"[14]

Proponents of inoculation had not set out to question religious belief, much less conventional medical thinking: they still relied on humoral treatments like bleeding and purging to prepare patients for inoculation and to relieve their symptoms during recovery. Neither side seemed to understand at first just how dramatic a change this new methodology represented. "The introduction of smallpox inoculation revealed the existence of a specific disease-causing substance that could be carried around in a box and cause the 'same' disease in every patient in succession," according to medical historian Margaret DeLacy. It had nothing to do with miasmas, corrupted bodily humors, or all the other wisdom of conventional practice. But people still barely knew whether to open the box, much less how to make sense of what was inside.[15]

THIS ABOMINABLE TOWN

Even as he publicly advocated inoculation, Cotton Mather waited too long to inoculate his own fifteen-year-old son. As the Boston epidemic intensified that September, Sammy barely survived what appeared by its timing and severity to be a naturally acquired infection. Abigail, an older daughter, also became infected, have remained unvariolated because she was about to give birth. Her newborn daughter died as Mather was preparing to baptize her. Abigail followed, two nights later. "A long and an hard Death was the Thing appointed for her," Mather wrote.

It was the same in households throughout the city, and for many families much worse: tradesmen and laborers desperate enough to risk inoculation typically could not afford the high cost to protect their children. Terror and class resentment, together with the lingering shadow of the witch trials, helped turn Mather into a target. By the end of September, smallpox had infected a quarter of Boston's population, and in October, death was everywhere about town. Then Mather brought his nephew and two others in from Roxbury to be inoculated at his home. But opponents considered it too dangerous to variolate even city residents, much less outsiders. In his diary, Mather wrote, "This abominable Town, treats me in a most malicious, and murderous Manner." The attempted bombing followed soon after. But the three Roxbury men, recuperating in Mather's former bedroom, were unhurt.

By the time the epidemic finally ended, more than six thousand residents, half of Boston, had come down with smallpox, and 844 had died. Older residents who had lived through past epidemics were probably already immune before the outbreak, according to medical historians Otho T. Beall and Richard H. Shryock. "The implication is that nearly all residents who had not already had the disease acquired it in the natural way in 1721." Boylston and two colleagues had managed to variolate just 287 people, though they took all comers, including some considered too frail for the procedure and others who may already have been infected naturally. Boylston tracked case outcomes and reported that six patients died. This 2 percent mortality rate compared with 15 percent mortality among the outbreak's natural smallpox victims. James Jurin, then secretary of the Royal Society, soon published a detailed accounting of results on both sides of the Atlantic. It was the first appearance of that essential tool in medical progress: a statistical comparison to evaluate a clinical trial. Improvements in technique would soon reduce the likelihood of death in variation from about one in forty-six to one in three hundred—a third of a percent—while the risk of ordinary smallpox stayed at or above 15 percent. These numbers proved persuasive. When another smallpox epidemic hit Boston in 1792, the response reversed: about 9,200 local residents took variolation, and only 232 suffered natural smallpox.[16]

AFTERMATH

None of the three men who introduced variolation to North America won much honor by it. Onesimus disappeared from the record after purchasing his freedom from Cotton Mather, and the business of stripping Africans of any credit was already underway in 1721. When an unnamed African-born informant could not say how his people had come by their knowledge of variolation, Boston minister Benjamin Colman concluded that no doubt "but GOD told it to poor Negroes to save their lives." In a wonderfully oblivious phrase, he added, "for they had not knowledge & skill as we have." At the same time, William Douglass was proposing to make inoculation a tool for exploiting Africans more profitably: while opposing inoculation as unsafe in Boston, he thought it might be "of great Use to the Guinea Traders," when smallpox came aboard the ship, "to inoculate the whole Cargo, and patch them up for a Market." Ship captains were soon using variolation to reduce losses in the trans-Atlantic trade.[17]

Zabdiel Boylston's reputation survived the deadly rhetoric of 1721. His medical practice prospered, and he was elected a Fellow of the Royal Society. Around Boston, streets, buildings, and a nearby town now bear the name Boylston, but mainly to honor his grandnephew, a wealthy merchant. The pioneer of inoculation lies beneath a broken gravestone in a cemetery in Brookline, Massachusetts.

Cotton Mather is of course also little honored. The surprise is that he continued to think cogently about contagion. He had started out years earlier with ideas that were half-demonic theory, half-humoral. But the epidemic of 1721 shifted him to an "animalcular" understanding of contagion. "Every Part of Matter is *Peopled*. Every *Green Leaf* swarms with *Inhabitants*," Mather wrote in *The Angel of Bethesda*, a quirky blend of medicine and religion completed in 1724. "The Surfaces of Animals are covered with other *Animals*," and "as there are Infinite Numbers of these, which the *Microscopes* bring to our View, so there may be inconceivable Myriads yett Smaller than these, which no glasses have yet reach'd unto. . . . The eggs of these Insects (and why not the *living Insects* too!) may insinuate themselves by the Air, and with our Aliments, yea, thro' the Pores of our skin; and soon gett into the Juices of our Bodies." In the proper conditions, "they soon multiply prodigiously; and may have *a greater Share in producing many of our Diseases than is commonly imagined.*"[18]

Mather openly borrowed his ideas from an obscure London physician named Benjamin Marten. His 1720 book *A New Theory of Consumptions* argued that a specific animalcule infecting the lungs was the cause of tuberculosis—and, by extension, that different specific animalcules caused other familiar diseases. Marten in turn was openly borrowing from other

European physicians, who believed, as one of them wrote, "*that Insects occasion most of the Diseases with which Mankind is attack'd.*" Both Mather and Marten also lifted the nicely literary bit about how "Every Part of Matter is *Peopled*" from the London essayist Joseph Addison, without credit. But Mather's book went unpublished, and nobody paid much attention to Benjamin Marten, who was forgotten even when identification of the bacterial cause of tuberculosis 160 years later proved him right.[19]

Mather, Marten, and the rest all credited the origin of animalcular thinking to the microscopic discoveries of Antoni van Leeuwenhoek, who was surprisingly still alive and available to consult about what it all meant. In May 1722, with the debate about variolation still raging, the Royal Society's James Jurin asked Leeuwenhoek to carry out two pertinent investigations: First, was Giovanni Bonomo correct? Were "insects found in the little Bladders of People troubled with the itch"? Second, would he "at [his] leisure, as Opportunity may offer, be pleas'd to observe, whether any Insects are to be found in the Pustules of those that are ill of the Small Pox, as some Persons have imagined"? The puzzling success with variolation, he explained, "has occasion'd Peoples' turning their thoughts more particularly to the manner of propagation of that distemper." Leeuwenhoek, then eighty-nine, agreed to take a look. But no suitable patient appears to have come to hand for either disease.[20]

When other microscopists failed to find animalcules in samples from patients with smallpox and other diseases, they began to back away from the idea of living things as agents of contagion. A technology for viewing viruses like the one that caused smallpox would not exist until the twentieth century. So even lynx-eyed Leeuwenhoek could have seen nothing. On the other hand, if researchers had examined *bacterial* diseases using improved microscopes or better techniques, they might have helped the animalcular idea develop more quickly. But Leeuwenhoek had remained true to his one real expression of ego, keeping his best microscopic methods to himself. At the end of August 1723, he died, age ninety, taking those secrets with him to the grave.

7 SLAYING THE SPECKLED MONSTER

The life of Edward Jenner can seem like a story about the unpredictable, even whimsical, nature of achievement. Jenner (1749–1823) did not set out to produce the single greatest advance in the history of medicine. On the contrary, he seems, for the first two-thirds of his life, to have wanted little more than a comfortable and modestly useful existence. As much as others angled for high position and public honor, Jenner shrank from them. Offered a place, at twenty-two, as a naturalist aboard HMS *Resolution* for the second voyage of the celebrated explorer James Cook, then at the height of his fame, Jenner demurred. He chose instead to retreat to the familiar charms of the British countryside and the study of hedgehogs and cuckoos. Offered a partnership in London, at twenty-six, with his friend and former teacher John Hunter, the greatest surgeon of the day, he politely declined. He preferred to remain a country doctor in Berkeley, Gloucestershire, his birthplace. A few months short of his fortieth birthday, and only a half-dozen years shy of the discovery that would save hundreds of millions of lives and win him worldwide acclaim, he admitted to being "still under the dominion of indolence." It is almost a parable in the futility of ambition.

Jenner had been orphaned at the age of six, reason enough for anyone to seek security in later life. But an older brother raised Edward like a son, and the family had sufficient landholdings to afford a generous living. After his conventional schooling ended at about age thirteen, Jenner served a six-year apprenticeship with a surgical practice in the village of Sodbury, on the edge of the Cotswolds, then went on to two years as John Hunter's student, living in the Hunter home in the center of London. He quickly developed a strong aversion to city life. But the Hunters, husband and wife, would become the great shapers of his adult mind.[1]

John Hunter (1728–1793) was a gruff Scotsman, a former carpenter with little conventional learning, but a driving interest in the natural world and in comparative anatomy. He dissected specimens of five hundred species, as well as "some thousands" of human cadavers obtained through the diligence of grave robbers. Comparisons of the analogous anatomic structures in different species helped make Hunter's surgery more precise—and more merciful in the era before reliable anesthesia.[2]

Jenner's skills as a naturalist no doubt endeared him to Hunter. Hunter recommended him in 1771 when botanist Joseph Banks needed help classifying specimens he'd brought back from the three-year journey of HMS *Endeavour*. Banks in turn offered Jenner the post aboard HMS *Resolution*. When Jenner returned instead to Gloucestershire, Hunter kept up the friendship, largely by mail, in brusque, affectionate letters, beginning, "Dear Jenner." One such letter in 1775 contained a line that has come to epitomize Hunter's approach to science and his influence on students. In response to Jenner's proposal for an experiment on hedgehogs, Hunter wrote (italics added): "I think your solution is just; but *why think, why not trie the experiment*."[3]

Anne Hunter was John's opposite, a poet and brilliant conversationalist who made the Hunter home a salon, attracting writers, musicians, and other influential men and women of the day. She published two volumes of poetry and collaborated with Franz Josef Haydn on the lyrics for several of his songs. Her influence in matters of art and music stayed with Jenner. He later formed a literary society in Cheltenham, where he practiced medicine during that spa town's "season," and he became a friend of poets Thomas Moore and Samuel Taylor Coleridge, among others.[4]

THE COUNTRY GENTLEMAN

As a young surgeon in Gloucestershire, Jenner found time to write his own poetry, though aiming only at what a friend called "harmless gentlemanly facetiousness." His "Address to a Robin" began, predictably, "Come, sweetest of the feather'd throng! / And sooth me with thy plaintive song." A local beer also evidently soothed:

> Come all ye bold Britons who love to be jolly
> And think that Starvation's a very great folly,
> Let's sing of the thing wch so much we admire,
> A good foaming pot, Boys, of Ladbroke's Entire.

Among other amusements, Jenner liked to host music parties, at which he sometimes performed on violin or flute. In the aftermath of Étienne Montgolfier's first human flight in Paris, he also experimented with ballooning. His balloons were too small to carry a passenger. But Jenner attached a poem by a friend, advising the reader who found the balloon of "A truth (which added years will make more clear) / 'That vain ambition is—an Air Balloon!'"[5]

A friend described the young doctor then as a country gentleman, "rather under the middle size . . . but active, and well-formed." He was also "peculiarly neat," dressed, the first time they met, in a broad-brimmed hat,

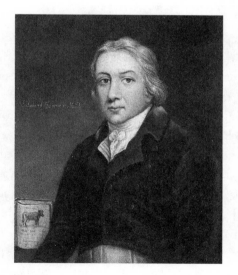

Figure 7.1
Though prone to indolence, Edward Jenner saved more lives than anyone who ever lived (Wellcome Collection).

"a blue coat and yellow buttons, buckskins, well-polished jockey boots, with handsome silver spurs" and "a smart whip with a silver handle." Another friend recalled that Jenner blended "activity of mind with indolence of person, and habits of procrastination." He had no innate aversion to a "more sustained and severe study" but lacked "discipline and regularity."[6]

As it happened, Jenner already possessed the critical knowledge to develop the world's first vaccine and save lives everywhere from the scourge of smallpox. He had acquired it at the age of nineteen, while still a medical apprentice in the Cotswolds. He had no clue yet how important that knowledge would become or what to do with it. But if he seems in retrospect to have become distracted from what we consider his true purpose, that's because we mistakenly assume that the path to great discoveries travels a straight line. In any case, we can hardly begrudge Jenner for finding such pleasure in the best years of his life, even if we seem now to hear legions of the dead rise up from their graves everywhere to cry out in one voice: "Try the experiment!"

THE CUCKOO AND THE COUNTRY DOCTOR

Jenner made a reputation in Gloucestershire, a friend recalled, as "a skilful surgeon and a great naturalist." He accomplished a lot during those decades of country doctoring. For the Gloucestershire Medical Society, he wrote a paper describing mitral stenosis, a hardening of the mitral valve in the heart, and distinguishing it from angina, a hardening of the coronary arteries. He also devised a technique for purifying a common medicine, with consistent results that were otherwise unobtainable. Hunter harried him by mail to capitalize on it, demanding, "Do you mean to take out a Patint? Do you mean to advertise it?" He even proposed a possible brand name, Jenner's Tartar Emetic. Jenner seems characteristically to have had no interest in profiting from his work.[7]

Under Hunter's direction, he devoted himself to the study of the European cuckoo's practice of laying its eggs in the nests of other birds. On hatching, the young cuckoo takes over the nest and induces its unwitting foster parents to give all their energy to the feeding of a nestling that is not their own. (This display of reproductive duplicity and parental gullibility is of course the origin of the word *cuckold*.) Jenner observed cuckoo behavior over the course of fourteen years before sending off a paper to the Royal Society in March 1787. Then he discovered that he'd gotten it wrong.

In his original version, he described a female hedge sparrow retaining the cuckoo in her nest but ejecting her own young, the accepted (if unnatural) explanation for the litter of eggshells and carcasses around such nests. That June, though, Jenner witnessed an actual eviction, with the hatchling cuckoo lifting a nestmate onto its back, then clambering up the side of the nest to the top, "where resting for a moment, it threw off its load with a jerk, and quite disengaged it from the nest." To be certain of this observation, Jenner made multiple experiments, watching hatchling cuckoos repeatedly evict eggs and nestlings he had placed into nests with them. He would repeat this pattern of a long, dilatory gestation followed by a dramatic breakthrough and experimental confirmation when he came to the discovery of vaccination.[8]

Jenner sent off a corrected manuscript, including a description of the broad depression in the cuckoo hatchling's back that facilitated its murderous work. Joseph Banks, by then president of the Royal Society, agreed to publish it in *Philosophical Transactions*, but also warned Jenner, via Hunter, that "there are many who can hardly believe it wholly." Vaccination opponents would later use Jenner's cuckoo work as a weapon to batter his credibility, with one prominent critic still complaining, more than a century later, that it was "a tissue of inconsistencies and absurdities." This anti-vaxxer cuckoo denialism persisted until 1921, 133 years after the original observation, when film footage of the behavior finally proved Jenner right.[9]

WHY NOT TRY THE EXPERIMENT?

Jenner's experience with smallpox began with his own variolation, as a "fine ruddy boy" of eight, in 1757. Because this form of inoculation was still entangled in traditional medical practices, it entailed six weeks of preparation during which he was repeatedly bled and purged, and put on a diet that left him "emaciated and feeble," all to "sweeten" the blood and bring the imaginary humors into a state of readiness. "After this barbarism of human-veterinary practice," his friend Rev. Thomas Fosbroke wrote, "he was removed to one of the then usual inoculation stables, and haltered up with others in a terrible state of disease, though none died." Jenner's own case was mild. But it took him six months to recover, and the ordeal left him acutely sensitive to sudden noises and jarrings. The sound of a fork falling on a plate "gives my brain a kind of death blow," Jenner wrote. Small wonder city life did not suit him.[10]

His first hint of a way around both smallpox and variolation came in 1768. The conventional story is that Jenner asked a milkmaid on a medical visit about smallpox and she replied, "I cannot take that disease, for I have had cow-pox." This minor affliction produced pustules on the udders of cows and could thus infect the hands and wrists of dairy farmers. The symptoms were typically mild, and "a vague opinion prevailed," Jenner later wrote, "that it was a preventive of the Small Pox." The milkmaid story fit a British cultural trope about the smooth skin of milkmaids and became part of the Jenner legend, though he mentioned no such encounter. Some historians have argued instead that Jenner acquired the vaccine idea second-hand from a country doctor named John Fewster, who practiced in the 1760s near Berkeley. But the evidence for this theory is flawed. Most of it comes from a London physician named George Pearson, an envious rival of Jenner. Some scholars also cite a Fewster publication—"*Cowpox and Its Ability to Prevent Smallpox*, unpublished paper read to the Medical Society of London, 1765"—which appears to exist only in their footnotes. In any case, Fewster himself thought cowpox was at best a medical curiosity because variolation was already a satisfactory means of controlling smallpox.[11]

For Jenner, on the other hand, the potential of cowpox as a preventive struck "with force and influence," according to Baron. Jenner raised the topic with John Hunter soon after becoming his student, and later showed him illustrations of the cowpox pustule. Hunter in turn discussed it with other physicians and sometimes included it in his lectures. But no one, including Jenner, seems to have done much with the idea. Baron attributed this to reports that cowpox sometimes afforded protection and sometimes didn't. London-centric thinking may also have been a factor. Jenner's "opinions were commonly regarded as the reveries of a rural enthusiast," according to his friend James Carrick Moore, a surgeon in London.[12]

These "reveries" recurred, however, whenever the rural patients Jenner variolated failed to display even the mildest symptoms of smallpox—and then turned out, on questioning, to have had cowpox. It's not clear why Jenner paid more attention to this phenomenon than other physicians did. Maybe it was the memory of his own terrible experience with variolation as a motherless eight-year-old. Maybe it was just a naturalist's predilection for looking, and looking, and looking again, until the key behavior occurs or the idea that has been sending down roots suddenly breaks through the soil and begins to put out leaves. In any case, Jenner mulled over what he was seeing. But he still had not made what one biographer called "the quantum leap from cowpox, the accidental protector, to cowpox, the transmissible preventive." Variolation—deliberately introducing a deadly human disease into healthy patients—was frightening enough. But deliberately infecting a patient with a disease from barnyard animals must have seemed unthinkable.

When Jenner finally acted, his immediate motivation seems to have been parental anxiety about protecting his own first child from smallpox. In December 1789, a girl who had nursed Edward Jr. came down a few days later with "an eruptive disease." The locals said it was swinepox, but Jenner apparently worried that his child and two young servants of a neighbor may have been exposed to smallpox. He took pus from the sick girl and used it to inoculate the three of them. When he subsequently tested them with a known specimen of smallpox—that is, with variolation—they had become resistant to the disease. Jenner by then regarded three veterinary diseases—swinepox, horsepox (or "grease"), and cowpox—as modified forms of smallpox. But he seems to have been uncertain whether he had initially inoculated the three with a mild version of smallpox—just another variolation—or with swinepox, a rather different thing, foreshadowing his eventual development of vaccination.[13]

He began to keep records of cases in which accidental exposure to cowpox protected patients against smallpox. He was learning to sort out the different pox types and also to distinguish cowpox from pustular cattle diseases that failed to produce protection against smallpox. Progress was slow because cowpox was an infrequent visitor to local dairies. Finally, in May 1796, a suitable case appeared within a short walk of Jenner's home in Berkeley.

Sarah Nelmes, daughter of a prosperous local farm family, had contracted cowpox while milking cows. Jenner took fluid from one of the resulting pustules and, on May 14, introduced it via two shallow incisions in the arm of James Phipps, the eight-year-old son of a local laborer. Phipps developed minor symptoms—headache, loss of appetite, a night of restlessness—then quickly recovered. Six weeks later, Jenner attempted variolation, "with variolous matter, immediately taken from a pustule," and found Phipps "secure from the contagion of the Small-pox." He exposed the child to smallpox again two months later, and repeatedly over the next two decades, always with the same result.

Although the word itself did not yet exist, this was the beginning of modern vaccination. It was such a momentous development that the names of Nelmes, Phipps, and even Blossom, the cow responsible for infecting Nelmes, still hold a place of honor in medical history. Blossom would in time be "turned out to end her days peaceably at Bradstone, a farm near Berkeley." But for Edward Jenner, the would-be fugitive from greatness, an enormous struggle still lay ahead.[14]

8 AN ANGEL'S TRUMPET

Early in 1797, Jenner submitted his cowpox work for publication in the Royal Society's *Philosophical Transactions*. He chose not to trade on his friendship with Sir Joseph Banks, then president of the Royal Society, nor could he rely on his friend and advocate John Hunter, who had died a few years earlier. A society functionary soon advised Banks that the cases Jenner had presented were "much too few to admit of Conclusions being drawn from them."

In fact, Jenner at that point had only one case of deliberate treatment with cowpox, the Phipps boy, backed up with multiple cases of people who had experienced cowpox accidentally and then, on testing by Jenner with variolation, proved to be resistant to smallpox. The society functionary thought those adult patients "were probably not naturally susceptible of that disease," perhaps having been exposed to smallpox earlier in their lives. If Jenner repeated his results on twenty or thirty children, the functionary said, "I might be led to change my opinion, at present however I want faith."[1]

Whether the Royal Society rejected the paper outright or merely sent it back for revisions, as it had done with Jenner's cuckoo paper, is unclear. Either way, "matters were managed somewhat uncourteously," according to Jenner's friend John Baron. Having won credit for his work on cuckoos, Jenner "ought not to risk his reputation," someone suggested, on an idea "so much at variance with established knowledge, and withal so incredible." Jenner, who could be thin-skinned, took it badly. As a result, the Royal Society lost the chance to publish "a contribution," Baron wrote, "which has done more for the relief of human misery than any work that man ever produced." Jenner turned away determined to pursue his experiments "with redoubled ardour."[2]

That long, bleak year passed without any further cases of cowpox in the local dairies. He tried to infect a cow with horsepox, to test a mistaken theory that cowpox originated when dairymen inadvertently got horsepox on their hands and transmitted it to cows. This experiment turned out to be "not so easily made as at first sight may be imagined," he admitted. But in March 1798, cowpox reappeared in the area on its own. Jenner proceeded to administer it to a dozen or so other patients, mostly children, including his eleven-month-old son, Robert. This time, he took the opportunity to attempt transmission from one patient's pustules to several other patients, and from their pustules to several more. After a suitable interval, he variolated some of these patients and found them resistant to smallpox. "These experiments afforded me much satisfaction," he wrote, in that "they proved that the [cowpox] matter, in passing from one human subject to another, through five gradations, lost none of its original properties." Keeping the cowpox alive from one arm to another, possibly without limit, was a key development. By reducing dependence on the chance appearance of a veterinary disease known only in western Europe, it promised to free this new method for use anywhere, at any time.[3]

Rather than crawl back to the Royal Society, Jenner published his work on his own in mid-1798, under the title *An Inquiry into the Causes and Effects of the Variolæ Vaccinæ*, with *variolae vaccinae* meaning "the smallpox of cows." The seventy-five-page pamphlet began with a thunderclap, on the zoological origin of many infectious diseases. "The deviation of Man," Jenner wrote, "from the state in which he was originally placed by Nature seems to have proved to him a prolific source of Diseases." The wolf, transformed into a lapdog, and the cat, drawn out of its native haunts, were "equally domesticated and caressed. The Cow, the Hog, the Sheep, and the Horse, are all, for a variety of purposes, brought under his care and dominion." As these domesticated animals had occupied our homes and our lives, their diseases had come to colonize our bodies, with "effects in some degree similar; but what renders the Cow-pox virus so extremely singular, is, that the person who has been thus affected is for ever after secure from the infection of the Small Pox."

Based on the patients he had treated, Jenner argued that cowpox provided three great advantages over variolation: "In the Cow-pox, no pustules appear," sparing patients even the significantly reduced outbreak common in variolation. Cowpox was not contagious, as variolation was now known to be. "So that a single individual in a family might at any time receive it without the risk of infecting the rest, or of spreading a distemper that fills a country with terror." And while variolation "sometimes, under the best management, proves fatal," Jenner wrote, he had "never known fatal effects [to] arise" with cowpox, "even when impressed in the most unfavourable manner." Above all, "it clearly appears that this disease leaves the constitution in a state of perfect security from the infection of the Small-pox."[4]

Serious issues would arise with these last two assertions. Jenner reported that one patient, a five-year-old boy, "was rendered unfit for inoculation"— that is, follow-up testing with variolation—"from having felt the effects of a contagious fever in a work-house." It was of course common for children to come down with fever in the harsh conditions of a workhouse and reasonable not to subject him to further testing. But Jenner failed to disclose until his second publication in 1799 that the boy had in fact died of the fever. The assertion that cowpox inoculation made the patient "for ever secure" from smallpox was also problematic. How could he know how long the protection would last?

Jenner also soon realized that cows were sometimes afflicted with pustules that a careless practitioner could mistake for cowpox, but which provided no protection whatsoever. He rushed to provide a detailed description of the type and timing of the "true" cowpox, publishing his *Further Observations on the Variolæ Vaccinæ* in April 1799, less than a year after his *Inquiry*, followed by *A Continuation of Facts and Observations Relative to the Variolæ Vaccinæ, or Cow Pox* in 1800. The compelling interest in smallpox attracted a wide readership. In a letter, Jane Austen described a dinner party in the Hampshire countryside where one couple took turns reading aloud from "Dr. Jenner's pamphlet on the cow pox" while another couple courted, and one guest slept.[5]

Missteps by others threatened the early success of Jenner's new method. In January 1799, cowpox appeared in a dairy on Gray's Inn Lane in London, and physician William Woodville summoned a group of influential figures to meet the next day at the dairy as witnesses. He brought along Jenner's *Inquiry*, to establish that the cowpox illustrated there matched the ones on the cows and their milkers. Then he took samples and used them to administer cowpox to fourteen patients. He sent an enthusiastic note about the test to Jenner, who replied in evident alarm. Woodville had treated these patients at his workplace, the London Smallpox Hospital, and might inadvertently have exposed them to the disease before the vaccine could protect them.

It was worse than that. Jenner typically waited six weeks for his vaccine to elicit an immune response before testing the effectiveness of the procedure with variolation. But Woodville did so within as little as three days after inoculation with cowpox. Predictably, a majority of test subjects developed the generalized eruptions seen with variolation, seeming to belie the assurances in Jenner's *Inquiry*. Woodville and an ally, George Pearson, a physician at St. George's Hospital, were already distributing potentially contaminated matter from such patients across England and the continent. Both physicians were advocates of the new method, however, and assured Jenner that they found the side effects "slighter" than those in variolation.[6]

Pearson was in fact so excited about the possibilities that he had rushed his own 120-page *Inquiry Concerning the History of the Cow Pox* into print just months after Jenner's publication. This booklet "was swollen with replies to a multitude of letters, which he had dispatched to the dairy counties in hopes of learning something," Jenner's friend James Carrick Moore later wrote. "But, by ill hap, his correspondents were as ignorant as himself; for not one of them had ever seen the Vaccine." The resulting "incoherent mass of misinformation formed a tottering basis for many sophistical deductions."

Early in his book, Pearson made the odd assertion that he entertained "not the most distant expectation of . . . the smallest share" in the honor due "on the score of discovery of facts." That honor, he piously declaimed, "belongs exclusively to Dr. Jenner; and I would not pluck a sprig of laurel from the wreath that decorates his brow." It reminded Moore of a murderer who cries "I didn't do it" before anyone has even thought to connect him to the crime. Pearson soon went on to establish the Institute for the Inoculation of the Vaccine-Pock in London and invited Jenner to become a dues-paying correspondent. Jenner replied angrily, knowing his own reputation would suffer "if the vaccine inoculation, from unguarded conduct, should sink into disrepute." Pearson's backers soon withdrew from the short-lived institute.[7]

Years later, when Parliament was considering whether to honor Jenner with a substantial grant for his work on the vaccine, Pearson, embittered, set out to block the move. He presented evidence that various people before Jenner had known about cowpox or even tried cowpox on family or friends to protect them from smallpox. But it was evident to all, except Pearson, that none of them had made these trials public, or conducted them so extensively, in such experimental detail, or with such concern for the public good, as had Jenner. Pearson was left to whine in a letter that Parliament had failed to offer even "an acknowledgement by honourable mention of services," instead setting the laurel wreath unplucked on Jenner's brow.[8]

Jenner's vaccine was otherwise winning friends everywhere. His allies urged him to move to London and establish a practice that they thought would bring in £10,000 a year, a fortune then. Jenner, who was forty-nine, made one last stand against London's notion of greatness. Having "sought the lowly and sequestered paths of life, the valley, and not the mountain," he confided to a friend, would it make sense, relatively late in life, to "hold myself up as an object for fortune and for fame?" The money hardly mattered; he and his family already had enough. As for fame, he called it "a gilded butt"—that is, a cask—"for ever pierced with the arrows of malignancy." And yet he was also "fearful that the practice [he had] recommended may fall into the hands of those who are incapable of conducting it." No doubt he was thinking of the Pearsons of the medical world. That fear would be his turning point. He took a house on Hertford Street in Mayfair and spent several months there each year, seeing patients and advancing the vaccination cause.[9]

VACCINE CLERK TO THE WORLD

In November 1798, Jenner had been unable to lay his hands on a single source of cowpox matter. But as news of his discovery spread, other physicians ransacked dairies for the stuff. Just one year later, Jenner could boast that more than five thousand in Britain had been "inoculated with vaccine virus," with "fresh and convincing evidence" of its power against smallpox "constantly flowing in." The clamor to put cowpox to work everywhere was, in the words of a later historian, "as if an Angel's trumpet had sounded over the earth." Jenner now became "vaccine clerk to the world," as he put it, propagating the cowpox vaccine at home and abroad via a rapidly expanding network of correspondents.[10]

In Vienna, physician Jean de Carro performed the first cowpox inoculation on the continent in May 1799, using vaccine sent by a friend in London. Jenner sent a further supply later that year, and de Carro was soon exporting vaccine to Poland, Germany, Hungary, and Russia, as well as to Constantinople, a small repayment for that city's gift of variolation. A physician in Milan found cowpox in local dairies there and wrote to Jenner in 1801 to report "more than eight thousand inoculations performed with the most happy success." In England and other places, the first vaccine skeptics also appeared, fearful that cowpox might cause people to develop cow-like tendencies, catch animal diseases, or even sprout horns. Satirist James Gillray responded with an 1802 cartoon depicting patients with miniature cattle erupting in place of noses, earlobes, and tongues.

In 1800, with Jenner's support, two physicians traveled with the British Mediterranean fleet, administering cowpox in every port of call. At Palermo, where eight thousand people had died of smallpox the previous year, they had to demonstrate the effectiveness of the new method to skeptical officials. But soon after, one of the doctors reported back to Jenner, "it was not unusual to see . . . a procession of men, women, and children conducted through the streets by a priest carrying a cross, come to be inoculated," with people calling it "a blessing from heaven, though discovered by one heretic and practiced by another." A doctor in Spain proposed making vaccination a sacrament, with priest and physician working in tandem to bless and protect children.[11]

Transporting the vaccine from one city to another, much less across continents and oceans, was challenging. An early method was to mail a lancet—a simple tool for making small incisions—with cowpox matter coated on the tip. When the cowpox liquid caused rusting, de Carro switched to ivory lancets. Jenner and other physicians also tried soaking cloth in the fluid from a cowpox pustule and posting the threads with instructions to eke out a small section of thread per patient, moistened and placed in an incision in the skin. Shipping cowpox matter pressed between glass plates was also common, sometimes dry, sometimes with the aim of keeping it wet by carefully sealing the edges.[12]

Jenner's first attempt to get cowpox to India failed when the ship sank en route. He sent another supply overland. But this seemed agonizingly slow to a colonial doctor in Madras who had lost "a beautiful little patient" to variolation and could no longer "take up a lancet for that purpose but with fear and trembling." When vaccine from Jenner finally got through, the dried cowpox turned out to have lost its potency. Jenner then urged the British government to recruit twenty volunteers on an eastbound ship to be inoculated one after another during the long voyage to India and ultimately deliver live cowpox arm to arm. Rebuffed, he proposed funding this means of delivery by private subscription and committed £1,000 to the effort.

In 1801, before that could happen, viable cowpox matter from de Carro made its hopscotch way from Constantinople to Baghdad to Basra to Bombay. "It gives me great pleasure to observe that the natives begin to acquire confidence in this practice," with two or three thousand children in Bombay already inoculated, a colonial doctor soon reported to Jenner. Predictably, his own children had been "the first in India to enjoy the protection of the cow-pox," an example soon "followed by every European family here."[13]

Jenner sent vaccine in 1798 to a friend who had become a clergyman-physician in Newfoundland, and a second batch circulated among his British colleagues before making the leap, in 1800, to the United States. There, Boston physician Benjamin Waterhouse successfully passed some of it along, on the third try, to Thomas Jefferson, who oversaw the inoculation of two hundred neighbors at Monticello, including people he had enslaved. He also devised a thermos-like device, a small flask within a larger flask filled with water, to transport vaccine, but seems not to have built it. As president, Jefferson gave vaccine to a visiting Native American delegation. Later, he sent vaccine west with the Lewis and Clark Expedition, with instructions to inform others they met of its "efficacy as a preservative from the small pox; and instruct & encourage them in the use of it."[14]

THE FIRST GLOBAL VACCINATION CAMPAIGN

Vaccine arrived in Spain in 1800, and King Carlos IV, who had suffered the devastation of smallpox in his own family, ordered an audacious maritime expedition to disseminate vaccination throughout the Spanish empire. The Royal Philanthropic Vaccine Expedition would become the first global public health initiative. It was remarkable for anticipating and devising solutions to problems that "were then without precedent but that would recur in many vaccination programs" up to the present day, according to medical historians Catherine Mark and José G. Rigau-Pérez.[15]

The ambition was to establish local and regional vaccine boards everywhere to maintain the vaccine supply and oversee its continued use, to train local vaccinators in proper technique, and to administer vaccine to the general public without charge. José Flores, a Guatemalan physician with years of experience practicing variolation, helped plan the expedition. He advocated using indigenous languages, working with trusted community leaders, and treating patients as gently as possible to encourage participation.

The expedition, under the command of physician Francisco Xavier de Balmis, sailed from the northwestern port of A Coruña in the 160-ton corvette *María Pita* in November 1803. To address the challenge of transporting the vaccine across the Atlantic, the ship carried twenty-two young boys from foundling homes, shepherded by the headmistress from one of the homes. Medical staff on board vaccinated one pair of boys at a time in succession over the course of the ten-week voyage, ensuring a supply of live vaccine on arrival in Puerto Rico. They also collected matter from the vaccination pustules en route and attempted to preserve it sealed between glass slides in a vacuum formed by a primitive pneumatic device.

Puerto Rico, it turned out, already had vaccine delivered by other means. Venezuela was less fortunate, and celebrated the arrival of vaccination with fireworks, concerts, and a Mass of thanksgiving. The expedition went on to introduce vaccine to Cuba, Mexico, and Central America. The Spanish foundlings then returned home, and twenty-six Mexican boys replaced them as the expedition pressed across the Pacific.

The expedition's surgeon, José Salvany, headed south on a separate leg of the humanitarian mission. His contingent carried the vaccine overland on a four-thousand-kilometer route, entailing years of discomfort and danger, to bring relief to present-day Colombia, Ecuador, Peru, and Bolivia. They vaccinated almost two hundred thousand people in South America before Salvany died of an apparent heart condition, age thirty-six, in Cochabamba, Bolivia, in July 1810. The main expedition had ended years earlier, after delivering vaccine to the Philippines and China, with the return to Spain of expedition leader Francisco Xavier de Balmis in 1806.

Modern scholars sometimes characterize such medical initiatives as little more than a device for advancing colonial enterprises and bringing indigenous populations under thumb. But given the deep fear at that time of smallpox as an inevitable fate, this interpretation may be too narrow. For Enlightenment elites, gaining protection for themselves and their families was an almost unimaginably profound relief, and the dream stirred of using science to protect cities, countries, even humanity. This was particularly true for doctors and nurses risking their lives in the expedition.

As in all human endeavors, though, the motives were mixed. King Carlos IV "apparently decided with his heart, rather than his pocket, on the need to send the expedition to America," launching it in the midst of major political and economic troubles, according to Mark and Rigau-Pérez. Faced with the considerable expense, his bureaucrats in Madrid then rationalized "that the benefit for the most severely affected populations, the Native Americans, would result in greater income for the Treasury." If they weren't dying of smallpox, they would be available to work in the mines.

THE LOATHSOME SMALLPOX

The speed with which the new method raced across the globe was stunning, at a time when the fastest travel was by horse or sailing vessel. But people still barely had a language to discuss the apparent miracle of prevention that was suddenly available to them. The idea that the body had an immune system did not yet exist to help explain what was happening, and the terminology—*cowpox inoculation*, *cowpoxing*, and, in the United States, *kinepox*—served mainly to emphasize that this process involved introducing an animal product into the human body.

And yet as early as 1801, Jenner could write in evident awe of the "immense" scope "that this inoculation has now taken." It was just five years from James Phipps, and from Jenner's own life as a little-known country doctor. It would be another two years before a British surgeon and vaccine advocate named Richard Dutton would take Jenner's *vaccinae* and coin the name by which the new methodology would become known in dozens of languages: *vaccination*. But already Jenner could write, "An hundred thousand persons, upon the smallest computation, have been inoculated in these realms," and an "incalculable" number in other countries. He predicted what would have been unthinkable a few years before: "It now becomes too manifest to admit of controversy, that the annihilation of the Small-Pox, the most dreadful scourge of the human species, must be the final result of this practice."[16]

He was not alone in thinking it. In an 1806 letter to Jenner, US President Thomas Jefferson wrote as if eradication of the disease—still 174 years in the future—were already history: "You have erased from the calendar of human afflictions one of its greatest. Yours is the comfortable reflection that mankind can never forget that you have lived. Future nations will know by history only that the loathsome small-pox has existed and by you has been extirpated."[17]

9 THE GREAT SANITARY AWAKENING

By the turn of the nineteenth century, the factories of the Industrial Revolution were already beginning to pack old cities with newcomers. Soaring urban populations would soon overwhelm the available housing and the adjacent untended, and often uncovered, cesspools. Entire families commonly huddled together in single rooms, often in windowless basements. Overflowing sewage at times made entire cities feel as if adrift atop a sea of human waste. Disease was the inevitable result.

The response to urban crowding and squalor came slowly because public health was then outside the purview of national governments. People also failed to recognize the developing scale of the problem, or they imagined that it would affect only the poor. When the urban sanitary awakening finally began, the French took the lead, establishing the first academic chair of public hygiene in 1794 and the first journal of public health in 1829. With their detailed firsthand accounts, pioneers of the new field helped establish the expectation in modern public health of personal involvement at the scene of an outbreak, regardless of hardship. Louis-René Villermé (1782–1863) produced a classic study of cotton mill workers, spending time with them on the job and in the streets and rooms where they eked out their lives. A. J. B. Parent-Duchâtelet (1790–1835) surveyed more than five thousand women for his massive work on prostitution. Victor Hugo later used this work to shape the character of Fantine in *Les Misérables*, correctly interpreting the data to put the blame for prostitution on dire poverty.[1]

PUTRID EXHALATIONS

Almost all the early sanitary reformers focused obsessively on smells, partly because they were everywhere—the acrid odors of factories, the backyard pigsties, the tonnage of droppings from horses and from livestock being driven to slaughterhouses, the rotting offal, the tanneries, the shallow graves of the dead, and the "vitiated air" of overcrowded and unventilated rooms.

Foul smells, or "putrid exhalations," were "poisons, as dangerous as mad dogs," a nineteenth century British sanitarian thundered, and yet "still allowed to be kept in close rooms, in cesspools, and in sewers, from which they prowl, in the light of day, and in the darkness of night, with impunity, to destroy mankind." This was partly an extension of the humoral obsession with miasmas, compounded by innate feelings of disgust. But both were now being updated with the discoveries of the scientific enlightenment. William Harvey had described the circulation of blood in 1628. Antoine Lavoisier had identified oxygen in 1778. Scottish physicist and chemist Joseph Black had described carbon dioxide in 1772 and demonstrated that it was a product of animal respiration. Medical thinkers set aside the idea of the lungs as primarily a means of releasing and balancing bodily humors. Instead, the developing picture of respiration and the exchange of vital gases led to a relentless focus on just what was being breathed. Faith in the protective power of fresh air was so strong that, when one hospital repeatedly ignored his orders to provide adequate ventilation, Parent-Duchâtelet had the windows smashed.[2]

Medical debate increasingly pitted contagionists against anticontagionists. The contagionists held that diseases spread from a sick person to a healthy one by way of some unknown infectious matter, on the air they exhaled, in bodily fluids, or on objects they touched. The anticontagionists countered that chemical substances in the air—effluvia, miasmas, poisons, foul odors—were the culprits.

AN OUTSTANDING BORE

The British ultimately proved more effective than the French at doing something about the stench, largely through the outsize influence of one peculiar man. Edwin Chadwick (1800–1890), now mostly forgotten, was a barrister, journalist, and social reformer. He had served as secretary to the wealthy and even more peculiar English philosopher Jeremy Bentham, who propounded the utilitarian idea that we should measure right or wrong by what produces "the greatest happiness for the greatest number." With this philosophy in mind, Chadwick campaigned aggressively and successfully from the late 1820s onward for the British government to intervene in matters of public health and welfare. His investigations made centralized systems for public water supply and sewerage a reality. He promoted essential urban services, including street cleaning, garbage removal, and also of course proper ventilation, as a natural antidote to foul smells. Chadwick's work transformed the character and well-being of cities not just in Britain but, by example, worldwide. Along the way, he helped to establish the basis for the modern liberal state. "Few men have done so much for their fellow-countrymen as Edwin Chadwick," biographer R. A. Lewis wrote, "and received in return so little thanks."[3]

This uncelebrated status is no doubt due both to the lowliness of his chief subject—the disposal of human waste—and to Chadwick's difficult personality. A sanitarian who was a friend described him in the heroic mode: "firm-set massive build . . . resolute expression . . . nose aquiline . . . the head altogether large, and to the phrenologist finely developed." But photographs from the period show a tall, round-faced figure, in moustache and muttonchops, hair smeared in hanks across his balding scalp, peering out from heavy-lidded eyes with something like judgment, if not disdain. Chadwick made a reputation for prodigious energy, and for his command of the facts of any issue he studied. But he was also humorless and uncompromising toward those who disagreed with him. He made little effort to hide his contempt for aristocratic domination or for foot-dragging by corrupt or indifferent politicians.[4]

He was also a bore, "a really outstanding specimen of bore in an age when the species flourished," according to the otherwise admiring biography by Lewis. "Mr. Chadwick is not an orator," a friend acknowledged. "When he first gets up to speak without book he looks an orator, but a few moments dispel the illusion; he bends forward, he speaks in a low voice, he disputes

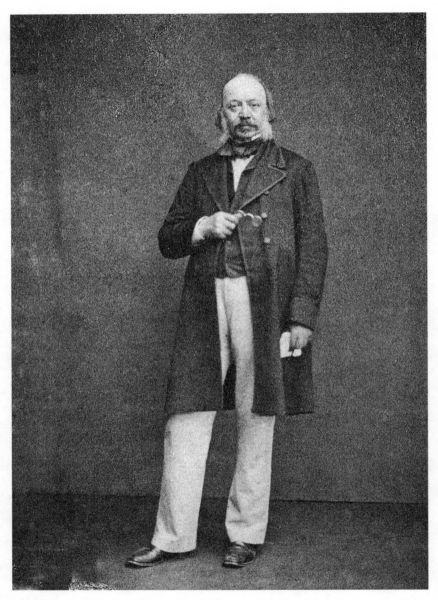

Figure 9.1
The sanitarian Edwin Chadwick (Wellcome Collection).

some points logically, then falls into confusion, then recovers his strain, goes back, and in fact if he speaks long, as he is wont, wearies the listener, and takes sometimes the points out of his own argument." But he possessed strengths far outweighing these weaknesses, among them his unrelenting diligence and attention to details, and his mastery of organization.[5]

BEING CHADWICKED

Chadwick made his first unfortunate public reputation working for a royal commission to modernize the system of relief for the poor. The resulting Poor Law Amendment Act of 1834, which he drafted, mandated the end of payments to the able-bodied poor, with the aim of bringing market forces to bear on underemployed workers lingering in rural areas. This accelerated flight from the farm to factory jobs in the city, thus inadvertently compounding urban squalor and desperation. The new law also established the notorious workhouse system, where those who continued to receive aid were required to take up residence in prison-like conditions, with children typically separated from their parents. Charles Dickens wrote *Oliver Twist* to expose this system's cruelties.[6]

It made Chadwick one of the most hated men in nineteenth-century Britain. The poor hated him not just for the Poor Law but for a subsequent law requiring civil registration of births, deaths, and marriages. They called it *being Chadwicked.* The keeping of vital statistics, particularly cause of death, would help save the lives of many of the people who at first resented it so bitterly. But it was easier to see the immediate intrusion than to anticipate the eventual benefit. At the same time, the rich and powerful hated Chadwick for threatening their preferred laissez-faire system with the shadow of centralized government authority.

In 1838, Chadwick turned his attention to public health, partly because Poor Law work had shown him the vulnerability of the urban poor to disease. That year, a devastating outbreak of typhus (a term that then included typhoid fever) sickened fourteen thousand people in London alone. In the aftermath, Chadwick arranged for the Poor Law Commissioners to have three prominent physicians investigate the link between public health and pauperism in London. The result, published in 1838, caused a sensation, particularly for its depiction of the city's unsanitary system of water supply by private companies. The commissioners then assigned Chadwick to conduct a similar investigation into the sanitary conditions in which the laboring classes lived nationwide. They provided no funding.

Chadwick undertook a prodigious correspondence with doctors and Poor Law officials across the country, asking them to answer a list of detailed questions. His passion for gathering evidence with his own eyes also made him a determined explorer into British slums, recording how the poor lived and died. In the process, he contracted typhus (or typhoid fever), which nearly killed him. The result was such a dire and unsparing picture of a nationwide public health emergency that his timorous employers demanded changes and ultimately declined to put their names on it.[7]

Thus one of the most important works in the history of public health carried only Edwin Chadwick's name when it appeared in 1842. The *Sanitary Report*—short for *Report on the Sanitary Condition of the Labouring Population of Great Britain*—was an odd publication to come from the government's own Stationery Office. It was "a masterpiece of protest literature," in the words of one historian, weaving together "the most lurid details and evocative descriptions, damning statistics and damaging examples." It sold one hundred thousand copies, more than any previous government publication.[8]

For most educated readers, the world of the urban newcomers of the Industrial Revolution had been as foreign as Calcutta. Chadwick's report led them deep into the squalor they had previously passed by with eyes and noses averted. On one perambulation through the narrow lanes and courtyards of a fever-ridden Glasgow neighborhood, he described open dung heaps piled high "with all [the] filth that the swarm of wretched inhabitants could give." Inside, people crowded "together to be warm; and in one bed, although in the middle of the day, several women were imprisoned under a blanket" because they had to share their only clothing with other women who had gone out for the day.

In London, there were cellars three feet deep in human excrement from overflowing cesspools, and houses in which "every article of food and drink must be covered," lest swarms of houseflies immediately attack it and render it unfit for use "from the strong taste of the dunghill left by the flies." From Stirling, Scotland, a correspondent wrote that "the filth of the gaol, containing on an average 65 prisoners, is floated down the public streets every second or third day, and emits, during the whole of its progress . . . the most offensive and disgusting odour," routinely joined by blood from the slaughterhouse.

Chadwick built his report as methodically as a legal brief. In the first section, he described the squalid residences of the working poor and the problems caused by crowding and lack of ventilation. He also showed how public arrangements worsened the health of workers, through inadequate water supply, lack of sewerage, and nonexistent street cleaning. Next, Chadwick focused on the devastating cost of existing sanitary conditions to the economy, in lives and workdays lost. He also made detailed recommendations, including public control of the water supply and sewerage systems, which needed to be properly pitched to flush wastes well away from crowded populations. (Sewage, he thought, could be harvested in farm areas for use as manure.) Finally, he presented evidence that sanitary measures could improve health and longevity at reasonable cost, and he reviewed the state of existing law and of the local authorities responsible for administering it.

The *Sanitary Report*'s angry rhetorical flourishes were calculated to startle the public out of its complacency: "The annual slaughter in England and Wales from preventible causes of typhus . . . appears to be double the amount of what was suffered by the Allied Armies in the battle of Waterloo." Chadwick also made shrewd use of medical statistics, a science then in its crude early stages. He compared the decreasing mortality in one East Anglia town that installed sewers with the rising death rate in a similar town nearby that continued to rely on open cesspools. Even more effective was a section with tables and maps showing the variation in death rates in different social classes within the same communities. In Bethnal Green, in London's East End, the average age of death for "gentlemen and persons engaged in professions, and their families" was forty-five, but for tradesmen it was twenty-six, and for "mechanics, servants, and labourers," just sixteen.

Chadwick's neighborhood-by-neighborhood, and street-by-street, comparisons foreshadowed the modern environmental justice movement. And he was plainly moved to moral outrage by the complacency with which the "better classes" tolerated and even tacitly applauded the endless dying. A common view held that a high death rate among the poor benefited society by providing a Malthusian check on population. To the contrary, Chadwick recounted a visit to a crowded neighborhood notorious for its high mortality rate. "Why, the undertaker is never absent from this place," he remarked to a local woman. She looked out over a courtyard full of underfed children and replied, "No, nor the midwife either." Chadwick wrote "that the ravages of epidemics and other diseases do not diminish but tend to increase the pressure of population."[9]

SEEKING THE CLEANLY PATH

Of all the converts in the wake of this sanitary jeremiad, perhaps the most surprising was Charles Dickens. In a September 1843 comment on Chadwick's work, Dickens had noted sharply, "I do differ from him, to the death, on his crack topic—the new Poor Law." But the sanitary awakening gradually won him over, and he began to adopt its ideas and even its language. Describing the habitats of the urban poor in his 1848 novel *Dombey and Sons*, for instance, he wrote, "If the noxious particles that rise from vitiated air, were palpable to the sight, we should see them lowering in a dense black cloud above such haunts, and rolling slowly on to corrupt the better portions of a town."[10]

That same year, Dickens launched his own weekly magazine, *Household Words*, as "the gentle mouthpiece of reform." Among other topics, it published a fictionalized account of London's "Troubled Water Question," taking Chadwick's view on the filthy water supplied by private companies, followed later by a series of articles on the full range of sanitary issues. Dickens at one point contributed an article of his own in which he sounded like Chadwick unchained, on the "intolerable ills" arising from the terrible living conditions of the poor: "A Board of Health can do much, but not near enough. Funds are wanted, and great powers are wanted; powers to over-ride little interests for the general good; powers to coerce the ignorant, obstinate and slothful and to punish all who, by any infraction of necessary laws, imperil the public health."[11]

No major legislation resulted at first from the *Sanitary Report*. Instead, Chadwick spent nine months preparing an appendix on one particularly offensive item in the catalog of foul smells: London was somehow packing fifty thousand corpses a year into just 218 acres of burial grounds. (Most were small children, which made for better packing.) The products of decomposition tainted the air and at times gave a "disagreeable" flavor to the water from nearby drinking wells. Characteristically for Chadwick, his report proposed remedies that relied heavily on government intervention. He wanted to prohibit burials in urban churchyards, replacing them with modern, suburban cemeteries. Prompt removal of the dead from homes, particularly in cases of infectious disease, would be mandatory, and regulations would minimize the cost of burial.[12]

The visceral horror of these reports took hold in the public mind. It aroused in politicians the need to be seen to be doing something, preferably without disturbing vested interests. A royal commission soon followed, chaired by the Duke of Buccleuch. He turned over much of the work to Chadwick, the acknowledged expert. But all thirteen eminent commissioners signed the two-part *Large Towns and Populous Districts* report, published in 1844 and 1845. It presented further evidence of the disease and degradation then commonplace among the poor. It also provided a remarkably comprehensive program for reforming towns and cities to improve the health of their residents.

The recommendations included provision of a constant supply of water to all homes and businesses, together with a system of sewers and drainage, all under the direction of a single administrative body for each locality. The aim was to provide a continuous "arterial-venous" flow of water, into cities for daily use, and out again, carrying away wastes. Local governments would have power over the removal of rubbish; widening, paving, and cleaning of streets and pedestrian walkways; the design, construction, and ventilation of buildings; and the appointment of a medical officer to inspect all such matters of public health. The report also recommended a way for local property owners to pay for these improvements without bankrupting themselves, by amortizing the costs over years or even decades. But the first, and clearly most important, recommendation was for a national authority to inspect and supervise sanitary improvements. This had always been Chadwick's ambition, given his faith in the value of a centralized civil service, aloof from petty local interests. It fit with the abundant evidence he had accumulated, at the local level, of indifference, incompetence, corruption, and favoritism of wealthy interests over the needs of the poor. The report was altogether a broad endorsement by the establishment for radical transformation in the way cities operated.[13]

It took another three years of political infighting to win approval of the Public Health Act of 1848, which established a weakened version of the central oversight body Chadwick had imagined. The law endowed all communities with a population of five thousand or more the exclusive power within their borders to provide water, sewerage, and street cleaning. The General Board of Health could, however, intervene and take over these responsibilities if the death rate was excessive, or if 10 percent of local ratepayers petitioned for intervention.[14]

By hard lobbying, Chadwick won appointment as the only salaried commissioner of the three assigned to run the General Board of Health. His six years in that post "were the happiest in his official career," according to biographer R. L. Lewis. At his office in the heart of Whitehall, he gladly worked twelve- or fourteen-hour days, "sending out his Inspectors to put chastened local authorities on the cleanly path of tubular sewerage and constant supply."[15]

This was bound to be hard work, against forces characterized by one historian as "parsimony compounded by ignorance and fear of engineering innovations." The reforms he was advocating were daunting in their scope for local officials and engineers who had never imagined water supply and sewer systems planned and built out across an entire town or city, much less across a natural topographic drainage. Then, as now, they resented outside interference and were capable of saying almost anything to defeat it. In 1846, a delegation questioned the Lord Mayor of London about the approaching threat of cholera. The squalor Chadwick had detailed remained entirely unchanged. But the lord mayor assured his interrogators that "there could be no sanitary improvement effected in the City of London." It was, he said, already "perfect." The cholera epidemic of 1848–1849 suggested otherwise, killing fifteen thousand London residents.[16]

SPARKS INTO FLAMES

In the General Board of Health's first five years of work under Chadwick, 284 towns petitioned to be recognized under the new Public Health Act. Drainage surveys—the first step toward a proper sewer system—were completed or in progress in 126 towns. Thirty-one municipalities had already finished their plans for water supply and drainage and had received approval from the board to seek the necessary financing. In some cases, work had begun. This no doubt seemed like a slow start to the notoriously impatient Chadwick. But it was still a novelty for any government to do anything at all about public health—much less do it at the mandatory expense of private property owners. The willingness of towns to go along was a measure of just how profoundly the conditions revealed by Chadwick's *Sanitary Report* had entered the public mind.

There had been one fiasco, on the first pipeline system installed under the Chadwick plan. Faulty construction and design caused the new sewer lines to leak into the new water line. An outbreak of typhoid fever precisely followed the line of the new work, with eighteen hundred cases and sixty dead, in a middle-class community of sixteen thousand. Remarkably, it wasn't fatal for the sanitary idea. Most other towns appeared to be satisfied with their new water and sewerage systems, which were "novel in design, cheap to construct, and efficient in operation, bringing the means of health and cleanliness down to a weekly charge of a few pence" per house, Lewis wrote. "But greater than the economy of money which resulted was the economy of life." The General Board of Health reported in 1853 that replacing cesspools with sewer pipelines in London's prosperous Lambeth Square had caused the annual death rate to fall from thirty to thirteen per thousand. Sanitary improvements had also halved the death rate in certain unnamed working-class areas. The board was no doubt cherry-picking its data. But it projected that the same improvements would prevent twenty-five thousand needless deaths per year if applied across London, and 170,000 across

England and Wales. The average age at death would climb from twenty-nine to about forty-eight.[17]

Unfortunately, Chadwick's career as an executive was destined to be brief. He had been making bitter enemies since Poor Law days, and too few friends. He had criticized physicians for dithering about the true cause of disease and promoting bogus cures. He had implied that civil engineers who disagreed with him were incompetent or corrupt. He had fought with undertakers and burial insurance schemes for robbing the poor, with private water companies for poisoning their customers in pursuit of short-term profit, and with shopkeepers and small businessmen for being fixated on keeping down their property taxes, even as the cost in human lives became more evident. Being adamantly in the right didn't necessarily help. Nor did his refusal to acknowledge when he was wrong.

In September 1849, the prime minister ousted Chadwick from a secondary position at the Metropolitan Commission of Sewers, then attempting to bring order to London's multiple unconnected systems for sewage removal. Failing to heed the warning, Chadwick kept at his habitual practice of "blowing sparks into flames," as a colleague put it. His opposition finally became a bonfire, and in 1854, Chadwick resigned from the General Board of Health, on the pretext of a physical breakdown. He would live another thirty-six years, and his influence on sanitary reform would spread to cities worldwide. But it was the end of Chadwick's career as a public servant.[18]

The *Times* rejoiced, with the sort of foolish bravado still sometimes seen in modern epidemics: "We prefer to take our chance of cholera and the rest than be bullied into health."[19]

10 FINDING PATHOGENS

Panic and rioting were the common response to news that cholera had arrived in a neighborhood. It wasn't just that it killed half its victims and did so with terrifying speed. There was also a special horror to the method of dying, with the body of a person who was in the prime of life at one moment seeming, in the next, to liquefy and flow out in endless vomiting and diarrhea. The victim soon collapsed, on a bed or the nearest patch of ground, helpless and with clothing often stripped away as useless before the uncontrollable loss of body fluids. Intense thirst followed. The eyes sank into the skull. Spasms and cramps wrenched the muscles. Breathing became labored, a desperate, gasping "air hunger," which gave way to shallow panting. People died with their minds seemingly intact, pale, staring, aghast, as the watery liquid was still being wrung from their guts onto the place where they lay. At the end, "rice water" evacuations from the intestines were clear and odorless, as if the disease itself had devised a more insidious way to infect those unwitting souls who laundered the bedclothes or who slept in the bed where a cholera victim had died.[1]

Or maybe hadn't died, after all. In the late stages of the disease, the coldness and color of the skin and the almost imperceptible pulse led some people to pronounce a death too hastily, perhaps because fear of cholera made them want to be rid of the corpse as quickly as possible. Or the opposite happened: the many stories of cadavers coming to life on the death cart, or even in the coffin, led people to cling to their loved ones beyond all reason.

"Our other plagues were home-bred, and part of ourselves, as it were," a Scottish physician later recalled. "We had acquired the habit of looking on them with comparative indifference; with a fatal indifference, indeed, inasmuch as it led us to believe that they could not be effectually subdued. But the cholera was something outlandish, unknown, monstrous; its tremendous ravages, so long foreseen and feared, so little to be explained, its insidious march over whole continents, its apparent defiance of all the known and conventional precautions against the spread of epidemic disease, invested it with a mystery and a terror which thoroughly took hold on the public mind, and seemed to recall the memory of the great epidemics of the middle ages. It was in a most emphatic sense felt to be a lesson from on High."[2]

When the first global cholera outbreak began in 1817 around the Bay of Bengal, it startled people even on that familiar turf by its ferocity. One British colonial official in Calcutta described it as "more fatal than at any former period" in living memory and capable of killing victims "in a few hours and sometimes in a few minutes." Another, in what is now Bangladesh, wrote that the "astonished and terrified" inhabitants "fled in crowds to the country as the only means of escaping impending death." In the course of a few weeks, ten thousand people died in that district.[3]

The rapidly increasing commercial and colonial trade sent this virulent strain racing south across open ocean to kill six thousand people in Mauritius. It hitchhiked to the Philippines in 1820, and a British expeditionary force delivered it to Oman in 1821. From there the disease tore across the Middle East and almost into Europe before finally wearing itself out in 1824. A second pandemic reared up in 1829, and people everywhere anxiously followed reports from the front lines as the dreaded disease steadily approached.

Faith in anticontagionist thinking was rapidly weakening. "It is very difficult to obtain from the advocates of the doctrine of non-contagion, any definite explanation of what they consider to be the nature of that malignant state of the air, or epidemic constitution of the atmosphere, that gives rise to the Plague," London physician William Macmichael wrote in 1825. "According to them it is neither extreme heat, nor extreme cold, nor dryness, nor moisture, nor is it any great change from one of these conditions to another."[4]

The failure to explain cholera, this monstrous new intruder, opened the eyes of some practitioners. They began to look around and think for themselves about the disease they were confronting. Evidence of its contagious nature drove an interest in what the French were beginning to call *pathogène*, materials or organisms of an indeterminate character that were *pathogenic*, or capable of causing disease.

MODERN CONTAMINATION CONTROL

Much of the early progress happened in diseases other than cholera—arguably ridiculous diseases, in Carlo Cogrossi's sense that they had little apparent connection to the leading human health threats of the day. History has accordingly scanted the researchers who did this work—among them, Agostino Bassi in Italy, James Paget in England, and Alfred Donné in France.

Bassi (1773–1856) was "a rather timid half-blind little farmer," in one writer's account, who worked alone, unsupported by any scholarly institution, and yet had the temerity to present his great discovery before a panel of nine faculty members from the University of Pavia. But Bassi was himself a graduate of Pavia, where he had studied with some of the leading lights of Italian science. He had gone on to become an important local official, before failing eyesight forced him to retire in his early forties to his family farm in Lodi, southeast of Milan. There, he published useful works applying science to agriculture. It is doubtful there was much forelock-tugging when he appeared in 1834 before the august faculty at Pavia.[5]

Silk production was a major industry in Italy then, and Bassi had been working to understand a mysterious disease killing the silkworms that were the means of production. This disease appeared in the silkworm nursery, seemingly out of nowhere, and caused the silkworms to become inactive and stop eating. They quickly died, their dried-out carcasses covered in a powdery substance.

Bassi spent eight years testing common assumptions about the disease, including the idea that it developed spontaneously, perhaps as an inherited trait. When that failed, he hypothesized that some "extraneous germ" must be entering and growing within the silkworms, "and I decided to follow the traces of this fatal thing, and to discover its true nature and its habits and all the ways by which it is introduced into the silkworm nursery, then into the silkworm causing in it this terrible disease." It took him another seventeen years. At first, he hoped to sell the results of a quarter century of self-funded research to some forward-thinking silk manufacturer. When no buyer materialized, he took his ideas public, via the University of Pavia.

Bassi identified a parasitic fungus as the cause of "the disease, death, and the subsequent hardening and bursting of the cadaver." To prove it, he took some of the powdery efflorescence from dead silkworms, containing the spores of the fungus, and injected it with a fine needle into healthy individuals at different stages of development. There, it sprouted and grew, drawing water and nutrients from the host, which it soon killed. Bassi also demonstrated how this powder could be carried into the silkworm nursery by dogs, cats, moles, and flies, as well as by air or water.[6]

"Perhaps some of my readers will respond with a smile to my doctrine . . . of living contagions," Bassi conceded, much as Cogrossi had done in presenting his "bizarre hypothesis" more than a century earlier. But this didn't stop him from stating the broad implications of what he had found: "The contagious causes which afflict animals . . . are to be considered as organic beings, subject in their growth and in their propagation to the same laws which govern all living beings in general, which grow and multiply by reason of the food which they receive."

Not content with having provided the first unmistakable proof of an "extraneous germ" causing disease, Bassi also proposed practical measures to keep the fungus from spreading. He called for disinfecting silkworm eggs purchased from outside sources, and also disinfecting equipment in the nursery, which should be well ventilated and designed to exclude houseflies and other intruders. Workers needed to practice basic hygiene and to keep the floor sprinkled with water in dry season to minimize dust. It was a remarkably modern program of contamination control.

Having won the imprimatur of the University of Pavia, Bassi finally published his silkworm work in 1835. At the time, according to medical historian Ralph H. Major, the great antiseptic pioneer Ignaz Semmelweis was just seventeen years old, antiseptic surgery advocate Joseph Lister just eight, Louis Pasteur thirteen, and Robert Koch, the cofounder of germ theory, not yet born. So why does history honor them and forget Bassi?[7]

One key element was lacking in Bassi's germ theory: He did not provide a complete identification of the germ, possibly because his vision was too far gone for him to see it through a microscope. Instead, later that year, a biologist in Milan provided a complete description of the fungus, which he named *Botrytis bassiana* in Bassi's honor. (It's now *Beauveria bassiana*, as a result of a taxonomic reorganization.) But there's a more likely explanation for Bassi's obscurity. The weight of scientific evidence had not yet sufficiently accumulated in 1835 for people to accept living microorganisms as the agents of disease. Germ theory was ready for the medical world. The medical world was not yet ready for germ theory.

LOOKING WITH A NATURALIST'S EYE

On February 2, that same year, at St. Bartholomew's Hospital in London, a first-year medical student and amateur botanist named James Paget (1814–1899) slipped back into the dissecting room following the autopsy of Paolo Bianchi, a forty-year-old laborer. "An immense number of minute whitish specks" had turned up scattered across Bianchi's muscles, particularly in the chest. These specks, commonly thought to be bits of bone, were familiar enough for experienced medical men to ignore, or mutter that their gritty texture made the scalpel work more difficult. But Paget was curious.[8]

"All the men in the dissecting-rooms, teachers included, 'saw' the little specks in the muscles," he recalled much later, when he had made his reputation as one of the founders of the science of pathology, "but I believe that I alone 'looked-at' them and 'observed' them: no one trained in natural history could have failed to do so." It was a product of "the habit of looking-out, and observing, and wishing to find new things, which I had acquired in my previous studies of botany." He took away a small tissue sample for closer examination. Using a rudimentary magnifying device, he saw that the specks were in fact cysts, each containing "a small worm coiled up." Because the hospital had no microscope, Paget carried his bit of the late Mr. Bianchi across town to the British Museum and made a closer inspection of "this peculiar animalcule" with a microscope belonging to the botanical collection. Four days after the autopsy, Paget presented his discovery to the hospital's student medical society and prepared to announce it in print.[9]

Like many newcomers before and after, however, he quickly found himself being preempted by the network of great men. Comparative anatomist Richard Owen, who held positions at both the British Museum *and* St. Bartholomew's, argued that the discovery would be more credible coming from him, rather than from a first-year medical student. Paget wisely extracted a promise that Owen would credit him for the discovery, and Owen, a notorious hijacker of other people's work, did so as ungenerously as he could manage. But much as promised, Owen's announcement of the discovery of *Trichina spiralis* later that same month created a sensation in the medical and scientific world.

In a letter to his brother, Paget was cautious about whether the "immense numbers" he had seen might ultimately be found to "accompany any particular disease." But, like Leeuwenhoek examining the living creatures in a drop of water, he could not conceal the thrill those immense numbers produced. "Fancy the body of a single individual supporting more separately existing creatures than the population of the whole world," Paget wrote, "and there must in this subject have been 10 times as many." In the manuscript of what was to have been his description, before Owen stepped in, he concluded, "it is scarcely possible to imagine such myriads of beings however insignificant their size, to infest the whole body of an individual, without producing some material effect on his condition." Other researchers would go on to describe the parasitic life cycle of *Trichina* (later renamed *Trichinella*) *spiralis* and demonstrate that its larvae, usually ingested in undercooked pork, cause the debilitating disease trichinosis in humans.[10]

THE RISE OF THE MICROSCOPE

Animalcules of one sort or another seemed to proliferate in midcentury. In Paris, the year after Paget's discovery, physician and microbiologist Alfred Donné (1801–1878) examined purulent matter from patients with sexually transmitted diseases and described the presence of a parasitic protozoan, also in "immense" numbers. Donné did not have the means to establish a role for this organism in venereal diseases. But it's now known as *Trichomonas vaginalis* and causes trichomoniasis, one of the most common sexually transmitted diseases.

Donné became an important advocate for microscopes in medical practice, over the objections of his traditionalist elders. At his own expense, he set up twenty microscopes in the lecture hall of the Medical Faculty of Paris and taught a course in their use. In 1844, he published a textbook about the microscope in medicine. Then he produced the first photographs of microscopic life and published eighty of them, reproduced as engravings, to supplement the textbook, a turning point in medical history.[11]

As microscopes rapidly improved and other researchers put them to work, they found animalcules everywhere, often in compromising circumstances: the fungus that causes favus, a skin disease of the scalp (Johann Lukas Schönlein, 1839); the first trypanosome, a protozoan, in the blood of a trout (Gabriel Valentin, 1841); a hookworm during the autopsy of a peasant woman (Angelo Dubini, 1843); an unnamed bacteria type in the blood of diseased sheep (Casimir Davaine and Pierre Rayer, 1850); and so on, almost without end. We tend to think of *germ theory*—the idea that specific microorganisms cause specific diseases—as a radical break, a lightning bolt striking out of a clear blue sky. In truth, it was more like a slow-growing plant. It had germinated in Fracastoro's time and then gone dormant for a time. Now, in the shadow of the cholera cloud, it was beginning to put out bright tendrils of new growth.

11 THE SEMMELWEIS REFLEX

The Vienna General Hospital in the mid-nineteenth century occupied a pleasant campus of two- and three-story buildings arranged around a grid of tree-filled courtyards. It provided the most advanced care then available, at no cost to its many charity patients. In the maternity service, the ambition was to bring in women from the streets to give birth, partly to reduce the likelihood of infanticide. But the hospital was also a death house for those women: One day a patient was healthy, cradling her baby in her arms. A day or two later, the shivering began. Stabbing pains radiated across her abdomen, her pulse raced, her breath went short, and in the end, in about half of such cases, she drew up her knees and quietly died. Often the new baby died too. It was called puerperal, or childbed, fever.

The hospital's maternity service could accommodate almost eight hundred patients, in two clinics. Medical students and midwives initially trained together, but in 1840, the maternity service assigned medical students (all male) to the first clinic and midwives (all female) to the second. Austrian-born Johann Klein, a dull conservative in his late fifties, headed the first clinic.

On July 1, 1846, Ignaz Semmelweis (1818–1865), a Hungarian obstetrician, became Klein's first assistant—essentially the chief resident—appointed on a two-year term to direct day-to-day operations. It was his twenty-eighth birthday, and a colleague depicted Semmelweis as "of a happy disposition, truthful and open-minded, extremely popular with friends and colleagues." He had not yet experienced young women roughly his own age—daughters, sisters, and mothers—routinely dying under his care.

It was common knowledge among women that being assigned to the first clinic meant a much greater risk of dying from childbed fever. Semmelweis was soon witnessing "scenes in which patients, kneeling and wringing their hands" begged "to be released in order to seek admission to the second section." Apart from the emotional toll, the situation was also professionally mortifying. "The disrespect displayed" by the hospital's other workers "made me so miserable," he wrote, "that life seemed worthless."[1]

Conventional theory attributed childbed fever to the usual suspects—an atmospheric condition, a cosmic alignment, the telluric forces of the underworld, the weather, or an excess of corrupted or vitiated air within the hospital itself. Blaming the victim was also common: She took too long in labor. She experienced imperfect contractions. She had too much blood in her circulation. She was immoral or guilty of "violent" mental emotions. "The high mortality," Semmelweis wrote, "was also attributed to the clinic's practice of admitting only single women in desperate circumstances." He was too discreet to say that poverty had reduced many of them to prostitution, just that "they were miserable and in great need, often malnourished, and may have attempted to induce miscarriages." But the same class of women were admitted to the second clinic, so that didn't explain the difference in mortality.

Semmelweis methodically investigated even the most trivial differences between the two clinics. At one point, he had patients switch from lying on their backs during delivery, the standard practice in the first clinic, to lying on their sides, the practice in the second clinic. It made no difference. He noticed that in the second clinic the priest was able to arrive to deliver last rites without disturbing other patients. But in the first clinic, he had to pass through five other patient rooms to reach the sick room, with a sacristan walking ahead and tolling a bell. This was demoralizing for Semmelweis, and probably terrifying for women uncertain if they would be the next to die. The priest agreed to come by a different route, without bells. The women died just the same. Semmelweis had been trained in the revealing power of statistics, and duly recorded the deaths with each passing month.

Surprisingly, hospital officials noted that the medical students in the first clinic were unmarried men, while the midwives in the second were women who had all given birth themselves and might perhaps be gentler in conducting internal examinations. Even more surprisingly, the hospital acted on this conjecture, by halving the number of medical students. (Klein targeted foreign students, regarding them as less trustworthy than good Austrians. The idea of accepting women as obstetrics students does not seem to have occurred.) In the immediate aftermath, the incidence of childbed fever in the first clinic dropped. But the effect turned out to be an illusion.

ONLY GOD KNOWS

That winter of 1846–1847, Semmelweis suddenly found himself out of a job when a predecessor came back to work in the first clinic. Semmelweis joined two friends on a visit to Venice, writing, "I hoped the Venetian art treasures would revive my mind and spirits, which had been so seriously affected by my experiences in the maternity hospital." Then his old job suddenly reopened, and at the end of March, Semmelweis was back at work in Vienna. There he soon realized that the higher mortality in the first clinic wasn't so much about the number of medical students. It was about the head of the first clinic, Johann Klein, and about Semmelweis himself.

The clue came from the death in his absence of Jakob Kolletschka, a close friend and teacher. Semmelweis reviewed the notes from Kolletschka's autopsy while he was "still animated by the art treasures of Venice," he wrote, and agitated by grief at the loss of a friend. "In this excited condition, I could see clearly that the disease from which Kolletschka died was identical to that from which so many hundred maternity patients had also died." Childbed fever was not, as widely believed, a disorder of the uterus, nor a disease of one gender. It was pyemia, a type of septicemia, which produces abscesses throughout the body. Semmelweis also knew exactly what caused Kolletschka's pyemia: A student had nicked his teacher's hand with a scalpel during an autopsy.

"Not the wound," Semmelweis wrote, "but contamination of the wound by the cadaverous particles caused his death . . . I was compelled to ask whether cadaverous particles had been introduced into the vascular systems of those patients whom I had seen die of this identical disease." He did not need to ask how: the midwives in the second clinic didn't participate in autopsies, but in the first clinic, autopsies were a routine training tool.

Doctors and medical students alike went back and forth between autopsies on women who had died of childbed fever and examinations of women in labor. They didn't wear gloves for either task, and even if routine handwashing in between had been required, it wouldn't have been "sufficient to remove all adhering cadaverous particles," Semmelweis wrote. Women in labor in the first clinic experienced on average five separate internal exams, in which inevitably "the hands, contaminated with cadaverous particles, are brought into contact with the genitals of these individuals, creating the possibility of resorption." Because they were charity patients in a teaching hospital, many more internal exams were possible—by multiple students, particularly in interesting cases or in first deliveries, where cervical dilation typically lasted longer.

The statistics Semmelweis had been keeping suddenly made sense. In the first clinic, the higher incidence of the disease in first-time mothers was a result of those extra examinations, especially in winter, when medical students were more diligent about spending time in the morgue and thus more likely to infect their patients. The statistics explained the lower mortality rate under a prior obstetrician who had prohibited use of cadavers by his students, and it explained the higher mortality when Johann Klein became chief obstetrician and reinstated training on cadavers. It even explained the surprising decrease in childbed deaths during the four months Semmelweis had been out of work and the increase upon his return. Unlike his temporary replacement, Semmelweis was diligent in using autopsies to train his students. "Only God knows the number of patients who went prematurely to their graves because of me," he later reflected. "I have examined corpses to an extent equaled by few other obstetricians." [2]

THE ANNIHILATING LOGIC OF HIS STATISTICS

With Klein's permission, Semmelweis instituted a remedy in May 1847, requiring doctors and students to wash their hands in chlorinated water before entering the maternity ward. The mortality rate in the first clinic soon dropped from 12 to just 3 percent—"below that of the patients in the second clinic." Semmelweis thought further washing between patients with soap and water would be adequate. But incidents that autumn changed his mind, particularly a case in which doctors and students examined a new mother in the first bed in the ward, then passed her infection on through subsequent internal exams, killing eleven of the twelve women in the ward. Semmelweis ordered antiseptic washing between exams. By 1848, the death rate in the first ward was down to 1.27 percent—just forty-five of the 3,556 patients. Roughly four hundred women went home with their babies who would have died only two years before.[3]

Semmelweis wasn't the first to propose antiseptic handwashing to stop doctors and nurses from transmitting childbed fever to their obstetric patients. Boston physician and poet Oliver Wendell Holmes (1809–1894) had done it a few years earlier, writing that the "*private pestilence*" caused by a single careless physician "should be looked upon not as a misfortune but a crime." ("But a gentleman's hands are clean," one physician protested, in a tone of wounded disbelief.) But in contrast to Holmes's anecdotal approach, Semmelweis delivered what a later physiologist called "the annihilating logic of his statistics," about deaths that had happened at his own hand. This would be harder for medical arrogance to ignore.[4]

In the leading Austrian medical journal, editor Ferdinand Hebra likened Semmelweis's work to Edward Jenner's vaccine for its power to save lives. Medical journals in other countries also reported the news, and some maternity hospitals adopted Semmelweis's methods. Others took offense at the idea that doctors could transmit deadly disease to their patients. Resistance also arose because his ideas forced physicians to think, many for the first time, that a particular disease could be the product of a single distinct cause. He was adamant about this unorthodox idea. He differed from British physicians who disputed his work "in this: in every case, without a single exception, I assume only one cause, namely decaying matter, and am convinced of this. The English physicians . . . recognize in addition all the old epidemic and endemic causes that have been believed to play a role in the origin of the disease."[5]

Medical thinking then was still thoroughly confused about how to identify a disease, according to Semmelweis biographers K. Codell Carter and Barbara R. Carter. The tendency was to categorize seemingly related symptoms as a disease, though these symptoms might in fact be completely unrelated in origin. An intense inability to swallow was "hydrophobia," whether the patient had suffered a blow to the throat or the bite of a rabid dog. As a result, "treatment was inconsistent and confusing; effective medical practice was all but impossible. Defining diseases so that each had only one specific cause was an essential step in the development of effective techniques for controlling any disease. Ignaz Semmelweis was among the first to adopt this approach."[6]

Resistance developed finally because Semmelweis became entangled in political disputes. Among his early backers at the Vienna General Hospital was his former teacher, Czech-born internist Josef Škoda, a popularizer of the stethoscope and a pioneer in the odd but informative business of thumping on various body parts to diagnose the state of health within. In an 1849 lecture describing the success of "Dr. Semmelweis's discovery," Škoda singled out a Prague maternity clinic under obstetrician Friedrich Wilhelm Scanzoni as an example of continued failure to save mothers and babies. Scanzoni was indignant. He replied that both chlorine washing and greater separation between the autopsy and delivery rooms had already been "applied and supervised with the greatest care" in the clinic. But they made no difference "until a more favourable genius epidemicus"—that is, a break in atmospheric conditions—"relieved us." Instead of prudently steering clear, Semmelweis entered into a prolonged feud with Scanzoni.

His allies also thrust him headfirst into the politics of his own workplace. The Vienna General Hospital's chief physician arranged for the Medical Society of Vienna to invite Semmelweis to speak, not thinking that this might jeopardize his relationship with his immediate boss, Johann Klein. Then Klein was left out of a commission created to investigate the death rate in the first clinic. When Semmelweis's term as chief resident expired, Klein withheld the customary two-year extension. He offered to let him stay on instead as a mere docent, with permission to work only on leather obstetric models, not cadavers, effectively ending his research.

Semmelweis quit in a fury and returned to his native Budapest. At obstetrics clinics there, he again demonstrated the lifesaving power of his antiseptic regimen. An Austrian medical journal published an account of this success in 1856. But the editor added a bizarre disclaimer: "We believe that this chlorine-washing theory has long outlived its usefulness. The experiences and statistical results of most maternity institutions protest against the views presented above. It is time we are no longer deceived by this theory."

In fact, the deception seems to have worked the other way around. At the Scanzoni clinic, a former intern there recalled, obstetricians had deliberately set out to provide "conclusive proof that the washings were entirely useless." Students shuttling back and forth between morgue and examining room merely dipped their fingertips "into an opaque fluid that had served the same purpose for many days and that was itself completely saturated with harmful matter." This phenomenon—blind resistance to new evidence that threatens old practices and beliefs—would become known as "the Semmelweis reflex." A better name might be "the Scanzoni reflex."[7]

NOT SETTLING DOWN

In 1857, at the age of thirty-nine, Semmelweis married Maria Weidenhoffer, the eighteen-year-old daughter of a wealthy Budapest merchant. They soon produced five children, suggesting a degree of domestic normalcy. Two died soon after birth, but that was normal too. Semmelweis maintained a busy practice and taught his antiseptic methods to young obstetricians at the University of Pest. He found time to compile his results and publish a book, *The Etiology, Concept, and Prophylaxis of Childbed Fever* (1861), expecting it to help save new mothers everywhere. But the reviews were dismissive, and the book, which included a seventy-five-page diatribe against Scanzoni, went largely unread.

Embittered, Semmelweis now turned the most vehement language on his adversaries. "I denounce you before God and the World as a murderer," he wrote to Scanzoni. Joseph Späth, an obstetrician at the University of Vienna, was participating in "a massacre," according to Semmelweis, who called for an end to "this homicide." Oliver Wendell Holmes had also characterized puerperal fever as "professional homicide." But calling out individual doctors by name was a step beyond. Semmelweis thought there was "no other means for checking the murder than unsparingly to unmask my opponents." It served instead to move his voice further to the margins and legitimize those who ignored it.[8]

At the Vienna General Hospital, Karl Braun, who had replaced Johann Klein, worked for the next fifteen years to prove Semmelweis wrong. He considered airborne microorganisms the real hazard, especially after a French chemist named Louis Pasteur implicated airborne microorganisms in spoilage of beer and wine in the late 1850s. Braun assigned obstetrician Karl Mayrhofer to search for microorganisms in the uterine discharges of childbed fever victims. Mayrhofer not only found and described what he called *vibrions* (from the Latin *vibrare*, to move by undulations), but also demonstrated their power to produce disease by spraying them into the genitals of newborn rabbits. For Braun, triumphant, this was powerful support for airborne transmission of disease. He persuaded the hospital to install an expensive new ventilation system as the best way to prevent childbed fever.

Mayrhofer meanwhile continued to tinker with his vibrions. In 1864, he announced that he had been unable to demonstrate how airborne transmission was possible. Instead, he had come to agree that transmission occurred on the unsanitized hands of attending physicians. He differed from Semmelweis only in defining the cause of the disease more precisely—not "decomposed animal-organic matter," but vibrions thriving in that matter. Either way, the remedy was the same: Handwashing in chlorinated water. Mayrhofer was soon out of his job at the Vienna General Hospital.

The adversaries Semmelweis had characterized as murderers now began to have second thoughts. After compiling his own statistical analysis, Joseph Späth acknowledged that Mayrhofer's work "can only be regarded as a further confirmation of Semmelweis's view." Even Scanzoni eventually found it necessary to acknowledge in 1867 that "puerperal fever is now almost unanimously considered to be an infectious disease." Swallowing hard, he added that "Semmelweis has rendered a great service to lying-in women in our hospitals."[9]

Semmelweis himself was unable to appreciate these belated conversions. Various authors would later diagnose him as a victim of manic depression, early onset Alzheimer's Disease, or perhaps tertiary syphilis, a common hazard for obstetricians then. In any case, his public and private behavior turned dramatically worse in the summer of 1865. Although he had "earlier lived for his family," he now seemed indifferent to them, according to a friend who gave him a medical exam late that July. He began to drink to excess. "He . . . established relationships with a prostitute and found nothing reprehensible therein." His conversation became embarrassing, even indecent. Semmelweis was suffering from a "disturbance of his mental state," the doctor wrote, soon after, and might benefit from "suitable supervision and medical care . . . in an institution for the mentally ill." Two other doctors added their names to this committal, without actually having examined Semmelweis. [10]

On July 29, 1865, Semmelweis boarded a train for Vienna, accompanied by his wife Maria and her uncle. He was under the impression that they would be continuing on to the spa at Gräfenberg, Germany. But at Vienna, according to the plan arranged by those around him, Semmelweis's friend Ferdinand Hebra met them at the train station. Hebra, who had once introduced Semmelweis to the world as a new Jenner, persuaded Semmelweis to delay his travels for a brief visit. He and Maria's uncle then walked him to a public insane asylum on the Lazarettgasse, a few minutes from Semmelweis's old clinic at the Vienna General Hospital. They left him in the asylum's garden, talking with a staff member, and slipped away.

Semmelweis remained in the asylum for the next two weeks. He attempted to escape and was severely beaten by guards, who confined him for a time in a straitjacket. An unsigned account, seemingly cobbled together after the fact, described his condition on nine days of his stay. It implied that Semmelweis had arrived at the asylum with an infected wound near the tip of the middle finger of his right hand, though no such injury had been evident to his wife or other recent companions.

The hand became swollen and gangrenous, and boils developed on his arms and legs. On August 12, he lay in bed all day, breathing loudly, "features fallen." No medical treatment appears to have taken place. In his book,

Semmelweis had envisioned a time when maternity hospitals everywhere would adopt his ideas and rid themselves forever of childbed fever. The certainty that this day "must inevitably sooner or later arrive will cheer my dying hour," he wrote. But there was no cheer in the horror of his dying. On August 13, his mouth hung open, "tongue hard as a board eyes glossy, half open." That evening, Semmelweis died, age forty-seven.

The asylum's medical report ended with a single, stark word: "pyemia?" It was the same disease that had killed so many young mothers before him.[11]

12 MAKING SENSE OF CHOLERA

In 1854, two scientists working independently were beginning to provide the first recognizably modern understanding of the most terrifying pandemic of the day. In England, physician John Snow (1813–1858) demonstrated that cholera was transmitted mainly in drinking water. And in Italy, anatomist Filippo Pacini (1812–1883) demonstrated exactly what the water was transmitting and how it caused cholera. In both cases, conventional medicine stood ready to bury their lifesaving discoveries—the Scanzoni reflex again—under a cloud of disbelief and indifference.

Filippo Pacini, the son of a shoemaker, was born in Pistoia, north of Florence. His parents dreamed of making him not just a priest but a bishop. An early interest in the natural world led him to medical school instead, as a scholarship student. There, in 1831, at age nineteen, Pacini made his first discovery, by the familiar means of looking more closely and doubting a teacher's explanation. "What are these?" Pacini supposedly asked during a dissection, indicating small, round bodies beneath the skin, attached to the ends of nerves. In the illustrations he later made, they look like a cluster of tiny potatoes, radiating out on their individual nerve-roots from a single stem.

"Small globules of fat tissue," his professor replied.

Doubtful, Pacini pursued the subject on his own, investing his savings in a crude microscope. Later, a local philanthropist gave him access to a more advanced microscope, and Pacini identified the "globules" as mechanoreceptors for sensing pressure and vibration. Pacini called them "tactile ganglia" or "new organs of touch." At the First Congress of Italian Scientists, his compatriots saw only "inessential and substantially negligible anatomical entities." But Pacini's work became known outside Italy after its publication in 1840, and a Swiss-German team coined the modern name *Pacinian corpuscles* in his honor.[1]

That recognition would not be repeated for the more significant discovery Pacini made in 1854. He had by then become an expert in the design and use of microscopes, at a time of dramatic technological improvements. But many Italian scientists still viewed the microscope "with varying degrees of suspicion," according to historian Claudio Pogliano. Some totally opposed its use and wanted to limit anatomical study to structures visible to the naked eye. Fear of the microscope's power to disprove medical orthodoxy was probably "why there seemed to be so many relentless *antimicroscopisti* around, who were deeply attached to the past and therefore advanced specious arguments in order to hinder the spread of the practice of microscopy." Pacini likened them to eunuchs attacking a better equipped rival. He successfully lobbied Leopold II, Grand Duke of Tuscany, for funding to design and build an advanced microscope together with Giovanni Battista Amici, then Europe's leading developer of optical instruments. But he had to fight with administrators to introduce the microscope in the classroom at the University of Pisa, and fight with them again over whether the microscope would go with him when he moved in 1847 to the University of Florence.[2]

In 1854, cholera was killing people with more ferocity than usual from Japan to Europe and across to the Americas. It was an ugly flare-up of the third pandemic, which had begun in 1846. When the disease appeared in Florence, Pacini performed autopsies on four victims, with detailed microscopic examination of blood, vomit, excrement, and intestinal fluids. The surface of the intestines looked, he wrote, as if "corroded by moths." The disease had torn away epithelial tissue and sheared off many of the *villi*, finger-like projections that function to absorb nutrients. When he pulled apart small clumps of mucus and shed tissue under the microscope, "myriads of vibrios emerged." He named them *Vibrio cholerae*, describing and illustrating them in an article published that December. He also identified them as the cause of cholera, though his evidence was circumstantial.[3]

"In spite of the most precise and meticulous search," he wrote, he had found nothing "capable of producing" the traumatic damage he had described except "the millions of *vibrios* that are found in the intestines." A few pages later, he resorted to uppercase type, as if to grip complacent readers by their lapels. He wasn't just talking about some unidentified contagious matter but an "ORGANIC, LIVING, SUBSTANCE OF A PARASITIC NATURE, WHICH CAN COMMUNICATE ITSELF, REPRODUCE ITSELF, AND THEREBY PRODUCE A SPECIFIC DISEASE."[4]

The discovery briefly attracted attention outside Italy. A notice in the medical press recognized Pacini as "the renowned discoverer" of the Pacinian corpuscles. But when it came to cholera, the writer wondered if Pacini had "actually mistaken an effect for a cause" or perhaps had "raised an incident to the unmerited position of an essential and fundamental feature." British medical researchers generally placed little value on microscopic evidence at that point. During the 1848–1849 cholera epidemic, physicians in Bristol had identified microscopic organisms, thought to be fungi, in the excretions of victims and in the drinking water of areas experiencing cholera. But investigators from the Royal College of Physicians refuted the idea. Pacini's paper in an obscure Italian journal did not lead them to reconsider the evidence.[5]

By 1866, when Pacini published an account of his further research, an unnamed writer in the same journal was more open-minded: "Dr. Pacini has observed that the operation of the parasites in cholera is primarily on the epithelium and villi, eroding the mucous membrane and laying bare the capillaries . . . the fact of the existence of parasites is based on Dr. Pacini's microscopical observations. . . . The treatise of Dr. Pacini is well written and keenly argued; on this account alone it is worthy of a perusal, apart from the originality of his observations."[6]

Pacini's work did not, however, get that perusal, though he elaborated on it in multiple publications. In Italy, his fellow scientists omitted Pacini when handing out awards in 1866 for meritorious work against cholera, and in 1881, the Accademia dei Lincei declined to honor him. Pacini took rejection badly, and the vehemence of his counterarguments only made further rejection more likely, as happened to Ignaz Semmelweis. Frustrated and embittered to the end of his life, Pacini remarked that his countrymen would accept his discovery only when they finally heard it being mouthed back to them by a foreigner. This prediction would prove dismayingly accurate.[7]

PROPOSING A MODE OF TRANSMISSION

Like Pacini, John Snow came from a family of modest means, the eldest of nine children of an unskilled laborer and his wife in York, England. At fourteen, he became apprenticed to a surgeon-apothecary in Newcastle-on-Tyne, a coastal town ninety miles to the north. There, in October 1831, cholera made its first dreaded appearance in Britain.

The surgeon, busy with patients in Newcastle, dispatched Snow to attend victims in the nearby mining village of Killingworth. He arrived to the spectacle of miners being brought up from the pit "after having had profuse discharges from the stomach and bowels, and when fast approaching to a state of collapse." For a lone and unsupervised nineteen-year-old, it must have been like being sent out to fight Ebola, without modern protective gear, and uncertain of what caused the disease, how to treat it effectively, or how to prevent it from spreading.[8]

Snow later moved to London to complete his medical education and set up general practice on his own in Soho. In 1847, he began to experiment with the new science of anesthesia, reducing the pain of surgery with ether, and later chloroform, administered through improved inhalers he developed. He became so trusted and successful as an anesthesiologist that Queen Victoria retained him to assist at the birth of her last two children, in 1853 and 1857.

Snow's decision in 1848 to undertake major epidemiological studies of cholera might seem like a surprising digression from this lucrative career path. But the outbreak occurred during a seasonal lull in elective surgery, and it was a chance to revisit that first daunting encounter with the disease at the start of his medical practice. He may also have become interested in cholera because some physicians, desperate for any remedy, had proposed using inhaled chloroform, his area of expertise. Other physicians had begun to discuss transmission of the disease via drinking water or contaminated food, which would also have interested him.[9]

Snow was a serious young man, organized, thorough, a teetotaler, and a bachelor. "He lived simply . . . on anchorite's fare," a friend later wrote. "He clothed plainly . . . kept no company, and found every amusement in his science books, his experiments . . . and in simple exercise." At seventeen, Snow had read *The Return to Nature; or, A Defence of the Vegetable Regimen* by John Frank Newton. Along with a vegetarian diet, the author recommended avoidance of "common water" because of contamination by "septic matter" in rivers, among other hazards. Of diseases generally, he thought that "the mischief, whatever shape it assume, proceeds from the alimentary canal." Snow knew this wasn't true of all diseases. But he became a vegetarian and drank only distilled water. He was thus predisposed to the theory he first laid out in 1849 in a thirty-two-page pamphlet titled *On the Mode of Communication of Cholera*.[10]

THE WHIRLPOOL OF CONJECTURE

Cholera then was unmatched in its ability to expose the haplessness of medical practice. "The question, What is cholera? is left unsolved," the *Lancet* acknowledged in 1853. "Concerning this, the fundamental point, all is darkness and confusion, vague theory, and a vain speculation. Is it a fungus, an insect, a miasm, an electrical disturbance, a deficiency of ozone, a morbid offscouring from the intestinal canal? We know nothing, we are at sea, in a whirlpool of conjecture."[11]

Anticontagionist physicians theorized that an "effluvium" entered the body via the lungs and poisoned the blood, causing it to thicken—hence the characteristic labored breathing and "cholera asphyxia." Snow, like Pacini, started out instead by focusing on the body parts most obviously affected by cholera, in the alimentary tract. He argued that the thickening of the blood occurred only later, as a side-effect from the dramatic loss of bodily fluids. Cholera would logically reach the alimentary tract in something that had been "swallowed accidentally," much as did the eggs of intestinal worms.

Detecting actual transmission would be difficult, Snow wrote. But he proposed that clear fluids from the final stages of cholera could contaminate the clothing and bedsheets of the victim, find their way onto the hands of caregivers, and thus be inadvertently swallowed. Cholera could also "be widely disseminated," he thought, "by the emptying of sewers into the drinking water of the community."

His 1849 pamphlet focused on an outbreak that July and August on Albion Terrace, in south London. Cholera struck there with "extraordinary mortality," he wrote, but, oddly, without causing any illness on neighboring streets. The affected homes were "the genteel suburban dwellings of a number of professional and tradespeople," with water from "a copious spring" piped to in-ground supply tanks in their back gardens. The first case of cholera was identified on July 28, in a woman who died after experiencing symptoms for three or four days. The disease soon spread to her neighbors, resulting in at least twenty deaths in ten houses by mid-August.[12]

A surveyor for the Commissioners of Sewers excavated the water system and identified the likely cause of the outbreak: every house had a cesspool in back, and some of them had overflowed and contaminated the entire water system. After briefly taking note, an inspector for the General Board of Health attributed the outbreak instead entirely to "offensive effluvia," some of it blown in over a distance of two hundred yards from the "sewer in Battersea fields," and some from the "stench" of the kitchen sinks of the Albion Terrace homes after a heavy rainstorm.[13]

In his pamphlet, Snow pointed out that there were several streets and rows of houses between Albion Terrace and Battersea Fields, all equally exposed to any wind-borne effluvia, yet none of them had experienced cholera. After countering other alleged insalubrities, he concluded, "It remains evident, then, that the only special and peculiar cause connected with the great calamity . . . was the state of the water, which was followed by the cholera in almost every house to which it extended whilst all the surrounding houses were quite free from it." The reality of drinking water contaminated with excrement was disturbing. But it was "much less dreary," he argued, than conventional anticontagionist thinking. "For what is so dismal as the idea of some invisible agent pervading the atmosphere, and spreading over the world?" Snow's argument made little headway with medical authorities. But even as he resumed his work as an anesthesiologist, he was thinking about ways to make the epidemiological evidence convincing.[14]

A NATURAL EXPERIMENT

In November 1853, Snow found the answer in a footnote to a report prepared by William Farr, the statistician for the General Register Office. Farr was hardly a natural ally for the idea of waterborne transmission of cholera. He was a proponent of a more scientific-sounding form of anticontagionism, called *zymotic theory*. It held that animal or plant decomposition could trigger fermentation within the body, a malfunctioning of the cells that spread to other cells and eventually manifested itself as disease. People in crowded and filthy conditions, especially those living in low-lying areas, were particularly susceptible. At the same time, Farr was a pioneering epidemiologist and entirely aware of the problems with London's water supply.[15]

It would have been hard to miss, for the stench alone. A cartoonist had dubbed water from the Thames "Monster Soup" a quarter-century earlier, and in 1848, a cartoonist in *Punch* had called the river "Dirty Father Thames." ("Filthy river, filthy river, / Foul from London to the Nore, / What

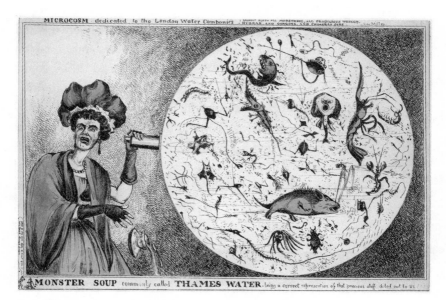

Figure 12.1

A microscopic view of the filthy stuff "doled out to us" by London water companies could put one off one's tea (W. Heath, 1828, Wellcome Collection).

art thou but one vast gutter, / One tremendous common shore?") It seemed only to become filthier with each passing year. One major supplier, the Southwark and Vauxhall Water Company (hereafter Southwark), still drew its water supply from a stretch of the river at Battersea Fields heavily polluted with raw sewage. A microbiologist who sampled the water in 1850 commented that some London residents "are made to consume, in some form or another, a portion of their own excrement, and moreover, to pay for the privilege." The other major supplier, Lambeth Water Company, had recently moved its intake twenty-two miles upriver to a site relatively free of urban pollution.[16]

"To estimate exactly . . . the effect of good or bad water supply," Farr wrote, "it is requisite to find two classes of inhabitants living on the same level, moving in equal space, enjoying an equal share of the means of subsistence, engaged in the same pursuits, but differing in this respect,—that one drinks water from Battersea, the other from Kew." He thought such an experiment unlikely in London because there were too many confounding variables. In particular, people with money generally lived on higher ground—elevation was key to Farr's thinking—and they obtained better drinking water, while the poor lived in low-lying areas and consumed less desirable water. But in the next issue of *Weekly Returns*, Farr added a footnote to a table of cholera mortality, apparently without realizing its significance: "In three cases (marked with an asterisk) the same districts are supplied by two companies." Snow seized on that footnote as the opportunity to conduct exactly the experiment Farr had suggested, and "on the grandest scale."[17]

He set to work when cholera returned to London in July 1854 and focused his initial research on two subdistricts in Kennington and Waterloo, on the south bank of the Thames. It seemed like an ideal natural experiment, with pipes of both the Southwark and Lambeth companies running down the same streets, each house having chosen its supply at the owner's whim. Snow consulted with Farr and obtained the addresses of cholera victims from the General Register Office.

It wouldn't be easy work. Homeowners often couldn't remember which company they used, and renters typically depended on what an absent landlord had chosen. Snow hit on the remedy of taking a sample from each residence with an unknown water source and testing it for sodium, on the theory that water supplied by Southwark, from mid-London, would be saltier than Lambeth's water from far upstream. He soon expanded the study to sixteen subdistricts supplied by the two companies. In 334 cases investigated during the first four weeks of the outbreak, he found fourteen times more deaths in Southwark-supplied homes than in those supplied by Lambeth. Later, after Snow had reviewed seven weeks of data and 860 cholera deaths, Southwark was only about eight or nine times more deadly. Even at that rate, though, the seemingly trivial decision about which water company to use had turned out, for many residents, to be a matter of life or death.[18]

13 THE BROAD STREET PUMP

Snow was still at work on the South London investigation when the cholera outbreak around Broad Street, near Golden Square, began. The first known victim was a baby named Frances Lewis at 40 Broad Street, who came down with vomiting and diarrhea. No one called it cholera at first. Intestinal disorders were commonplace, and the cholera outbreak seemed to be safely confined to South London, across the river. But later that Thursday, August 31, 1854, scores of her neighbors developed unmistakable cholera symptoms, and a tailor living just downstairs became the first death. Baby Frances followed at 11:00 a.m. Saturday. The dead were soon piling up in almost every house in the neighborhood.

Snow would later describe it as probably "the most terrible outbreak of cholera which ever occurred in this kingdom." He knew the neighborhood intimately, having lived nearby since first coming to London, and he immediately suspected the popular Broad Street pump, adjacent to number 40. Experience had taught Snow that intense, highly localized cholera outbreaks often began from a single water source, and he could identify no other possible cause common to the deaths in the neighborhood. Over the course of ten days, the outbreak would kill more than five hundred people within 250 yards from that spot.[1]

According to the medical legend that has risen up around the Broad Street pump, Snow proceeded single-handedly, and at great personal risk, to investigate door-to-door in the neighborhood, carefully mapping where people died of cholera and where they obtained water. The rectangular black marks stacked up like coffins at each address, and clustered unmistakably around the public water pump on Broad Street. Snow then presented his findings to local officials, who quickly removed the pump handle. In some versions, he removed the pump handle himself to end the outbreak, and his striking proof of how cholera is transmitted ushered in a revolution in medical thinking.

This "anecdote resembling an urban legend," as historians have termed it, began to accumulate in the 1930s. Wade Hampton Frost, an epidemiologist at Johns Hopkins University, resurrected Snow from historical oblivion as "a nearly perfect model" of epidemiological detective work. The aim was to elevate epidemiology to the stature then being enjoyed by laboratory science. From there, Snow's popular reputation grew to the point that a 2003 survey by the journal *Hospital Doctor* named him the "greatest doctor" of all time. (Hippocrates came in second.)[2]

The myths about Snow include the idea that the "spot maps" he made were the key to discovering the source of the outbreak. In fact, he did not draw his first map until December 1854, months after forming his analysis of the outbreak. Also mythical is the idea that Snow worked as a lone hero in the fight against the Golden Square outbreak. William Farr and his staff at the General Register Office, as well as many local physicians and clergy, shared essential information. But it was Snow who drove the inquiry in the direction we now recognize as correct. By Thursday, September 7, he had determined that more than 80 percent of the first victims had used the Broad Street pump. There had been no cholera, Snow argued, "except among the persons who were in the habit of drinking the water of the above-mentioned pump-well."[3]

Some deaths noted by Snow occurred miles away from the pump, but in ways that added both credibility and poignance to his argument. On Friday, September 1, a man hurrying up from Brighton to visit his stricken brother arrived too late even to see the corpse. He stayed in the area only long enough for "a hasty and scant luncheon of rumpsteak, taking with it a small tumbler of brandy and water, the water being from the Broad Street pump." Two days later he was dead. A woman in Hampstead had moved out of the neighborhood months earlier. But she still preferred water from the Broad Street pump, which had a reputation for carbonated freshness. Her sons ran a percussion cap company at 38 Broad Street and had a cart making daily deliveries in Hampstead. So they routinely sent a bottle of the water to her new home. She drank it on Thursday, August 31 and was dead on Saturday, September 2. The brothers also kept two tubs full of water from the Broad Street pump for their workers, and eighteen of them died during the outbreak. None died at a nearby brewery, which had its own well and provided its seventy workers a daily allowance of malt.

On the evening of September 7, Snow presented his findings and a recommendation to the sanitary committee of St. James's Westminster Parish. The committee ordered the Broad Street pump handle to be removed the next day. But it's another myth to say that this put an end to the outbreak. Snow knew that fatal attacks had already begun to subside, in part because so many terrified residents had fled the area. (Oddly, those who remained objected loudly to the loss of the pump water. Their other sources of water were apparently more offensive. When the pump handle was eventually restored, one skeptic commented ironically: "Loud and long the exulting shouts of children working the handle in wantonness of exuberant joy!")[4]

DIGGING DEEPER

The case against the Broad Street pump benefited from detective work by Rev. Henry Whitehead (1825–1896), curate of St Luke's Church, just off Broad Street. While Snow was busy with his continuing research in South London, Whitehead spent every waking hour tending the sick and dying in his parish. He started out as an anticontagionist and a believer in outdated ideas about atmospheric contamination. He opposed Snow's theory about the pump, "which scarcely anyone believed." In fact, an excavation of the pump well late that November found it "free from any fissures or other communication with drains or sewers by which such matters could possibly be conveyed into the waters." Moreover, chemical and microscopic analyses had failed to detect anything "capable of acting as a predisposing, cooperating, or specific agent in the production" of cholera. But Whitehead would soon become less confident about "clearing the character of the pump."[5]

In January 1855, Snow published a revised version of his 1849 pamphlet *On the Mode of Communication of Cholera*, now greatly expanded to cover the 1854 outbreaks in both South London and Golden Square. He printed three hundred copies of the book at his own expense and sold just fifty-six. Reading it, Whitehead realized for the first time that Snow was attributing the cholera outbreak not to some general impurity of the well water, but to "special contamination of it from the evacuations of cholera patients, which he conjectured must have reached the well from the sewer or a cesspool."[6]

Whitehead went on to make two critical discoveries. While searching through records at the General Register Office, he happened to notice the account of the death on September 2 of a five-month-old girl at 40 Broad Street, the house closest to the pump. He may perhaps have recalled the infant, Frances Lewis, as the first known case in the outbreak. But what really caught his attention—and he italicized it—was the note that her attack had begun "*four days previous to death.*" This suggested that the cholera outbreak had begun not on Thursday, August 31, as generally thought, but on Monday, August 28, long enough for the pathogen to have spread and to explain the wildfire breakout of the disease that Thursday and Friday. Whitehead "hastened off at once" to the house on Broad Street, where the baby's mother confirmed the timing. She also told Whitehead that she had soaked the sick child's soiled nappies in buckets of water, which she emptied in the back garden of the house, as well as into a "*cesspool in the front area.*"

Whitehead arranged for a new excavation that April focused on the area between the house and the well. The cesspool turned out to be constructed of bricks that came loose to the touch. Its drain line out to the sewer in the street lacked the pitch for proper flow and was located less than three feet from the brick wall of the well. Evidence of "continuous passage of fluid through the sides of the cesspool" and "channeled furrows observable from inside the well" together confirmed that the well itself had become an auxiliary cesspool. Whitehead had identified not just the index case for the outbreak, but also the means by which her infection had spread through the entire neighborhood, killing, by his count, nearly seven hundred people.[7]

This might sound like a compelling demonstration that cholera was primarily a waterborne disease. It seemed that way to the Cholera Inquiry Committee appointed by St. James Parish, with both Snow and Whitehead as members. In June, the committee unanimously agreed that the outbreak "was in some manner attributable to the use of the impure water of the well in Broad Street." But Snow's evidence may seem convincing to us now because we know he would ultimately be proved correct: cholera *is* primarily a waterborne disease. We also have a natural bias for winners. Both factors cloud our judgement and lead us to treat his critics as fools. But the critics and contemporary public health officials were right, some modern scholars argue, to remain unpersuaded by what they knew at the time.[8]

It was entirely reasonable, for instance, to question Snow's reliance on the sodium test in South London to distinguish one water company from the other. In a review published that April, the physician and medical professor Edmund A. Parkes doubted "whether the source of supply could safely be inferred from a chemical test alone." Too often, he added, Snow assumed waterborne transmission of cholera, instead of providing persuasive evidence for it, and he neglected to give serious consideration to alternative explanations. When several people on Albion Terrace contracted cholera even though they had not drunk the contaminated water, for instance, Snow theorized that they had ingested the contagion some other way, in the course of nursing patients, or from food previously prepared with contaminated water. But "the point," Parkes objected, "is to prove the fact of water being the agent, and not to assume it, and then to seek for some other explanation of those cases for which the presumed contamination cannot account."

Snow's tendency to interpret facts in ways favorable to his argument was most obvious at the Broad Street pump. The best evidence for his argument lay in Whitehead's discovery of the Frances Lewis case and its direct connection to the leaking cesspool practically on top of the pump well. But Snow necessarily omitted this evidence because he published his book in January, just five months after the outbreak—and four months before Whitehead actually made his discoveries. Parkes, reviewing Snow's book in between those two events, called Snow "an honest and conscientious observer." But the evidence he had produced at best "rendered the transmission of cholera by water an hypothesis worthy of inquiry."[9]

Unlike Pacini and Semmelweis, Snow remained professional in the face of criticism. But he also alienated potential converts by a political miscalculation. In the aftermath of the cholera outbreak, a Parliamentary committee moved to regulate tanners, bone-boilers, gas works, and other "offensive trades" whose putrid effluvia still seemed like the true cause of disease. Having heard of Snow's cholera theory, the trades in question asked him to testify on their behalf.

It was reasonable for Snow to defend them from the charge that their operations caused cholera or other infectious diseases. But in doing so, Snow linked his theory in the public mind with businesses that were increasingly considered obnoxious: they stank, in the heart of cities where other people were trying to live and work. Snow acknowledged that noxious smells in extreme concentrations could cause vomiting or even death. But he added that they did "not cause disease; those poisons do not reproduce themselves in the constitution."[10]

The members of the committee responded with mounting incredulity. "Are the Committee to understand," a member inquired, that no matter how foul smelling "the effluvia that comes from bone-boiling establishments may be, yet you consider that it is not prejudicial in any way to the health of the inhabitants of the district?"

"That is my opinion," Snow replied.

Another member followed up: "Assuming that there is a large number of horses in a state of decomposition, from which of course there would be very offensive effluvia, as far as the sense of smell is concerned, do you apprehend that that would not be prejudicial to the health of the inhabitants round?"

Again, Snow replied, "I believe not."

This testimony made it easy for critics to dismiss Snow's theory based on the company he kept. In an unsigned editorial, Thomas Wakley, the quarrelsome founder of the *Lancet*, called Snow the perfect witness for "'vested interests' in the production of pestilent vapours, miasms, and loathsome abominations of every kind." These "unsavoury persons," he added, fattened "upon the injury of their neighbours" and "came in a crowd, reeking with putrid grease, redolent of stinking bones, fresh from seething heaps of stercoraceous [that is, fecal] deposits, to lay their 'case' before the Committee."

Snow's testimony merely reinforced Wakley's faith in the theory of localized noncontagion, whose effects he could see and smell on a daily basis with his own offended senses. It would be "very difficult to persuade us," he promised, that gases with "lethal powers" in extreme concentration are not also "injurious to health, when in a state of dilution . . . and we presume that there is hardly a practitioner of experience and average powers of observation who does not daily observe the same thing." Wakley concluded "that the well whence Dr. Snow draws all sanitary truth is the main sewer. . . . In riding his hobby very hard, he has fallen down through a gully-hole and has never since been able to get out again."[11]

The best public health authorities could say about Snow's work was that he had provided evidence furthering the sanitary cause. John Simon, a physician, had replaced Edwin Chadwick as the leading voice of the British sanitary movement. In a June 1858 report, he provided an accurate summary of Snow's "peculiar doctrine" about cholera, including the idea that "an increase of the swallowed germ of disease takes place in the interior of the stomach and bowels." But "against this doctrine," Simon wrote, "almost insuperable arguments have been stated." Simon acknowledged Snow's "most zealous labours." But he credited him only with providing "valuable evidence of the danger of drinking fecalized water" in a cholera outbreak. It was hardly the birth of germ theory.[12]

That same year, the French Academy of Science offered a prize of 100,000 francs to the person who discovered the cause of cholera or provided a cure. Among the 153 applications, one came in from John Snow on his 1854 epidemiological demonstration of waterborne transmission of cholera, and another from Filippo Pacini on his 1854 discovery of *Vibrio cholerae*. The committee passed over both, offering small prizes instead to a physician who dosed cholera patients with calomel and to a Russian who recommended inoculating them with smallpox pus. Soon after, as John Snow was working on a new book about anesthesia, he suffered a massive stroke and died of its effects, age forty-five.[13]

When cholera returned to London in 1866, much of the epidemiological detective work fell to William Farr, the same statistic-minded physician who had deemed it impossible "to estimate exactly the effect of good or bad water supply" on public health in London—and whose footnote had unintentionally encouraged Snow to prove otherwise.

"Dirty Father Thames" was becoming somewhat less dirty. An extensive sewerage system designed and being built by civil engineer Joseph Bazalgette had begun to move sewage miles downriver, with the aim of dispersing effluvia from the centers of population. By law, the water supply companies had meanwhile moved their intakes miles upriver and applied filtration, to minimize the potential for "fecalized" drinking water. These improvements paid off. A cholera outbreak that year still killed about six thousand people in London. But that was down from nearly fifteen thousand in 1848–1849.

This time the dead were also narrowly concentrated in East London— "just the locality," Bazalgette confirmed in a letter to Farr, where "our main drainage works are not complete," raising suspicion that the drinking water there had been contaminated by sewage. Farr soon discovered that the deaths occurred mainly among residents supplied by the East London Waterworks Company, and hardly anywhere else. "It has been so for two weeks," Farr wrote in a letter to a colleague at the end of July, "and quite reminds me of the Southwark slaughter." He was thinking of his old sparring partner John Snow's work in South London.

Farr's suspicions made their way into the *Weekly Return* of August 2, 1866, eliciting a furious denial from the engineer of the East London company. Writing in the *Times*, he asserted "that not a drop of unfiltered water has for several years past been supplied by the company for any purpose." In reply, two local residents wrote to report eels—one of them nine inches long—delivered via the company's water pipes. "Can an eel pass through a filter bed?" one of them wondered.

An epidemiologist for the Privy Council investigated the outbreak and called in Henry Whitehead for help, having recently read Whitehead's account of the Broad Street pump investigation. Together, they identified faults in the filtration protocol of the East London Waterworks, and also located a middle-aged couple whose cholera appeared to be the source by which the company's supply first became contaminated. Under questioning at a hearing that December, the same engineer who had asserted that the company had not delivered "a drop of unfiltered water" confessed that he had given "an implied sanction" to draw on unfiltered water in certain conditions, and that those conditions had applied during the cholera outbreak.[14]

Farr announced himself a convert to Snow's cholera theory. Much of London agreed and seethed with outrage at the callous behavior of the East London company, whose customers suffered 93 percent of that year's cholera deaths. The *Lancet*, which had consigned Snow to a gully-hole a decade earlier, now pronounced him "a great public benefactor" whose research was "among the most fruitful in modern medicine." British sanitarian John Simon, who had previously seen "insuperable arguments" against Snow's theory, withheld his public approval until 1873. But then, in a report about the transmission of cholera, Simon declared that "the whole pathological argument" he was making grew out of cogent facts "to which the late Dr. John Snow . . . had the great merit of forcing medical attention: an attention at first quite incredulous, but which, at least for the last fifteen years, as facts have accumulated, has gradually been changing into conviction."[15]

Acceptance came slower among medical authorities outside Britain. In much of Europe, the thinking of hygienist Max von Pettenkofer held sway. He was an advocate of clean air and water, but also routinely ridiculed what he dubbed "the one-and-only drinking-water faith," arguing that cholera poison could produce the disease only in combination with certain conditions of soil, locality, and season. He was so sure of it that in October 1892, he took a sample of *Vibrio cholerae* from a dying patient and, in one of the more foolish acts of autoexperimentation on record, drank it. Pettenkofer lived and claimed to have experienced only mild diarrhea. It won him a place in the history of cholera discovery—mainly in the role of clown.[16]

In the end, the fight against cholera was—and remains—a collaborative effort, with no shortage of heroes. John Snow was undoubtedly one of them, for having a brilliant insight and the courage to pursue it in the face of public condemnation. But Henry Whitehead unexpectedly proved to be a better epidemiological detective, and William Farr a better statistician. Both also displayed more than their share of courage. So did Filippo Pacini, for discovering and understanding *Vibrio cholerae* thirty years before other scientists were willing to accept it as a reality. Even the perennially quarrelsome Edwin Chadwick, who went to his death in 1890 still devoutly believing in effluvia theory, deserves honor. The effort he helped launch to improve sewer systems and clean water supplies had a more profound effect on public health in the developed nations of the nineteenth century than all the work of more medically advanced thinkers combined. (They would catch up in the century ahead.)

This is how discovery happens, with good ideas and bad clanging together, heroes and clowns doing combat, wrong ideas producing right results, and science sometimes advancing one funeral at a time, but also sometimes regressing.

It is a messy business, and we owe our lives to it.

14 LOUIS PASTEUR: THE RISING

Infectious disease was still a mysterious force that swept through every life, out of nowhere, strewing carnage in its wake. Louis Pasteur (1822–1895) would break open that mystery and begin to parse out its deadly elements. But first, like everyone else, he would suffer its effects. He saw one sister die of tuberculosis, and another become mentally disabled as a result of an unspecified cerebral fever (meningitis, measles, or whooping cough are all possible candidates). Two of his daughters died in separate incidents of typhoid fever. A son barely survived the disease.

Like Leeuwenhoek, Pasteur was not at first driven by a compulsion to understand why this should be so. He did not set out to become a physician or study disease. In truth, he felt so uneasy with the subject matter that in his late thirties, when the work for which he was already famous began to bend in that direction, he found it necessary to audit a college physiology course taught by a colleague. Physicians who opposed his thinking often loudly noted his lack of medical credentials. And yet it was the revolutionary impact of his work on medicine and the treatment of disease that would in time rank Pasteur as one of the great names in human history, the cofounder of germ theory and the developer of the first effective vaccines since Edward Jenner more than eighty years earlier.[1]

Pasteur's reputation has come down in recent decades from medical demigod to something like "mortal but still glorious." Since the 1995 publication of a sharply critical biography based on Pasteur's laboratory notebooks, *The Private Science of Louis Pasteur* by Gerald L. Geison, it has become apparent that Pasteur appropriated the work of subordinates and rivals, usually without credit, and sometimes misrepresented his evidence. A more favorable biography published at about the same time, *Louis Pasteur*, by the French immunologist Patrice Debré, acknowledged some of the same behaviors: "For although he conveyed the impression of working all by himself," Debré wrote, "he was adept at choosing his collaborators and building on the work of his predecessors. Quite a few of his hypotheses were dictated to him by his time; indeed, it sometimes seems as if Pasteur merely verified the findings described by others and then appropriated them." But with good reason, Debré added: "Yet it was precisely when he picked up demonstrations that had been, as it were, left to lie fallow, that he proved to be most innovative. The salient feature of his genius was his synthetic ability."

By all accounts, Pasteur was not an attractive person to know. "Let us all work; it is the only fun there is," he once wrote to a colleague. Assistants who joined in this fun were obliged to maintain a monastic silence in the laboratory and carry out experiments precisely according to his careful protocol. But he seldom told them the intended goal, nor did he express any interest in their ideas or opinions. "Pasteur does not want anyone next to him. He trusts only himself," an assistant wrote. "What he wants, what he needs, is the most complete concentration on his own powers."

He could be charming in cultivating high-ranking individuals in academia or government with the power to advance his career. He could also be an entertaining orator when taking his case to the public. But he was relentlessly argumentative, and heaped disdain on lesser souls who dared to disagree with him. "Permit me to tell you, Monsieur le marquis, without acrimony and with all the deference due to your sense of honor, . . ." he wrote to one critic, "that you do not know the first thing about my research, its results, the firm principles it has established, and the practical importance it has already acquired. You have not read most of my publications, and as for those that have come into your hands, you have not understood them."

Ethical lapses and difficult personality aside, the medical world clearly needed Pasteur. It needed his self-confidence, his arrogance, his flamboyant instinct for publicity. It needed his painstaking experimentation combined with his scientific ingenuity to break away from its slavish two-thousand-year devotion to humoral theory, filth theory, and anticontagionism. It needed Pasteur's bone-crushing rhetoric to make germ theory real and to make it impossible for his many battered, squirming adversaries to escape with their thinking unchanged.[2]

LEFTIES AND RIGHTIES

Pasteur had grown up in the village of Arbois, near the Jura Mountains on the French border with Switzerland. His father, Jean-Joseph Pasteur, pursued one of those foul-smelling occupations the effluvia-minded found so disturbing. He was a tanner, a business that entailed salting raw animal skins, liming them, stripping off hair, grease, and fat (sometimes with the help of maggots), hosing them off, and soaking them in tannic acid, among other processes. The tanning vats occupied the ground floor of the family's three-story stone house, with the wastes presumably carried away by the River Cuisance flowing past the back garden.

His father's work inevitably exposed young Louis Pasteur to the stench. (Homesick during his first time away from home for school, he lamented, "If I could only smell the odor of the tannery.") But it also exposed him to the many chemical processes involved in the work, perhaps influencing his later choice to specialize in chemistry. His father, who had served three bloody years in Napoleon's army, also instilled in his son a fervent belief in the glory of France and the possibility of individual greatness. Where Pasteur *père* wore the red ribbon of the *Légion d'honneur* for heroism in combat, Pasteur *fils* would wear the *Légion d'honneur* for heroic scientific discoveries.

The choice of chemistry meant that Pasteur avoided the orthodoxy in which medical students of his own age were steeped as a standard part of their education. While they learned the ancient art of bleeding their patients, he was beginning to see the world through the microscope—and also the polarimeter, the goniometer, and other tools of the newfangled science of microbiology. This outsider perspective would be a key to his transformative effect on medicine and on the understanding of infectious disease.

Around the beginning of 1848, in his first independent research, Pasteur began to study minute chemical crystals having mostly to do with winemaking.

(As was often the case, Pasteur's industrial research would ultimately matter to medicine too.) Tartaric acid is the primary acid in grapes and some other fruits, and may be familiar to wine drinkers in the form of tiny crystals, like sugar granules, in the bottom of a glass, or on a cork. Among other commercial uses, it is also one of the main components of baking powder. Paratartaric acid was a material produced by inadvertently overheating tartaric acid.

Decades earlier, French physicist Jean-Baptiste Biot had conducted experiments demonstrating that when polarized light passes through certain substances in liquid solution, the plane of the light can rotate either left or right. Such substances are *optically active*, in the language of chemistry. But what puzzled Biot, Pasteur, and other chemists was the discovery in the 1840s that two seemingly identical forms of a substance could nonetheless differ in their optical activity. A liquid solution of tartaric acid rotates the plane of polarized light to the right; chemists call it *right-handed*. But its twin paratartaric acid has no effect at all; it is optically inactive. And yet the two forms, or isomers, of the acid appeared to have the same chemical composition, crystalline form, and specific weight.[3]

Pasteur set out to solve this mystery by studying individual tartaric acid crystals in minute detail with a *goniometer*, an optical tool for measuring the length and angle of different facets of a crystal. He soon discovered that one facet of the crystal was minutely different from the other facets and could plausibly pull polarized light to the right—hence the right-handedness of tartaric acid. The logical expectation, when he moved on to the paratartaric acid crystal, was that it would turn out to be entirely symmetrical, and thus pull the light neither right nor left. But to his surprise, Pasteur again found a minute difference in one facet, making the crystal asymmetric.

Pasteur looked closer, with a characteristic combination of persistence and painstaking attention to detail. He eventually found that paratartaric acid crystals had both right- and left-handed forms. When he meticulously separated the crystals of each type with tweezers, the right-handed isomers predictably pulled light to the right, and the left-handed ones to the left. Mixed together, each negated the optical effect of the other.[4]

This ability of some molecules to produce dissymmetric forms—meaning that you cannot perfectly superimpose one isomer on its opposite, much as your right hand cannot fit easily into a left-handed glove—is now known as *chirality*, from the Greek word *kheir* for "hand." It was one of the most important discoveries in the history of chemistry, and the beginning of stereochemistry, or chemistry in 3D. Biot—by then the grand old man of French science, haggard, with hanks of gray hair flying out to the sides—summoned the young man to repeat the experiment in his presence. After Pasteur had successfully demonstrated the effect with the two different isomers of paratartaric acid, he recalled, "the illustrious old man, visibly moved, took me by the arm and said: 'My dear boy, I have loved science so much all my life that this stirs my heart.'"

Chirality would turn out to affect substances beyond tartaric acid and behaviors other than bending polarized light. Pasteur theorized that it "plays a considerable role in the most intimate laws of the organization of living organisms and intervenes in the most hidden of their physiological processes," and he was right. Later researchers would demonstrate that the shape of different isomers could affect how they fit into the binding sites for smell in the human nose, or taste on the human tongue. So in the modern food industry, for instance, the sugary taste of left-handed l-aspartame makes it valuable as an artificial sweetener. But its right-handed twin d-aspartame has no taste at all. In medicine, d-penicillamine, sold under the name Cuprimine, is considered one of the safest and most effective drugs for kidney stones, rheumatoid arthritis, and other conditions. But its left-handed twin l-penicillamine is toxic.

For Pasteur, it wasn't enough to make such an important discovery. He also deduced that molecules that were optically active all came from plants or animals. Substances lacking optical activity were of mineral origin. Chirality, he proposed, was a defining feature of organic matter—that is, of life itself.[5]

FERMENTATION: THE RISING

Throughout his career, Pasteur demonstrated a genius for building on discoveries and extending them by bold leaps of intuition into whole new fields. He continually advanced, as a fellow scientist put it in 1856, "from the theoretical conception that imagines a fact to the experiment that demonstrates it, and from that demonstration to new speculative views . . . in a continual sequence of corollaries and verification."

At about that time, Pasteur switched from the basic science of chirality to the seemingly humdrum concerns of industrialists in the northern city of Lille. Work on applied science was one of the mandates of the position he had assumed as dean of a new university there, and it fit Pasteur's own concerns as a chemist and the son of a tanner. A distiller there sought his help on problems he was having in the production of beet root alcohol. The fermentation vats smelled bad and the alcohol had an off taste. In the spring of 1856, Pasteur set up a laboratory on site and went to work in earnest. His course load at that point consisted of a single weekly lecture, and his wife Marie Pasteur worried that "he has lots of time, which he uses and abuses, I can assure you." But the work fit naturally with one of his brilliant intuitions.[6]

Advanced scientific thinking then held that fermentation was a simple chemical process. Antoine Lavoisier had reduced it in the eighteenth century to a formula describing the conversion of sugar into an equal weight of alcohol and carbonic acid, but omitting any role for yeast. Pioneering nineteenth-century chemists like Justus von Liebig in Germany added yeast, but merely as a chemical catalyst. They regarded the idea that fermentation was a product of living things as hopelessly antique.[7]

Pasteur, on the other hand, had a hunch that fermentation was the business of living organisms, in part because Biot, who had become his mentor, had mentioned to him that a certain amyl alcohol was optically active. Researchers in France and Germany had already independently described yeast as a biological organism in 1837, only to be ignored. This was a fate unlikely to befall Louis Pasteur. He quickly confirmed their findings on the growth of yeast through the fermentation process. He also identified the cause of the local distiller's tainted batches of beet-root alcohol—bacterial contamination producing lactic acid. The remedy was to heat the beet juice to destroy the *Lactobacillus* contaminant, then reseed with the correct yeast varieties. Again, many researchers might have stopped at that.[8]

Pasteur proceeded instead to go well beyond his predecessors in his refined analysis of every stage of the fermentation process. In place of the "modern" idea of fermentation as a purely chemical process, he presented detailed evidence that it was a biological phenomenon. As yeast grows and reproduces, the sugar and other nutrients in the brew provide it with essential energy and become converted in the process to alcohol, carbonic acid, and other products. Pasteur presented his evidence in characteristically bold language, and enlisted the backing of the French scientific hierarchy for his findings. He engaged in long debates with Liebig over the nature of fermentation, and at one point even challenged him to a sort of scientific duel, a battle of experiments, though under circumstances highly favorable to a certain French scientist. Later, he traveled to Liebig's home in Munich and actually doorstepped the poor man. (Liebig did not invite Pasteur in for a *weisswurst* and a chat.)[9]

In the course of this fermentation research, Pasteur developed many of the key insights that would become the basis for his future work in microbiology—among them, according to biographer Gerald Geison: the idea that specific microorganisms produce specific types of fermentation, and that different types of microorganisms compete for nutrients in the fermenting medium; the recognition that chemical features of the fermenting medium could promote or inhibit growth of the microorganism, and that the microorganisms in fermentations were largely airborne in origin; and the development of techniques for isolating and purifying a specific microorganism.[10]

Pasteur was characteristically always seeing the larger implications and the possibilities for greatness. Even in his first speech on fermentation, in April 1857, he was already suggesting that the study of microorganisms might eventually contribute to the understanding of infectious diseases. (Liebig had argued, on the contrary, that decay and putrefaction produced the chemical changes underlying these diseases.) He also interrupted his description of the "spontaneous" appearance of lactobacillus in a batch to state explicitly "that this has nothing to do with spontaneous generation." That was a separate topic that would engage him in his next great public combat.[11]

THESE MYSTERIOUS AGENTS

Much as Pasteur's work on chirality had led him to fermentation, fermentation in turn naturally led him to spontaneous generation. Among the questions that arose from this research, he wrote in 1860, the one that commanded his attention was the origin of the microorganisms: "Where do they come from, these mysterious agents, so feeble in appearance yet so powerful in reality . . . ? This is the problem that has led me to study the so-called spontaneous generations." Colleagues urged Pasteur not to become entangled in a topic perennially distorted by strong emotions and imprecise experimentation. Pasteur agreed that it was "only a digression." But he said he "wanted to arrive at an opinion on the question of spontaneous generation," the better to argue in favor of his ideas on fermentation.[12]

He became openly engaged with the debate early in 1859 when a naturalist in Normandy challenged his assertion that microorganisms in fermentations are airborne in origin. Félix Pouchet (1800–1872) was a physician and an accomplished scientist, who had produced numerous studies of plant and animal biology. In 1859, he published a 762-page book making the case for spontaneous generation. For the Academy of Sciences, "the question of the so-called spontaneous generations" had also become more urgent, given the increasing importance of microorganisms. That year, it offered the Alhumbert Prize for the winner of a competition to produce "well executed experiments" illuminating their origin.[13]

Pouchet's strategy was to repeat experiments by notable predecessors in the spontaneous generation debate, but with "a substantially higher degree of precision." For these experiments, he heated water in sealed flasks to the boiling point and let them cool. Then he submerged the sealed end in a mercury bath, opened it, and inserted a tube or small flask to add sterilized air and nutrients to the mix. He performed these manipulations under the surface of the mercury to eliminate any possibility of airborne contamination. And yet, he reported, a mass of microorganisms inevitably developed within the flask. Ergo, spontaneous generation.[14]

Looking to see where Pouchet had gone wrong, Pasteur soon realized that mercury does not in fact exclude air or microorganisms. Chemists describe mercury as a *nonwetting liquid*, meaning it does not wet glass or other surfaces because the cohesive forces *within* droplets are greater than the adhesive forces *between* droplets. That means dust and airborne germs can find their way onto and between droplets. Moreover, Pasteur wrote, a thin gap—he called it a *sheath*—between the mercury and the glass surface made it easier for these contaminants to enter the flask. Pouchet wasn't about to concede the point. He replied that air couldn't contain all the different microorganisms Pasteur was suggesting. "It would form a dense fog," Pasteur said, in a mocking paraphrase of his rival. "Like iron."[15]

The next stage in the debate looks in retrospect rather like a Monty Python skit, with the two scientists undertaking separate expeditions into the mountains to capture air samples and bring them back to the lab for analysis. Pouchet thought he'd show that spontaneous generation occurs even in the purest atmosphere. Pasteur thought he'd show that spontaneous generation wouldn't occur when he tested thin mountain air where microorganisms were likely to be scarce or nonexistent. He did his mountaineering in jacket, tie, and pince-nez, as if for a day in the laboratory. He hired a guide to take him up onto the glacier on Mont Blanc, together with a donkey bearing small glass flasks and an alcohol-fueled blowtorch for sealing up air samples. Pouchet responded by climbing even higher.

The dispute dragged on and turned ugly, with Pouchet quoting Voltaire's remark about a critic: "I worry about him only enough to spit on him." Newspapers became caught up in the scientific showdown and in the existence and possible ubiquity of microorganisms. Questions also loomed about the origins of life, especially after the French translation of Charles Darwin's *On the Origin of Species* appeared in 1862. But the mountaintop combat ended with each of the two scientists believing what he had started out believing, persuading no one.[16]

SWAN NECKS AND MAGICAL MICE

Pasteur's decisive experiment—or at least the one that drove Pouchet from the field—has become celebrated for "the swan-neck flask." Based on a suggestion from a colleague, Pasteur devised a flask with its thin neck drawn out to the side in an elegant S-shape and left open. Then he boiled liquid in the flask, and left it exposed in this fashion to the air. In test after test, he reported, the sterilized liquid remained free of microorganisms days or months later, even when he substituted urine, blood, or milk for water. Dust and germs were "without doubt" trapped along the way by the "sinuosities and inclinations" of the narrow throat, Pasteur wrote. It was an impressive display, especially when Pasteur broke off a neck, inserted it into the flask, and demonstrated that the liquid soon turned cloudy with microorganisms.[17]

In 1862, the Alhumbert Prize jury at the Academy of Sciences duly awarded its prize to Pasteur. The bickering between Pasteur and Pouchet continued, however, and in 1864, the academy appointed a committee to have them repeat their experiments at the same time in a Paris laboratory. Negotiations continued up to the day of the proposed duel. At the last minute, however, Pouchet abandoned the field, no doubt in part because he recognized that the jury was loaded in Pasteur's favor. He would continue to argue the case for the rest of his life. But for the scientific community at large, spontaneous generation was now a dead idea.

The Pouchet-Pasteur dispute has lived on as a source of continuing debate among science historians. Revisionists argue that Pasteur succeeded mainly by outtalking and otherwise outmaneuvering Pouchet. According to biographer Gerald L. Geison, Pasteur also engaged in a form of data manipulation, counting only those experiments that fit his hypothesis and writing "unsuccessful" experiments out of the record. Other historians argue that the scientific community correctly judged the outcome based on the experimental evidence available to them. And, as in almost every debate of his career, Pasteur's experiments were more carefully thought-out and executed than those of his opponents.[18]

It is at least undeniable that Pasteur outtalked Pouchet. On April 7, 1864, he delivered a celebrated lecture on spontaneous generation before an audience that included the great and the good of Paris society—among them Princess Mathilde Bonaparte, novelists Alexandre Dumas and George Sand, the press, and the medical faculty at the Sorbonne, where a lecture hall served as the venue for this event. Pasteur began by rehearsing the history of the spontaneous generation idea, dwelling on its more ridiculous manifestations. The seventeenth-century scholar Jan Baptist van Helmont, for instance, had asserted that a dirty shirt left to ferment with grains of wheat in a pot would transform the wheat into mice after about twenty-one days—adult mice, at that, both male and female. Pouchet's spontaneous generation experiment, he said, was as bad as van Helmont's pot of dirty linen. "I shall show you where the mice came in." He proceeded to lay out Pouchet's error with the mercury, in all its mortifying detail.

The high point of the talk came later, with special effects. First, Pasteur reminded his listeners of watching dust motes dance in the beam of sunlight slanting down in a darkened room through the slats of a window shutter. We don't otherwise notice them, he said, because full sunlight overwhelms them, much as by day we cannot see the stars in the sky. Then he called for the lecture hall to become night. When the lights were down, a single beam of gaslight rose up from the stage, and in it Pasteur pointed out the constant and capricious movements of the dust. "So, gentlemen," he announced, "there is dust everywhere in this room." He was still focused on refuting Pouchet. But in passing, almost casually, Pasteur flicked at the more momentous implications of his work: the particles of dust in his beam of light "should not be trivialized," he said, "for sometimes they carry the germs of disease and death: typhus, cholera, yellow fever, and many other plagues."[19]

Pasteur was wrong about those three diseases; other scientists, put on the scent by his lead, would later demonstrate that cholera is transmitted mainly by water, and the other two diseases by insects. But about the microbial origin of infectious diseases he was of course absolutely correct, and ready to stake his reputation on it. He had declared as much to the emperor, Napoleon III, on being elected to the Academy of Sciences the year before. His "whole ambition," he confided, "was to arrive at an understanding of the causes of putrid and contagious diseases." The emperor had not only approved, according to Pasteur, but also declared his own belief that some animalcules might well play a role in the development of these diseases.[20]

The idea was in the air.

15   THE SUBTLE FOE

Despite his declared ambition, Pasteur did not move on directly to research on human diseases. Silkworms, chickens, pigs, and sheep would be his subjects for the next two decades, until a desperate, deeply risky attack on a human disease near the end of his career. But at least one physician almost immediately recognized some implications of Pasteur's work for human medical care. Joseph Lister (1827–1912), a surgeon at the University of Glasgow, was walking home one evening early in 1865 with Thomas Anderson, a physician turned professor of chemistry. The topic of conversation was the putrefaction of wounds in the aftermath of surgery, and Anderson suggested that Lister read a couple of recent papers by a certain French chemist. The first was Pasteur's 1861 article on airborne germs in the spontaneous generation debate, the other his 1863 paper about the role of microorganisms in putrefaction.

Lister had grown up with a front-row seat on the rising science of microbiology. His father, Joseph Jackson Lister, a wine merchant, naturalist, and amateur optician, had reconceived the design of microscopes in ways that, after 1830, quickly became universal. These improvements enabled microscopes to bring objects into sharp focus, without the blobby, iridescent edges that had plagued earlier microscope design. They made it possible for researchers to develop the new science of *histology*—the study of minute animal and plant tissue structures—as well as the burgeoning science of bacteriology.[1]

Young Joseph Lister in turn put the microscope to work as a surgeon, to study wound infections. In the aftermath of amputations, compound fractures, and other major operations, it was routine to watch helplessly as a third or more of the patients died. Sepsis and gangrene were common killers. Infection was so routine, even in the most successful cases, that many surgeons regarded "laudable pus" as part of the cure. ("Ichorous pus," on the other hand, was the kind that killed you.) The patient laid out on the operating room table, a surgeon remarked at the time, has a greater risk of death than an English soldier on the battlefield at Waterloo.[2]

Reading Pasteur, Lister made the leap from fermentation to infection. The new research cast "a flood of light," he wrote, on the question of how the atmosphere produces decomposition. It wasn't the work of oxygen or other "gaseous constituents" of the air, as commonly thought. Instead, the air carried suspended in it "minute particles . . . which are the germs of various low forms of life." These germs had been "long since revealed by the microscope, and regarded as merely accidental concomitants of putrescence." But Pasteur had now shown them "to be its essential cause." By analogy with the way Pasteur had prevented putrescence in his experimental flasks by heating them and then protecting them from atmospheric contamination, Lister now thought it might likewise be possible to prevent putrescence in a wound by carefully applying an antiseptic. "In pursuing this object," he wrote, in another article for the *Lancet*, later in 1867, "we are guided by the 'germ-theory,' which supplies us with a knowledge of the nature and habits of the subtle foe we have to contend with; and without a firm belief in the truth of that theory, perplexity and blunders must be of frequent occurrence."[3]

For his antiseptic, Lister turned to carbolic acid, a coal-tar derivative, also known as phenol, or German creosote. Other surgeons had tried it before, in the American Civil War and on the Continent, where a German chemist had first identified its antiseptic powers in the 1830s. But their methods were haphazard and ineffective. Lister was motivated instead, oddly, by the industrial city of Carlisle's use of carbolic acid to treat sewage, "not only preventing all odour from the lands irrigated with the refuse material," but also preventing the intestinal parasites otherwise common in cattle grazing on such lands.[4]

Lister's first attempt to apply the treatment directly to a surgical wound was "unsuccessful." (He didn't specify if this meant the patient died. Perhaps it did not need saying.) But on August 12, 1865, he repaired a compound fracture of an eleven-year-old boy named James Greenlees whose leg had been run over by a cart. Lister reset the broken bones and washed the open wound with a solution of carbolic acid in linseed oil, then dressed it with a blend of putty and carbolic acid, under a tinfoil covering. Six weeks later, Greenlees walked out of the hospital on two healthy legs.[5]

By the time of his articles in the *Lancet*, Lister could report treatment of eleven compound fractures. One had ended in amputation, and one in death, though not by infection. The other nine patients had recovered, five of them without a trace of infection. The mortality rate was half his usual 18 percent in such cases, and a colleague noted that Lister had never seen so many of his patients free from infection, adding, "Indeed, I doubt if he had ever seen one." Lister also applied his carbolic acid in treating patients with infected abscesses, and the immediate success with those cases provided additional support for his antiseptic idea. "Upon these principles," Lister concluded, "a really trustworthy treatment for compound fractures and other severe contused wounds has been established for the first time, so far as I am aware, in the history of surgery."[6]

The British community did not rush to embrace Lister's methods. "The presence of these germs is not proved," Thomas Nunnelley, a prominent surgeon, lectured the 1869 meeting of the British Medical Association, "and probably, with safety, we may go much further, and deny their existence in the number and universality maintained by Pasteur and Lister." Other critics preferred *aseptic* methods, meaning absolute cleanliness in the operation itself, and regarded *antiseptic* methods as aimed at cleaning up damage better to be avoided in the first place. Lawson Tait, a young surgeon of the "cleanliness-and-cold-water-school," complained that in a dozen compound fractures he treated, the only cases with suppuration "were two in which I employed the acid paste exactly as recommended by Mr. Lister."[7]

Filth and gore were still as common in the operating theater as agony had been a few decades earlier, before the arrival of anesthetics. Most surgeons regarded cleanliness as out of place. "It was considered to be finicking and affected," Frederick Treves later recalled, of his start as a surgeon in the

1870s. "An executioner might as well manicure his nails before chopping off a head. The surgeon operated in a . . . frock coat of black cloth . . . stiff with the blood and the filth of years. The more sodden it was the more forcibly did it bear evidence to the surgeon's prowess." Lister fit this conventional model. The operating coat he wore at least into the 1880s was suitably "stiff and glazed with blood," though in fairness, his was of *blue* cloth. He boasted in an 1875 talk that his patients "have the dirtiest wounds and sores in the world," but it did not matter because of the blessing of carbolic acid.[8]

Other surgeons simply did not like carbolic acid. They still prided themselves on speed and efficiency in their work, and the preparation of wound coverings according to Lister's ever-shifting prescriptions took too much time. Moreover, carbolic acid was harsh stuff and could irritate the wound. It also irritated the hands and mucus membranes of surgeons, especially after 1871, when Lister devised a sprayer to cast a steady carbolic acid mist across the operating area. At times, this left the incision obscured under a haze of carbolic acid. It also left ugly brown splotches on the surgeons' hands, leaving them for once feeling not just dirty, but dirty and embarrassed.

Lister came to the antiseptic fight with several important advantages over his adversaries. Along with an intellectually rich upbringing, his family had provided him with an income to ease his entry into the world and support his interests. He was well-connected both socially and professionally. As a surgical student at the University of Edinburgh, he married Agnes Syme, whose father James was a widely respected and influential professor of surgery. "Lister therefore inherited his place in the upper middle ranks of the rigid Victorian class system, just as he inherited his butler from his father," according to one late-twentieth-century physician's attempt to recreate that social world. That writer also thought Lister "used his wife unmercifully as his secretary and assistant, often into the late hours of the night, and she appears to have been totally subservient."[9]

For one of Lister's students, on the other hand, Agnes Syme was an "almost equal" partner in his extensive laboratory research to develop better antiseptics. The medical laboratory they maintained in their home, with plumbing, a gas supply for Bunsen burners, an autoclave for sterilizing instruments, and other equipment, became her domain. The marriage produced no children, and servants spared her from the burden of housework. Instead, she became an unpaid and uncredited brain trust for his work.[10]

Her precise contribution is unknown—for instance, in the production in 1877 of the first pure bacterial culture ever. The intent of that experiment was to demonstrate the power of even a single bacterium to produce some of the dramatic effects suggested by germ theory. The two researchers couldn't deliberately introduce a pathogen into human test subjects to show that it produced the expected disease. Instead, they followed the long tradition of treating fermentation as an analogy for putrefaction—that is, infection. Taking a bacterium known to produce fermentation and curdling in milk, now known as *Lactococcus lactis*, the Listers hit on the strategy of repeatedly diluting a specimen to the point that there would be only a single *L. lactis* bacterium in a specific volume.

By introducing a single-bacterium sample into each of a series of test flasks filled with fresh milk, the Listers demonstrated that it quickly multiplied and curdled the milk, much as a single pathogen could reproduce in the human body and cause a systemic disease. It was a powerful demonstration of germ theory. But we have no way of knowing whether the laboratory innovation that made it possible—now known as the "limiting dilution method"—was his idea or hers. Lister didn't mention her in his paper on the experiment, though he used the word "I" forty-seven times over eight pages. Perhaps, given the gender politics of that time, he thought mentioning a female research partner might have undermined his credibility. What's clear, in any case, according to medical historian Ruth Richardson, is that "the evolution of the thoughtful technique that underpinned Lister's extraordinary surgical advances and bacteriological work was elaborated at home." It's worth adding that Joseph and Agnes Lister appear to have loved each other, though they shared a distaste for the unseemly business of expressing emotions. Friends considered it a perfect marriage.[11]

Being so abundantly supported by wife and family no doubt helped Lister endure and even benefit from the decades of criticism and debate about his methods. Semmelweis, his predecessor in the antiseptic cause, had wasted his rage in blind, flailing attacks that hurt himself more than anyone else. Pasteur somehow refashioned his rage into precisely targeted and utterly devastating rhetorical attacks, and also used it as a motive for pushing to new heights of discovery. Lister instead managed for the most part to deal with his critics politely, though firmly, with what one biographer characterized as a "cool, introspective submersion of his emotions."[12]

This must have been maddening for the likes of Lawson Tait, who took time away from his surgery to publish thirteen separate attacks on Listerism over the course of more than twenty years. One approach he pursued in arguing for his "cleanliness-and-cold-water-school" was to publish detailed statistical accounts of his own surgeries and demand that Lister do the same. Lister ignored him and dismissed the usefulness of statistics. Because other surgeons weighed in on both sides of the debate, the *Lancet* eventually suggested a rigorous experimental test, with a statistical comparison of results in two similar clinics, one practicing aseptic and the other antiseptic methods. Lister ignored that idea too.[13]

What also infuriated critics like Tait was Lister's knack for gradually absorbing useful criticisms into his methodology as if they had been his own ideas in the first place. As germ theory became more widely accepted, for instance, other surgeons began to think that both antiseptic and aseptic methods might work better together than as rival ideologies. Surgical gloves, masks, and gowns gradually came into wider use. Lister resisted at first. But he and his backers later spun these innovations as part of his original conception of antiseptic surgery. In a spluttering outburst in the *Lancet*, Tait called the idea "that antiseptics really mean absolute cleanliness . . . a mere perversion" of what Lister's antiseptic doctrine had in fact stood for. Despite these attacks, Lister steadily rose in stature and his name became synonymous with both antiseptic and aseptic surgical practices, while Tait himself survived mainly as a minor character spinning furiously within his archenemy's triumphant narrative.[14]

16 THE MYSTERY OF THE CURSED MEADOWS

In 1873, in a rural corner of what was then the German Empire, a dreaded disease broke out in sheep, cattle, and horses. The usual first sign of an outbreak was a sheep apart from the flock, unable to hold up its head, or a cow falling listlessly behind the herd. Victims trembled with fever. They staggered. They became breathless and bled from their orifices, quickly followed by collapse and death. It could happen so fast that the first thing a farmer noticed were the animals lying in a field, with bloated bellies and legs sticking straight up in the air. Anthrax killed livestock by the countless thousands each year in the nineteenth century. No one knew where it came from, what to do to prevent it, or how to control it once it had begun. Inhaled or gastrointestinal forms also occurred in humans and sometimes led to death. A form that blackened human skin gave anthrax its name, from the Greek word for coal. But livestock were the usual victims.[1]

Robert Koch (1843–1910) was a young physician living in Wollstein, Germany (now Wolsztyn, Poland). Since opening his practice a year earlier, he had made a reputation with local residents for kindliness and good medical care. He was also a doting father who liked to share his enthusiasm for the natural world with his young daughter. But he was hardly the "simple country doctor" of some accounts. A photograph of him from that era shows a serious young man in wire-rimmed eyeglasses, staring off into the imagined future, unsmiling, with his mouth concealed behind a moustache like a thick hedge. The effect was earnest and determined.

With the first free cash set aside from his practice, another doctor might have bought a decent carriage for making house calls in all weather and at all hours. Instead, Koch acquired a microscope of the highest quality available. (It may have been a gift from his wife Emmy. She merely said it "was obtained" through careful saving, adding, "How happy Robert was!") He was myopic, like Antoni van Leeuwenhoek and Louis Pasteur before him. The inclination to focus on objects near at hand was perhaps part of what attracted all three of them to the microscope. Koch used his to study algae, protozoa, and other natural curiosities, and also matters of public health and hygiene. The outbreak gave him the opportunity to examine the blood of a sheep killed by anthrax.

Over the next three years, working part-time in a homemade laboratory, Koch would not only identify the pathogen responsible for anthrax, he would also detail its complete life cycle. Where Louis Pasteur had made the great intuitive leap from fermentation to germ theory, Koch would for the first time lay out step by step how germ theory worked. If Pasteur "was a master architect of scientific medicine," one writer later remarked, "Koch was a master builder." He would go on from anthrax to identify the causes of some of the deadliest and most terrifying diseases known to humanity. Over the next few decades, the methods he developed would enable followers and rivals alike to identify an astonishing rogues' gallery of deadly pathogens and begin to target them for prevention and treatment.[2]

Koch remains surprisingly little-known today outside Germany. Only two or three serious English-language biographies exist, compared with at least three dozen Pasteur biographies, children's books, and even comic books. *Pasteurization* has become part of our everyday language. Koch's name meanwhile is less familiar, even in medical circles, than that of R. J. Petri, a Koch assistant who invented a useful piece of laboratory glassware, the petri dish.

Among the possible reasons for this neglect: Koch cured no diseases, though he made cures by other researchers possible. Worse, at the height of his fame, he raised the hope of a cure for tuberculosis in terminally ill people worldwide, then embarrassingly failed to deliver. Anti-German feelings may have further detracted from Koch's reputation in the twentieth century. Koch also lost support in his late forties when his affair with a beautiful actress half his age became public and he divorced his wife to marry her. Heinrich Mann,

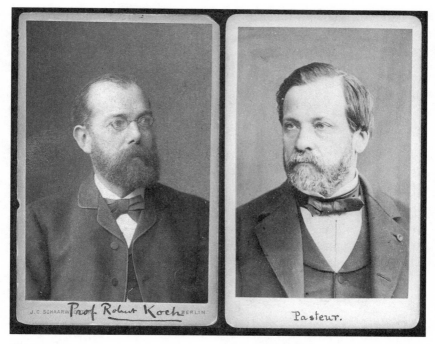

Figure 16.1

Koch (left) and Pasteur (right) cofounded germ theory and fought bitterly over it (New York Academy of Medicine).

elder brother of Thomas, spun this scandal into his novel *Professor Unrat* (The dirty professor). It became the basis for Josef von Sternberg's 1930 film *The Blue Angel*, with Marlene Dietrich in the role of seductress.

HUMBOLDTIAN DREAMS

Koch had grown up in the hilly, Harz Mountain country of northern Germany. His father was the administrator of a mine in Clausthal, and the family occupied a large, handsome house on the town square. Robert was the third of thirteen children, eleven of whom survived to become adults, another mark of the family's prosperity. An uncle on his mother's side became his great influence, taking him on hikes into the countryside and introducing him to the natural world. Young Robert learned to collect and classify beetles, butterflies, and other wildlife, with the help of a magnifying glass. The same uncle also introduced him to photography, at a time when capturing an image required patient chemistry as much as art. Koch went off to the University of Göttingen in 1862, intent on a career like that of his hero, the great Prussian naturalist and explorer Alexander von Humboldt.

The switch to medicine was a practical choice. But the enthusiasm, and some of the ideas and skills, of a naturalist carried over. Koch became familiar with the microscope and used it to conduct prize-winning research. One of his teachers, the physician and anatomist Jakob Henle, had published an 1840 paper arguing for microorganisms as a cause of disease, but Henle had given up studying infectious disease by the 1860s, and it played no part in his teaching. "Bacteriology did not exist at that time," Koch later recalled. He would have to invent the field himself.[3]

THE CURSED FIELDS

In Wollstein, Robert, Emmy, and their daughter, Gertrud, lived in a five-room apartment, with one room given over for seeing patients. A curtain divided off part of that room for a small laboratory with his microscope and photographic gear. There, in the course of his research, Koch examined blood from a sheep killed by anthrax. The sample contained relatively large, rod-like organisms, or, on closer examination, chains of segmented rods, linked in a line like box cars in a train. In favorable conditions, these organisms reproduced by dividing. The repeated doubling in number could quickly lead to devastating effects on a host.

There was, however, a deadly mystery about anthrax. In most diseases then known, contagion seemed to involve transmission of the disease only from one individual to another. But outbreaks of anthrax sometimes occurred when no new animal had entered a flock, in fields where no cases of the disease had happened for years or even decades past. The French called them *champs maudits*, or cursed fields. Koch's practice of patient and persistent watching would finally explain the curse.

On April 12, 1874, Koch saw something unusual happening beneath the lens of his microscope and jotted it down in his lab notes. The anthrax bacteria he had been studying seemed to be swelling up. They "become shinier, thicker, and much longer," he wrote. This was different from the usual bacterial reproductive method of simply dividing in two. Intrigued, Koch began to devote more time to his research. On occasion, his wife Emmy had to screen patients, sending home those who could get by without medical attention, and diverting others to a neighboring doctor.[4]

In late 1875, the police asked Koch, in his role as the local public health inspector, to examine an animal that had died in another anthrax outbreak. This new supply of bacteria gave his work a fresh start. He had begun to use rabbits in his research and discovered that the anthrax bacteria flourished in a rabbit's cornea, the clear outer layer of the eye. That gave Koch an idea: A rabbit is easier to work with than sheep, but it's still a highly inconvenient growth medium for careful microbiological study. To examine the anthrax bacterium in detail, he needed to see it outside the infected animal, in an artificial culture, on a piece of glass he could put under the lens of his microscope. Having seen anthrax proliferate in the rabbit's corneal fluid, he drew a small amount of this liquid onto a glass plate and found that he could make it work as a growth medium. This technique of using an artificial medium to culture bacteria would become an essential tool for all of microbiology, especially as Koch and his associates refined it over the next decade.

For now, though, he was able to resume his study of that unusual phase of the anthrax bacteria's reproductive development. What no one knew until then is that when conditions turn bad, anthrax bacteria can produce a sort of escape pod. Instead of repeatedly dividing in two, the bacterium develops a small capsule, called an *endospore*, encased in a tough shell. Later, the outer membrane of the bacterium vanishes, and free-living spores emerge. It may have been easier for Koch to recognize what was happening beneath the lens of his microscope because he had previously observed this process, called *sporulation*, in algae or fungi.

Next, Koch observed that the anthrax spores could survive in the soil in a dormant state and "remain for weeks without changing." To demonstrate that these spores could still infect animals after a period of dormancy, he injected the spores into experimental mice, quickly giving rise to a new and deadly population of anthrax bacteria. Finally, to be certain of his result and also to maintain a population of the bacteria for his studies, he injected anthrax material from one mouse into another, and from that mouse into another, and so on, in a series that in one case extended to twenty mice. (They were wild mice, incidentally, because meeker laboratory mice did not exist then. To handle them, he used an old bullet extractor from his time as a physician in the Franco-German War.) It would turn out that anthrax spores could survive in the soil in a dormant state not just for weeks, but for years or even decades. This was the answer to the mystery of the cursed fields—that is, the ability of anthrax to appear seemingly out of nowhere.

Koch conducted most of this research within a month or so of receiving that diseased animal in 1875. Despite the speed and directness with which he worked, none of it was easy. Every bacterial species has specific requirements—for instance, for preferred nutrients or for ambient temperature at different stages in its life. Different species require different staining techniques to enhance their visibility under a microscope. Koch encountered these variations and devised solutions on his own, in that corner of his examining room, often with makeshift equipment. To maintain a specimen at the right temperature, for instance, a modern researcher relies on a precisely calibrated benchtop incubator powered by electricity. But there wasn't any household electricity in 1876. Instead, according to biographer Thomas D. Brock, Koch found he could maintain the correct temperature by placing a slide culture on top of a piece of filter paper, on top of a flat dish filled with moist sand, on top of an open kerosene flame. Once he figured out the correct height of the flame, it was necessary only to refill the kerosene reservoir once a day.

Despite the complications, his new ability to peer into the inner world of tiny microbial creatures, and to track their behaviors and life histories as if they were elephants out on the African savanna, must have thrilled the naturalist in him and gratified his Humboldtian dreams. Koch generally maintained a scientific reserve in his work, but he could not help noting "the remarkable spectacle of actually watching the bacillus grow." In April 1876, he wrote a letter humbly seeking an audience with Ferdinand Cohn at the University of Breslau to explain his work. It was a smart choice: Cohn was not just a prominent botanist and microbiologist but also an early proponent of bacterial taxonomy. He named species at a time when many biologists still thought of all bacteria as an undifferentiated mass, or as slight variations on a single form.

Cohn extended an invitation, and on the last Sunday of the month, Koch boarded the train at 1:00 a.m. for the nine-hour ride to Breslau. He was carrying a satchel of laboratory equipment and a vial of blood from the spleen of a mouse, a freshly deceased anthrax victim. At the university that afternoon, Cohn and an assistant looked on as Koch set up his cultures in a growth medium of fluid from the eye of a slaughterhouse cow. Back at the laboratory next morning, Cohn peered through his microscope at the development of these cultures and listened with growing interest as Koch walked him through the experiments he had made. When each of them realized the other had also witnessed the little miracle of spore formation—Cohn in a harmless species he named *Bacillus subtilis*—they shared a joyous moment of mutual recognition, an echo of their original epiphanies. What most impressed Cohn, though, was the care and thoroughness of Koch's work. Word of the remarkable newcomer began to spread. On the third day, prominent figures from around the campus came in to be part of the moment, to be part of history.

"Now leave everything as it is, and go to Koch," one of them excitedly urged his assistants. "This man has made a magnificent discovery, which for simplicity and the precision of the methods employed, is all the more deserving of admiration, as Koch has been shut off completely from all scientific associations. He has done everything himself and with absolute completeness. There is nothing more to be done. I regard this as the greatest discovery in the field of pathology, and believe that Koch will again surprise us and put us all to shame by further discoveries."[5]

Within a few months, Cohn was on a previously scheduled visit in England and Scotland, where he met with Charles Darwin and other leading scientists. The great Irish polymath John Tyndall took a special interest in Koch's discovery. He would become a key figure in making Koch's work known to the English-speaking world, beginning in October 1876, when Cohn's own journal published Koch's paper, "The Etiology of Anthrax, Based on the Life Cycle of *Bacillus anthracis*."

What that paper described wasn't just the complete life history of a bacterial species. By repeatedly inoculating the bacteria from one mouse to another, in each case producing the symptoms of anthrax, Koch had proved the long-contested reality of contagion, and he had demonstrated beyond reasonable doubt that *Bacillus anthracis* was the agent of that contagion.

What he had demonstrated, in short, was the germ theory of disease.

17 A NEW VACCINE

By the mid-1870s, Pasteur was already a great name not just for his work on the germ theory of disease, but for discoveries that had saved the wine and silk industries of France from various microbial blights. He managed a large, well-funded laboratory amid the universities and hospitals of Paris, assisted by scientists who would themselves become great names in the history of medicine. They might have wished to be doing research directly on human diseases, especially after one of them, Émile Roux, lost his wife to tuberculosis in 1879, and another, Émile Duclaux, lost his wife to puerperal fever in 1880. But veterinary diseases, primarily anthrax and chicken cholera, provided a safer model for working out Pasteur's ideas, while also serving his interest in science beneficial to French industry.

What Pasteur now wanted was to develop the first new vaccines since Edward Jenner. He was aiming not merely to equal the greatest figure in the history of disease prevention, but to surpass him, devising a way to expand the vaccine idea from smallpox to the broadest range of deadly diseases. Pasteur had begun his vaccine research on anthrax in 1877. He added chicken cholera as a possible vaccine candidate soon after, when another researcher managed to culture the bacterial cause of that disease. Unlike anthrax, chicken cholera wasn't a common problem for agriculture. But when it struck, it could decimate a flock.

The key step in developing a vaccine happened, ostensibly by accident, in the summer of 1879, while Pasteur was away from Paris for a long break at the house where he had grown up in Arbois. On his return to the laboratory in October, his assistants reported that cultures of chicken cholera bacteria left unattended over the summer no longer produced disease when injected into a group of test animals. Another scientist might simply have discarded the weakened bacterial cultures.[1]

Instead, according to the traditional account, Pasteur had one of his dazzling intuitions. He was of course aware that people who survive certain virulent diseases, like measles or smallpox, become protected against a future recurrence of that disease. He also knew that Jenner's smallpox vaccine somehow artificially elicited this same phenomenon of acquired immunity. And he had heard the theory that it worked because cowpox was just a weaker version of smallpox, strong enough to trigger the immune response but not to cause the disease. The wheels turned in Pasteur's head. His assistants had injected the accidentally weakened bacterial culture into a group of test animals, thinking it would produce the disease, only to find that it didn't. Pasteur took it a step further: What if the weakened bacteria actually elicited immunity to chicken cholera? He thought for a moment and then supposedly exclaimed, "Do you not see that these animals have been vaccinated?" A simple test—injecting them with the live pathogen—would prove it.[2]

There is, however, an alternative version of this episode. It's based on two separate studies of Pasteur's unpublished laboratory notebooks, long kept private by order of Pasteur himself, but finally made available to scholars in the 1970s. The historians Antonio Cadeddu in the 1980s and Gerald Geison in his 1995 book *The Private Science of Louis Pasteur* both argued that the decision to leave the chicken cholera cultures unattended for several months was anything but accidental, and that the ingenious idea to make a vaccine with the resulting weakened, or attenuated, bacteria came not from Pasteur, but from Émile Roux, a key assistant. This alternative account is less romantic than the traditional story. But, if true, it would fit better with how scientific discoveries seem to happen, not as the lightning-stroke insight of one brilliant mind, but as a result of wheels turning in many minds.[3]

Émile Roux (1853–1933) had joined the laboratory in 1878 and quickly demonstrated what Cadeddu called "an extremely independent mind" and a willingness to take "initiatives outside the teacher's directives," though he combined these traits with a lifelong dedication to the Pasteur legend.

(A student later lamented that Roux was unwilling to commit his intimate knowledge of Pasteur to paper, though he sometimes touched on the master's failings in conversation.) The vaccine, in Geison's analysis, was "the still-imperfect outcome of an extensive and twisting program of research in which an independent set of experiments by Roux played a crucial role." The exact details of those experiments are unknown, because Roux was literally working off the books: Pasteur had taken his laboratory notebooks with him to record his own experiments during his summer sojourn in Arbois.[4]

According to both Cadeddu and Geison, Roux had been experimenting with oxygen to make chicken broth less acidic and thus a better medium to

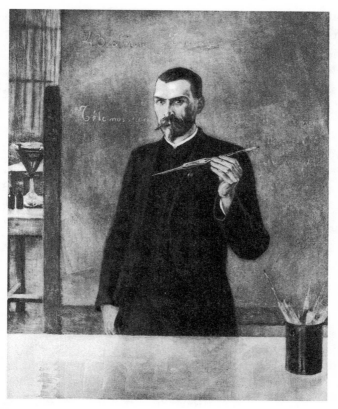

Figure 17.1
Émile Roux served as a private genius behind Pasteur's public face (Wellcome Collection).

culture the chicken cholera bacteria, which he was deliberately working to weaken at the same time. Roux injected a sample of the theoretically weakened bacteria into chickens and, as he hoped, no disease resulted. Pasteur wanted to test immediately to see if the chickens had become immune in the process. But Roux advised him to wait. As the only physician on his staff, he knew from his experience with smallpox vaccine that it took time for an immune response to develop. When Roux subsequently injected the same chickens with a fully virulent strain of chicken cholera, the birds in fact survived unharmed. Pasteur then announced the discovery of attenuation of chicken cholera to the Academy of Medicine in February 1880. He followed up soon after with a description of the chicken cholera vaccine his laboratory had developed as the practical outcome of this research. It was the first new vaccine in the eighty-four years since Jenner's smallpox vaccine—with credit due, in the revisionist interpretation, more to Roux than to Pasteur.[5]

In his published account that October, Pasteur theorized that exposure to oxygen had weakened the pathogen during the extended period in culture, an idea he attributed in his laboratory notebook to Roux. The more likely modern understanding of why the vaccine worked, according to microbiologist Thomas D. Brock, is that leaving the cultures undisturbed had altered the conditions for natural selection to operate: When Pasteur or Roux took fresh material from recent victims of chicken cholera, they were selecting for the virulent bacterial strains that dominate in the natural environment of a victim's body. When they left the bacteria to grow in culture, however, virulent strains lost their selective advantage, allowing less virulent, or even harmless, strains to thrive.[6]

THE TWISTED PATH TO AN ANTHRAX VACCINE

Based on the mistaken belief in the success of oxygen exposure, Pasteur raised the tantalizing prospect of being able to develop vaccines against the microbial causes of other deadly diseases. Henri Toussaint (1847–1890), a young veterinary professor in Toulouse, had meanwhile already developed an anthrax vaccine of his own and announced the news to the Academy of Medicine in August 1880, via Henri Bouley, a friend who was a member.

Some academicians dismissed the thirty-three-year-old veterinarian as an upstart, particularly because he had the audacity to hide his methodology in a sealed envelope, a practice that had drawn a reprimand a few months earlier when Pasteur himself had tried it in announcing attenuation. From Arbois, Pasteur wrote to Bouley "in astonishment and admiration before M. Toussaint's discovery; in admiration that it was made and in astonishment that it could be made."[7]

Toussaint had taken blood from an infected animal, removed the fibrin to prevent clotting, and then killed the pathogen by heating his sample for ten minutes at 131 degrees Fahrenheit (55°C). Pasteur, however, believed that only a live attenuated vaccine could elicit immunity. This would turn out to be another serious mistake. But bear in mind that the science of immunology did not yet exist, and the understanding of vaccines had advanced hardly at all since Jenner's day. Pasteur's theory was that the body of a potential host contains only trace amounts of the specific nutrients a pathogen requires. He thought a weakened but still living version of the pathogen would consume those trace amounts, preventing the regular pathogen from ever taking hold. This might have seemed like a logical idea in the laboratory context of bacterial cultures, where a supply of the proper nutrients determined survival.

Toussaint's rationale for using a killed anthrax vaccine was equally contorted, and also wrong. And he was encountering major difficulties in a small field test of his vaccine: Of twenty sheep he injected, four died immediately. The others became badly sick, though they survived and appeared at least temporarily immune. Toussaint's friend Bouley soon stopped by the Pasteur laboratory in Paris for a chat.

Roux told him that the laboratory's own tests of Toussaint's methods suggested that any apparent immunity may have resulted only because weakened bacteria had survived the heat treatment. The Toussaint vaccine also sometimes caused full-blown anthrax infections, or killed animals outright, Roux said. Bouley then confided that there was more to Toussaint's method than previously disclosed: he also weakened the vaccine material with carbolic acid, the same antiseptic Joseph Lister was promoting in surgery. In a letter to Pasteur the same day, Bouley expressed concern that Toussaint's vaccine as currently prepared only "temporarily anesthetized" the bacteria and "would be a vaccine full of 'treachery,' since it would be capable of recovering its potency with time." He also told Pasteur in confidence that Toussaint had now become convinced of the need to make a live vaccine.

Bouley revisited the Pasteur laboratory later that August, this time accompanied by Toussaint. They were seeking a virulent anthrax culture for further testing on vaccinated animals. On yet another visit, Toussaint asked Roux to inspect a vaccine sample to ensure that it was free of living bacteria. Roux again found living bacteria, as well as various contaminants he described in a letter to Pasteur as the result of careless laboratory technique.

These meetings alerted Roux to the possible value of an antiseptic of some kind in producing a better live anthrax vaccine. Microbiologist Charles Chamberland (1851–1908), who had joined Pasteur's laboratory in 1875, was already working on different ways to weaken anthrax bacteria, including an experiment a month earlier exposing them to gasoline fumes, then a common sanitizer for laboratory equipment. Roux now wrote to Pasteur: "Could it be that the anthrax cultures in many of the flasks we have at the laboratory would show themselves to be benign for sheep and give them immunity—notably the cultures of the spores that Chamberland has left exposed for some time to gasoline vapors?"

At the end of February 1881, after what must have been a flurry of research that fall and winter, Pasteur reported the development of a vaccine against anthrax. He followed up in late March with news of a successful trial in sheep. Because of his outsized reputation for delivering valuable results, this announcement attracted immediate public excitement—perhaps more excitement than Pasteur intended. Hippolyte Rossignol, a veterinarian in Pouilly-Le-Fort who was a germ theory skeptic, challenged him to a public demonstration.

By that point, Pasteur's tests with various vaccine strains weakened by oxygen exposure—the method he was publicly backing—had produced only limited success in a small number of test animals. But admitting uncertainty, in Geison's analysis, would have exposed Pasteur "to charges that he, like Toussaint, had made his announcement prematurely." It would also have been a blow to Pasteur's "richly deserved reputation" for rising to any scientific challenge, in any public arena, armed for combat.[8]

GOING PUBLIC AT POUILLY-LE-FORT

On Thursday, April 28, while Roux and Chamberland were away on vacation, Pasteur agreed to the proposed terms for a rigorous test of his discovery in Pouilly-Le-Fort. The local branch of the Society of French Farmers would provide sixty sheep for the test, which was to take place on Rossignol's own large and prosperous farm. Pasteur was to vaccinate twenty-five sheep in two doses delivered over twelve days. After a waiting period for the vaccine to take effect, the original twenty-five, plus another twenty-five unvaccinated sheep, would receive an injection of deadly anthrax bacteria. Start to finish, the experiment would take five weeks. Deep into hubristic overreach, Pasteur delivered what he later admitted was the "boldly prophetic," even "brash," prediction that only the vaccinated sheep would survive. Ten remaining sheep would go without any injections and serve as a control group for the experiment.[9]

In a note beginning, "My dear Roux," Pasteur wrote that same day to inform his vacationing assistant that a public test of the vaccine would begin on May 5—that is, the following Thursday, just one week from his having signed the protocol. "I very much wish you to return by May 3 or 4 at the latest. This is a big and important event. We must have a serious talk about it before we begin. All my very best."[10]

Roux and Chamberland hurried back to Paris. In their work for Pasteur, they had been diligently pursuing the combination of oxygen exposure and heat to weaken anthrax bacteria, trying to make different test strains into more reliable vaccines. But they had also resumed experimenting on the side—apparently against Pasteur's wishes—with alternative weakening agents. Their most recent test using an anthrax strain weakened with potassium bichromate, a highly toxic antiseptic, had produced the intended immunity and hadn't killed any animals outright. While the sample was embarrassingly small—just two sheep—it represented an improvement over their latest test with an oxygen-weakened strain. Pasteur gave the nod to push ahead with the alternative.[11]

On May 5, as agreed, Pasteur's team presented itself at Rossignol's farm. So did a large crowd of observers brought out by the spectacle of the great

Pasteur putting his genius to a barnyard test. There were last-minute negotiations: two sheep were too weak for the experiment, and two goats took
their place, while an ox stood in for a frail cow in an auxiliary test group
of ten cattle. Chamberland and Louis Thuillier, a young assistant, immobilized each of the animals in turn, while Roux handled the big glass-and-
silver Pravaz syringe to administer the vaccine. Rossignol stood by, looking
simultaneously proud to host the great event and also duly skeptical of the
putative vaccine. Physicians in their stovepipe hats conferred learnedly, and
farmers in wooden clogs traded off-color jokes as if at a country fair. Pasteur
presided over all with "Olympian calm," according to Debré, and delivered
an impromptu lecture on bacteria, disease, and the great potential of vaccines. The second round of vaccinations took place on May 17. Then there
was nothing to do but wait for the injection of all animals with a deadly strain
of anthrax on Tuesday, May 31. One of Pasteur's most determined critics
from the Academy joined the crowd on the appointed day. He challenged
Pasteur to deliver a dose of anthrax triple the amount originally agreed on
and, to prevent any fiddling, to inject a vaccinated and an unvaccinated
animal in turn throughout. Pasteur agreed, of course, and at no point did
he "waver from his calm," Debré wrote. "He seemed so sure of himself that
even his collaborators were impressed. Yet those who knew him well might
have wondered, for when Pasteur knew that he was right, he was not calm
but combative and sometimes outright aggressive."[12]

The final result of the experiment would not be apparent until Thursday, June 2. The night before, a telegram arrived alerting the laboratory
that one of the vaccinated ewes appeared to be in trouble and unlikely to
survive. Pasteur snapped, according to a later account of the incident. "In a
rush, he saw the consequences of a failure for his ideas, his laboratory, himself." He couldn't believe that the vaccine itself might be at fault. It had to
be an error in carrying out the experiment. Émile Roux, the only one of his
assistants present, "bore the avalanche" of Pasteur's disappointed fury. "They
say it was brutal. Madame Pasteur tried to calm her husband." Finally, failing, she pointed to the clock and reminded him that he needed to rest for
the early morning train to Pouilly-le-Fort. Pasteur "leapt from his seat and
declared that he would not go, that it would be impossible for him to bear

the confusion, the public shame. Since Roux was the author of the disaster, Roux alone would endure it."[13]

In the morning, Pasteur continued to fret. At 9:00 a.m., another telegram arrived at the laboratory with the news: all the vaccinated animals appeared to be in good health, while their unvaccinated counterparts now lay dead or dying. "I had a little moment of emotion that made me see all the colors of the rainbow," Madame Pasteur admitted, in a letter to her daughter. God knows, she had earned it.

They boarded the train on schedule, and when they arrived at Pouilly-le-Fort, a crowd had already gathered to celebrate the great genius of the day. Pasteur rose in his carriage to accept the accolade of former skeptics who were now disciples. "Ah, you men of little faith!" he cried out, gleeful in his triumph. "Now you see it." At 2:00 p.m., twenty-three of the unvaccinated animals in the main experimental group were dead, the *Times* of London reported next day, and at 3:00 p.m., the last two followed. The same pigheaded critic who had insisted on tripling the virulent dose now pronounced himself persuaded, and with a convert's zeal, even offered to be vaccinated and then injected with the same dose of anthrax. Roux and Chamberland, the true heroes of the day, stayed quietly in the background, and Marie Pasteur reported, rather tartly, "There were cordial embraces all around amidst the guinea pigs."[14]

Pasteur realized how much he owed his assistants. When he published his account of the experiment at Pouilly-le-Fort, the byline said "Louis Pasteur (with the collaboration of Mr. Chamberland and Mr. Roux)." But that report carefully omitted any description of the vaccine itself, leaving readers to infer that he succeeded with the oxygen-attenuated method he had previously advocated. In Geison's interpretation, Pasteur wanted to avoid any mention of antiseptic attenuation because it might remind people that Toussaint had used the same method for his vaccine. He might equally have been buying time to perfect his methodology in private.[15]

Two months later, at a medical congress in London, Pasteur rose to give "the term vaccination an enlarged meaning" and to "consecrate" it "as an homage to the merit and immense services rendered by one of the greatest men of England, your Jenner. What joy for me to glorify this immortal name on the very soil of the noble and hospitable city of London." It was a bold assertion of his own place in history.[16]

Pasteur was undoubtedly egotistical, arrogant, even unsavory in some of his behaviors. But even Geison had to admit that Pasteur was a great communicator of his science. By putting his laboratory's work to a barnyard test amid the dung-spattered farmers at Pouilly-le-Fort, he had made his vaccine an international triumph. "Pasteur's sensitivity to the concerns of his audience, his ability to win them over to his side, even his skillful exploitation of the external advantages he enjoyed, show that he was in fact a 'better' scientist than Toussaint."[17]

Better in truth than almost any scientist then living, with the possible exception of Robert Koch.

18 THE BIBLE OF BACTERIOLOGY

In the aftermath of his landmark publication on anthrax, Robert Koch turned his attention not to grand theories or miracle cures, but to minutia. His aim now was to see what was happening in certain specific infections, and to see it far more clearly than anyone had done before. While Pasteur raced to wow the world with his new vaccine, Koch focused on microphotography. Thinking about it even now, the heart sinks a little. It seems like such an underwhelming career move. "I would be exceedingly grateful," he wrote early on to a photographic equipment supplier, "if you would inform me as to whether it would be possible to obtain good photographs of tiny transparent objects."

He had no funding, other than a country doctor's meager earnings. His research still took place on his own, in a corner of his examining room, in between tending patients with all their familiar complaints. And yet the techniques Koch devised over the next few years, the minutia, would largely invent the science of microbiology, spawn a generation of microbe hunters, and open the door to the greatest epoch of disease discovery and prevention in human history.

Photography appealed to Koch on several counts. When he applied his camera to the microscope, he found that the photographic emulsion captured microorganisms that had escaped even his highly attentive eye. (With anthrax, the relatively large size of *Bacillus anthracis* made it easy to see and describe in all its stages of development. But it was different when he came to the various miniscule varieties of *Micrococcus*.) A photograph also proved to be more accurate than a drawing and less prone to human misinterpretation in rendering the complexity of microbiological life. "I am absolutely certain that a bad photograph of a living organism," he wrote, "is a hundred times better than a misleading or possibly inaccurate drawing."[1]

Koch was in fact interested only in the best possible photographs, with a view to publishing them. He employed a horizontal box camera-and-microscope setup, at a window in the same corner of the examining room that held his laboratory. A clock-operated heliostat tracked the sun and reflected its rays through the specimen Koch intended to photograph. Having set up and focused the image, Koch then had to go to a dark box in a corner of the kitchen, paint a light-sensitive emulsion onto a glass plate, carry the plate back in a lightproof wooden box, and insert the plate into the camera. His wife stayed outside and served as "cloud chaser," to alert him to sudden changes in light as he was about to shoot the photograph. After all that, the only way to tell if the image had actually stayed in focus was to develop the negative. He could produce at best one or two photographs per hour.[2]

He published the results in 1877, together with a detailed how-to account for other researchers interested in working with the techniques he had devised. He started with a drop of liquid containing bacteria on a glass slide, dried it, and protected it with a thin glass cover slip. "I saw to my astonishment," he wrote, that, unlike some other microorganisms, "bacteria do not collapse and become deformed upon drying." He also described a way around the "tiny transparent objects" problem, with a new technique for staining bacteria with aniline dyes, an extract of coal tars. These dyes had been invented in the 1850s by a British researcher seeking an alternative to quinine as an antimalarial. Instead, aniline dyes soon produced such a flowering of new colors in women's dresses that *Punch* called it "mauve measles." Less fashionably, a pathologist at Breslau named Karl Weigert devised a way to stain bacteria with these dyes. He allowed Koch to include the technique in his article, ahead of his own publication.[3]

In addition to his own genius, some of Koch's groundbreaking discoveries were partly a result of being in the right place at the right time. In 1878, he and Weigert visited the Carl Zeiss Company, a leading manufacturer of microscopes. There, co-owner Ernst Abbe showed them two innovations for which he had not yet found a market. First, the Abbe condenser, positioned below the microscope stage, concentrated the light source—sunlight—and enabled the operator to optimize the brightness and evenness of illumination passing through a specimen. Koch had been frustrated until then in identifying the pathogens responsible for wound infections. But with the condenser, he wrote, "everywhere in the diseased body micrococci were visible."[4]

Abbe also introduced them to the oil-immersion lens, for improving resolution at higher magnifications. It depended on a fine oil coating applied to both the lens and the specimen. The optimal recipe, a mix of cedar and fennel seed oil, had only emerged after Abbe and a collaborator had worked their way through three hundred different types of oil. Koch reported that "in the same slides which had previously shown nothing, the smallest bacteria are now visible with such clarity and definition that they are very easy to see and to distinguish from other colored objects." He could now describe pathogenic bacteria by size and shape and begin to categorize them taxonomically. He was soon conducting experiments in animals to show that specific bacteria caused specific types of wound infection, including pyemia, which had killed Ignaz Semmelweis and the new mothers he studied. Other scientists followed his lead, after Koch published an eighty-page book with photographs on the microbes in wound infections.[5]

In July 1880, at thirty-seven, Koch left daily medical practice to head his own bacteriological laboratory at the newly organized Imperial Health Office in Berlin. There, working elbow to elbow with two assistants in a small room with one window, he quickly developed another critical improvement. Although corneal fluid had proved successful as a growth medium with anthrax, a liquid medium was too susceptible to contamination by other microbes, which could swirl together in "a tangled mixture of different shapes and sizes." Koch suspected the same problems afflicted "the Pasteur school in its noteworthy but blindly zealous researches."

To be certain which specific bacteria caused a particular disease, Koch needed to grow bacteria instead on a solid medium, with just one bacterial type per culture. He found his first solid medium, according to a homey legend, when someone left a slice of boiled potato in the laboratory. As Koch was about to toss it in the trash, he took another look and recognized spots of bacterial growth. Examination under his microscope revealed that each spot consisted of a single bacterial type. If he carefully removed a spot and transferred it to another potato slice, under sterile conditions, he could grow it as a pure culture. The story is true, but it wasn't an accident. Koch learned the potato slice technique from another German researcher who had devised it a few years earlier for work on fungi.

Many of the bacteria that cause deadly diseases in animals were unenthusiastic about growing on a potato slice, however. Koch set out to devise a more suitable solid medium on the same basic principles. After many futile experiments, he eventually found that if he took gelatin, and treated it with potassium or sodium to reduce acidity, heated and filtered it to remove impurities, then heated it again to kill any surviving microorganisms, and mixed the gelatin at a rate of about 3 percent into whatever nutrient worked for a particular pathogen, then he had the beginnings of a solid medium. It was, however, *only* the beginning. The next step was to spread the gelatin-nutrient mixture on a sterilized microscope slide, using a sterilized pipette, and leave a stack of such slides in a moist chamber for several days to dry. Koch then sterilized a needle or platinum wire and used it to pick up a tiny amount of the material he wanted to test—for instance, a drop of blood from an animal with septicemia—and streak it in three to six lines across the dry gelatin-nutrient surface of a slide. The slide went under a bell jar to protect it from contamination and sat there for a few days to grow at 68–77 degrees Fahrenheit (20–25°C). Koch could then examine the lines under a microscope to identify a pure culture of the probable target organism, which he could transfer to other slides prepared with the same gelatin-nutrient mix to grow them in pure culture almost indefinitely for whatever experiments he needed to undertake.[6]

It was a long way from the homey potato slice. But it made Koch's 1881 paper introducing this method the "bible of bacteriology," according to Koch biographer Thomas D. Brock. What became known as the *plate method* is still standard in microbiology today. That summer, at an international medical conference in London, the holy trinity of germ theory were briefly together in the same room when Joseph Lister brought Louis Pasteur to a laboratory session at which Koch demonstrated both the plate method and his technique for staining bacteria. Pasteur, though fiercely anti-German, was moved to congratulate Koch, saying, "C'est un grand progrès, Monsieur."[7]

By making it relatively easy to obtain a pure culture of almost any bacteria, the plate method removed a major roadblock to understanding what role these tiny organisms played in infectious disease. New language had already begun to acknowledge that *microbes*, a word first popularized in an 1878 speech to the French Academy of Medicine, played *some* role in disease. The word *pathogenic*, or capable of producing disease, had made the leap from its French origins into English, German, and other languages, sharply spiking from the mid-1870s onward. But skeptics could still debate whether such a thing as a specific type or species of microorganism even existed. They theorized instead that bacteria somehow shape-shifted to cause different diseases. As late as 1877, one Swiss botanist complained that, after ten years and thousands of bacterial specimens, he had been "completely unable to distinguish even two distinct species."[8]

Koch clearly found it exasperating. "From the very beginning of bacteriological research . . . right up to the present time," he complained in his 1881 paper, "there has been a tendency to take all of the different kinds of bacteria and throw them into one pile, and make one or at most several species from them." Now he was delivering the microbiological definition to change that. He proposed that bacteria capable of retaining their distinctive characteristics "*when they are cultured on the same medium and under the same conditions, through many transfers or many generations . . . should be designated as species, varieties, forms, or other suitable designations.*"[9]

Researchers who used Koch's innovative techniques, particularly the plate method, could now isolate different types of bacteria in pure culture, study them in detail, and work through the differences that might justify calling them separate species. As a result, resistance to the idea of distinct bacterial types largely evaporated. For the first time since Antoni van Leeuwenhoek hinted at the tantalizing possibility two hundred years earlier, medical researchers could begin to see into the world of pathogens.

And knowing our enemies would become the basis for saving ourselves from them.

19 DEFINING THE INDEFINABLE SOMETHING

Koch's sense of confidence and his ambition "to work as hard as [he could] for science" were now both on the rise. Almost immediately on returning from the August 1881 conference in London, he set out to understand the single biggest killer among all infectious diseases: tuberculosis. Other diseases were more dramatic. But deaths from smallpox had declined dramatically as a result of vaccination. Cholera was also fading away, if only in the developed world, as sanitary reform took effect from the 1860s onward. Plague had become an infrequent intruder, though still terrifying.

Tuberculosis had none of the apocalyptic associations of those outbreaks. It was merely a full-time resident, quietly at work, year in and year out, with its debilitating pulmonary effects made worse by the suffocating air pollution of nineteenth-century industrial cities. Koch estimated that one person in seven died of tuberculosis. Among adults, it was more like one in every three or four, a New York physician added a few years later, and the average age of death was just thirty-two. "The robber of youth," as it was known, killed parents at the moment their child-rearing labor was most in need.[1]

There was nothing pretty about the dying either, though the notion persisted that tuberculosis was somehow romantic, or even erotic. Lord Byron sometimes fed only on water, vinegar, and rice, to attain the desired emaciated look, according to his friend, Irish poet Thomas Moore. Admiring himself fondly in the mirror one time, he mused, "I look pale; I should like to die of a consumption." When Moore raised one eyebrow, Byron explained, "Because the ladies would all say, 'Look at that poor Byron, how interesting he looks in dying.'"[2]

In reality, what the human body experienced in consumption, or tuberculosis, was a prolonged and polymorphous siege. Various forms of the disease could target the liver, the gastrointestinal tract, the membranes around the spine and brain, the tissue layers around the heart, or the lining of the abdominal cavity. One common form caused swollen lymph nodes in the neck. (Called *scrofula*, it was decidedly not erotic.) Another form attacked the skeleton, causing severe back pain and stiffness. A genital form could swell the testicles and cause pelvic or urinary pain in either sex. And a cutaneous form could cause wart-like, mulberry-colored lesions, none of this being the sort of "interesting" Byron had in mind.

Pulmonary tuberculosis was the most common form of the disease. Edgar Allan Poe, who tended his beloved wife for five years until her death at twenty-four, called it a "horrible never-ending oscillation between hope & despair." Virginia Poe suffered all the usual symptoms, including fatigue, fever, night sweats, and weight loss. She was ravaged by violent coughing jags, which typically produced thick, green, foul-smelling mucus. Once, at a dinner party with friends at their home, she was singing and playing the harp after dinner, dressed in white, and looking "delicately, morbidly angelic," according to one account. At a high note, she suddenly stopped, clutching her throat, "and a wave of crimson blood rushed down over her breast." The same thing occurred "again—again—and even again at varying intervals," Poe later wrote. "Each time I felt the agonies of her death—and at each succession of the disorder I loved her more dearly and clung to her life with more desperate pertinacity."[3]

Some victims suffered a "galloping" form of tuberculosis, like the one John Keats contracted sometime between the summer of 1818 and early 1820. It killed him on February 23, 1821, when he was just twenty-six. For others, like the essayist Ralph Waldo Emerson, the disease dragged on across a normal lifespan. He referred to it, at twenty-five, as "the mouse in my chest." It was still softly gnawing when he died at seventy-eight. Emerson also called tuberculosis the "family scourge," and its tendency to cluster in families—novelists Charlotte, Emily, and Anne Brontë all died from it—led many people to think it was an inherited disorder. The idea that tuberculosis might be a type of cancer was also commonplace, because of the lesions, abscesses, and other deformities it could produce. The idea that tuberculosis might be an infectious disease became more common after 1865, when a French physician injected material from a human tuberculosis victim into a rabbit, causing the organ damage characteristic of tuberculosis. But until Robert Koch went to work in 1881, the specific cause of the disease remained unknown.[4]

PATIENCE

The tuberculosis pathogen eluded the groundbreaking techniques he had perfected in other infections. It was difficult to grow in culture, and, even if you managed to grow it, difficult to see. Giving up on this deadly puzzle would have been easy, for someone lacking Koch's "extreme patience" and "*strong faith* . . . in the parasitic nature of tuberculosis" according to biographer Thomas D. Brock. It would take all the microbiological know-how and ingenuity he had acquired in his makeshift laboratory in Wollstein.[5]

Among other issues, the pathogen would not grow at room temperature. But when Koch tried to grow it in an incubator at body temperature, the gelatin on his plates melted, destroying the culture. He switched at first to a culture of blood serum sterilized and solidified by heating in test tubes kept on a slant, with the slant intended to create a larger surface for bacterial growth. After introducing a sample of tuberculosis material, Koch then incubated his test tubes. He knew that the tuberculosis pathogen was slow growing. So if bacterial growth occurred in the first week, that meant something else must have contaminated the sample, consigning it to the trash. But if a different kind of bacterial growth developed after ten days, that merited study.

Two innovations helped refine the technique for growing pure tuberculosis cultures, with far-reaching benefits for future research. Angelina Hesse, a talented research technician and medical illustrator, heard about the problem with gelatin melting at high temperatures from her physician husband, then working on sabbatical in Koch's laboratory. From her childhood in New York City, she recalled a Dutch neighbor who taught her about using agar to solidify jellies and puddings. The neighbor had learned the technique during her own childhood in Java, where agar-agar was a gelling product derived from certain red algae. Testing by Koch soon proved that agar, combined with a meat broth or other nutrient, remained solid at much higher temperatures. To protect agar cultures from contamination, Julius Petri, a laboratory assistant, then devised a shallow, flat-bottomed glass dish, with a slightly larger glass dish fitted on top as a lid. Even today, almost 150 years later, agar and the petri dish remain among the indispensable tools of microbiology.

Unfortunately, the tuberculosis bacteria at first proved impossible to see, much less photograph. Koch's usual staining methods didn't work because, as we now know, these bacteria are contained within an unusual hard, waxy surface layer. Prolonged staining with methylene blue soon made the bacteria visible for the first time, but not clearly enough. After repeated trial and error, Koch turned to a new counterstaining technique developed by Karl Weigert, developer of the aniline stain he had used to describe anthrax bacteria. Counterstaining meant adding another color stain, in this case vesuvin, to develop greater contrast among the different parts of a sample. Under his microscope, Koch could now see the tuberculosis bacteria as tiny rods standing out in bright, transparent blue against a drab brown background.[6]

Next Koch needed to show that these bacteria were present in every case of tuberculosis and that the same bacteria reliably produced the disease in healthy experimental animals. He had the good fortune to work with guinea pigs, which turned out to be far more susceptible than rabbits to the tuberculosis pathogen. Using standard sterile procedures, he injected different strains of the bacteria into small test groups of guinea pigs. As a result, he reported, "the animals become progressively weaker and die after four to six weeks." Dissection revealed the same sort of organ damage seen in human tuberculosis victims.[7]

A CHARACTERISTIC BACTERIUM

On the evening of March 24, 1882, Koch presented his findings in a paper modestly titled, "Concerning Tuberculosis." It was just seven months since his return from London full of determination to take on the disease. The venue was a small meeting room at the University of Berlin, and it was packed with distinguished scientists in anticipation of his results. This would be Koch's first public presentation, outside of a laboratory setting, at age thirty-nine. Where Pasteur had made himself a master of oratorical panache, Koch spoke in a thin, reedy voice and was nervous and faltering at first. He dwelt on technical details, starting with a step-by-step recipe for staining. He described in the plainest language what this had allowed him to see: "The bacteria visualized by this technique show many distinct characteristics. They are rod-shaped and belong therefore to the group of Bacilli. They are very thin and are only one-fourth to one-half as long as the diameter of a red blood cell, but can occasionally reach a length as long as the diameter of a red cell."[8]

These bacteria were scarce at certain times and abundant at others. They were also extremely difficult to see without his specialized staining methods. But the bacteria were always present in all forms of the disease. "I consider it as proven that in all tuberculous conditions of man and animals," he declared, "there exists a characteristic bacterium which I have designated as the tubercle bacillus, which has specific properties which allow it to be distinguished from all other microorganisms." Being present didn't prove these bacteria cause the disease, he acknowledged. But he then described how his inoculations of test animals produced the same disease in every case. "All of these facts taken together lead to the conclusion," he said, "that the bacilli which are present in the tuberculous substances not only accompany the tuberculosis process, but are the cause of it. In the bacillus we have, therefore, the actual tubercle virus."[9]

He described the implications of this discovery for public health—the need to sanitize clothing and bedding of tuberculosis patients, the importance of spitting as a possible means of transmitting the disease organism, the dangers of meat or milk contaminated with the bacteria. In place of vague theories about atmospheric emanations, these had now become practical matters to be addressed with the tools of modern medical science. "In the future, in our fight against this terrible plague on humanity," he said, "we will no longer be dealing with an indefinable Something. Instead we have a distinct parasite whose living conditions are for the most part known, and still subject to further study."[10]

No one clapped when he finished. Instead, the audience sat in stunned silence for a moment, thinking perhaps of loved ones lost to tuberculosis, or their own lives potentially saved. They began to file up and quietly shake Koch's hand. Physician and chemist Paul Ehrlich (1854–1915), twenty-eight, was in the audience that night. Years later, well into his own Nobel Prize–winning career, he still recalled it as "the most important experience of my scientific life."

That night, Koch, who knew Ehrlich as a useful ally, sent him off with a pure culture of the tuberculosis bacteria. Ehrlich took it straight to his laboratory and began tinkering with the staining formula. Late that night, satisfied that his improvements showed the bacteria more clearly, he set the slides on top of a cold stove to dry. Next morning, he was momentarily horrified when he came into work to see that someone had already lit the stove. But the accidental heating made things even more visible. Ehrlich passed on his results to Koch and published them soon after. Koch later credited Ehrlich's improvements with making it routine for physicians to diagnose tuberculosis from a saliva sample.[11]

In London, the *Times* announced Koch's great discovery on April 22. The *New York Times* speculated on May 3 that work to develop a vaccine would certainly follow. Another article two days later praised Koch's "beautiful theory" for holding out "the hope that tuberculous consumption may in time become almost unknown." When that happened, it said, "Prof. KOCH's name will go down to posterity side by side with that of JENNER." Evidently embarrassed at being late to announce "one of the great scientific discoveries of the age," the *Times* ran an editorial that mocked newsmen for using "the wings of the lightning" to report the doings of "princely noodles and fat, vulgar Duchesses" while leaving "Dr. Koch and his *bacilli* to chance it in the ocean mails."[12]

DUST AND ITS DANGERS

Soon Robert Koch was a household name in much of the world. Germ theory also gained a permanent hold on the public mind, by way of the deadliest disease of the day. People were already conscious of the sanitary reform push for uncontaminated drinking water, proper sewage disposal, and greater cleanliness in public spaces. But the realization that tuberculosis could lurk on the breath of any passing stranger, or the kiss of a family member, led to more profound changes in the ways people went about their daily lives.

Public spitting, formerly regarded by some men as a minor art form, was now literally sickening. "Spitting is dangerous, indecent and against the law," an American tuberculosis campaign advertisement warned. A sign on an Irish railroad line gently pleaded: "PLEASE DO NOT SPIT IN THE CARRIAGES. IT IS OFFENSIVE TO OTHER PASSENGERS AND IS STATED BY THE MEDICAL PROFESSION TO BE A SOURCE OF SERIOUS DISEASE." Fear that lengthy Victorian dresses and cloaks could sweep up germs and carry them into the home soon caused hemlines to rise several inches off the ground. "Rainy Day" clubs promoted the abbreviated "rainy daisy" skirt as less likely to suffer a wet hemline from bad weather or more obnoxious causes.

Dust likewise posed new terrors. The 1890 book *Dust and Its Dangers* warned "that *every person suffering from consumption of the lungs may be expectorating every day myriads of living and virulent tubercle bacilli.*" Tuberculosis ran in families not because it was a hereditary disease, author and pathologist T. Mitchell Prudden wrote, but because "house-mates have unwittingly poisoned one another, usually, no doubt, through the dust." The common practice of feather-dusting only stirred up dangerous particles, making them available for inhalation. Prudden recommended moist dust cloths instead. "Carpets and heavy hangings and upholstery," he wrote, "all insure the more or less persistent retention of dust particles in rooms," along with whatever harmful germs happened to be present.[13]

Ornate muttonchops and handlebars lost their old magic for the same reason, according to historian Frank M. Snowden. "Bacteria could nestle amidst the whiskers, only to fall into other people's food or onto their lips during a kiss. Indeed, some public health authorities advised that kissing was excessively dangerous and should be avoided altogether." Persistent coughing became suspicious, "even unpatriotic," behavior, and tuberculosis victims struggled "to obtain lodgings, employment, or insurance." Their value as potential spouses also plummeted as the deliciously languid turned out to be dreadfully contagious. Carl Flügge at the University of Breslau soon demonstrated that coughing produces an aerosol spray of droplets capable of carrying the tuberculosis pathogen—or, by implication, a host of other pathogens then being recognized for the first time.[14]

The realization that they could sicken those around them caused many tuberculosis victims to modify their behavior. If bed-bound, they coughed into disposable paper cups or tissues, rather than into cloth handkerchiefs. If mobile, they carried small flasks, like personal spittoons, to avoid spitting in public spaces. Those who could afford it withdrew to a sanitorium, partly in the hope that clean mountain air and new therapeutic methods would bring about the elusive cure—but also to die without taking the family down with them.

Fear of germs also affected family life more broadly. "Infants should be kissed, if at all, upon the cheek or forehead, but the less even of this the better," advised Luther Emmett Holt in the 1914 edition of *The Care and Feeding of Children*, the parenting bible until the mid-twentieth century. A kiss could communicate "tuberculosis, diphtheria, syphilis, and many other grave diseases." A chillier, more remote style of child-rearing, averse to physical displays of affection, became standard in many middle-class homes.[15]

In the decades following Koch's 1882 discovery, the number of tuberculosis cases and deaths declined significantly in some areas—notably Britain (not including Ireland). But it had been mysteriously declining there at least since the start of the nineteenth century. Some medical historians have attributed this long-term decline to higher wages, better nutrition, or improved living conditions. Others have argued that sanitary reform helped, by causing improvements in drainage, water supply, and building ventilation. Still others have proposed that natural selection was causing the pathogen to become less virulent. Koch himself thought "the considerable number" of specialized hospitals for tuberculosis in Britain contributed to the decline. Some modern scholars have also argued that the increasing tendency to isolate tuberculosis patients may have reduced the rate of infection.[16]

THE WAY FORWARD

The other monumental effect of Koch's tuberculosis discovery was that it inspired so many other disease researchers to follow. To make the way forward unmistakable, Koch soon promulgated influential rules for pathogen discovery. Koch's postulates, as they became known, laid out four essential steps for proving that a particular microbe caused a particular disease: (1) Demonstrate that the microbe exists abundantly in individuals suffering the disease, but not in their healthy counterparts. (2) Isolate the microbe from diseased individuals and grow it in a pure culture. (3) Introduce the cultured microbe into healthy experimental animals, thereby causing the same disease. And (4) isolate the microbe again from these test cases and demonstrate that it is the same as the original microbe.[17]

These postulates came with serious issues. During a typhoid outbreak in 1902, Koch would discover that, contrary to the first postulate, some people could be "carriers" and covert spreaders of an infectious pathogen without suffering any visible symptoms themselves. Koch would also find that, for certain diseases, there was no susceptible test species for carrying out steps three and four, other than humans. These lapses aside, Koch's postulates, and the example of tuberculosis discovery, opened a rough path for a new generation of microbe hunters. Over the next twenty years, they would go on to identify the pathogen responsible for such ancient afflictions as diphtheria, typhoid, tetanus, plague, dysentery, various types of diarrhea, meningitis, and botulism, among others. For many such "indefinable Somethings," now defined down to genus and species, it was the beginning of the end of their power over humanity.

20 (RE)DISCOVERING CHOLERA

After the deadliest disease of the century came the most terrifying. Cholera broke out in the Mediterranean port of Damietta, Egypt, near the mouth of the Suez Canal in May 1883, and became widespread by late June. The *British Medical Journal* reported multiple theories then circulating about the outbreak: it was of "local origin *de novo* at Damietta," or it had evolved there from typhoid or another disease, or it was a sporadic occurrence of a form of the disease that had existed in Egypt since 1865. The idea that a British steamer passing through the Suez Canal might have introduced cholera came only sixth on the list, and with a finger pointed to an ethnically convenient scapegoat, either a Muslim crew member or an unnamed Bombay merchant. The final theory was that it wasn't cholera at all but some sort of "choloroid disease." By July, in any case, it was killing five hundred people a day in Cairo.[1]

That month, Louis Pasteur dispatched a volunteer team, including Émile Roux and Louis Thuillier (1856–1883), to find and describe the pathogen. They arrived in Alexandria on August 15, just twenty days after the French government authorized the expedition. Pasteur, who was sixty years old and partly disabled by a stroke, remained at his summer place in Arbois. But he sent homework, earnestly wishing for team members to "all attentively read my two volumes on the diseases of the silkworm in their entirety," on the theory that "there must be major analogies" with cholera. Not to be outdone, the Germans ordered Koch to lead his own team, which arrived in Port Said on August 23 and quickly moved on to Alexandria.[2]

The relationship between the two great germ theory researchers had sharply deteriorated over the two years since Pasteur had praised Koch's laboratory technique as "un grand progrès." Koch started it with a lengthy 1881 attack on Pasteur's anthrax vaccine. Koch believed bacteria were fixed in character and thus not subject to the sort of change implied by attenuation. He was also sharply critical of Pasteur's methods—notably, the reliance on bacteria cultured in a liquid medium and treated in ways that did not reliably kill anthrax spores. "Of these conclusions of Pasteur on the etiology of anthrax," Koch wrote, "there is little which is new, and that which is new is erroneous. . . . Up to now, Pasteur's work on anthrax has led to nothing." The grudge was also clearly personal. In the past, Pasteur had acknowledged Koch's work in describing the anthrax pathogen. But now, Koch complained, he "speaks as if nothing is known about anthrax etiology and sends things into the world as new discoveries that have long been proven and agreed upon."

Pasteur responded by arranging for Thuillier to demonstrate the anthrax vaccine before an independent commission in Germany. Mistrusting German customs inspectors, Pasteur sent the vaccine by diplomatic pouch, and explained to the French ambassador, "We must do everything to win our victory at Salamis." The trial went well enough for the vaccine to become an accepted veterinary treatment in Germany, meaning that the royalties would flow gratifyingly back to France and the Pasteur laboratory. But in the course of his travels, Thuillier was also able to spend an hour touring Koch's laboratory—and report to Pasteur the unsettling news of his rival's latest triumph, the discovery of the cause of tuberculosis. (Koch was "a bit of a rustic," Thuillier thought, and also "ignorant of parliamentary language.")

A face-to-face confrontation had taken place in 1882 at a public health congress in Geneva. Koch and his team took seats in the first row to listen as Pasteur delivered a stiff response to their criticisms of his vaccine. A German-speaking friend was translating for Koch, and at a certain point, when Pasteur referred to Koch's work as *receuil Allemand*, meaning the collection of German works, the friend heard it as *orgueil Allemand*, meaning German arrogance. Koch immediately rose up and protested until Pasteur, twenty years older and glowering back with all the arrogance he could muster, silenced him. The audience was of course appalled at this clash of the titans, which did not end with the lecture. Koch's written response, published soon after, was scathing, repeating the old slur that Pasteur was "not even a physician," and asserting that those celebrating Pasteur as a second Jenner should recall that Jenner achieved his triumph in human beings, not sheep. Pasteur replied in the same tone, calling Koch a newcomer to research and a debtor to French science. There things stood in the summer of 1883, as the warring parties faced off on the coast of Egypt.[3]

A FEW DROPS OF BLOOD

The French, based at the European Hospital, soon examined twenty-four cholera victims and set to work with rubber tubes to feed samples of their excreta into guinea pigs, rabbits, mice, chickens, pigeons, quails, a jay, a turkey, pigs, cats, dogs, and a monkey. No cholera-like disease ensued. They had come "prepared mainly for microscopic observations and animal inoculations," according to Thomas D. Brock. The Germans, on the other hand, came with "*everything* needed to fulfill Koch's postulates." Their equipment list included, among other things, a large supply of laboratory glassware and chemicals, at least eight varieties of dye for microscopic preparations, a microtome slicer for cutting razor-thin sections of tissue, an apparatus for freezing these sections, a steam sterilizer, Bunsen burners, a drying oven, scalpels, scissors, forceps, syringes, and fifty mice. But for the Germans, as for the French, neither the mice nor any other animal species proved to be a suitable model for cholera.[4]

On September 17, 1883, Koch sent off the first of six reports to the German Minister of the Interior. These reports promptly appeared in the German press and were widely reported abroad. They gave a kind of serial drama to the hunt to understand this terrifying killer. In their first three-and-a-half weeks in the field, Koch wrote, his team had examined a dozen living cholera patients and ten who had recently died. Autopsy tissue samples from lungs, spleen, kidneys, and liver all proved free of a likely pathogen, as did the blood. A potential culprit had turned up, however, in the walls of the small intestine in cholera victims, but not in those who had died of other diseases. Whether it was the cause of cholera, or merely an effect, was so far unknown.[5]

For the French team, the news was far less encouraging. The same day Koch sent off his first report, Louis Thuillier began to experience intermittent stomach trouble. He remained "lively and in good spirits," according to Roux, and that evening he went for a swim in the ocean. But the next morning, a Tuesday, he woke at three, announced that he was feeling poorly, and collapsed on the floor. Diarrhea and vomiting followed, and it became clear that he had come down with cholera. His colleagues treated him with the standard ineffectual remedies of the day, including energetic rubbing of arms and legs, subcutaneous injections of ether, and iced champagne to drink. After a day-long struggle to breathe—cholera's familiar, gasping "air hunger"—Thuillier was dead, age twenty-seven. It was a stark reminder of the danger all of them faced in their work, at home as well as abroad. Koch and his team attended the funeral, and he "spoke very beautifully about the memory of our dear departed friend," Roux wrote to Pasteur. The Germans placed laurel wreaths on the coffin, with Koch saying they were "suitable for one who deserves such glory." Koch also served as a pallbearer. Pasteur took the news of the death badly when it reached him in Arbois. "The only way to console myself about this death is to think of our dear fatherland and of what he has done for it," Pasteur wrote, to an old teacher. To an assistant, characteristically, he added, "We must work." Later, after a day of brooding silence, he exclaimed, "I just hope they have not forgotten to take a few drops of blood."

The cholera outbreak began to wane, and the disheartened French team soon returned home. The disease persisted in a few outlying villages. But the Germans found that attempting to perform autopsies there would only enrage survivors. Koch sent off a request to Berlin for permission to move the expedition to India, where a steady supply of cholera cases seemed assured. While awaiting a reply, he and his team found time to savor the experience of travel. As a boy, Koch had dreamed of becoming a naturalist and venturing into unknown territory like his idol, Prussian explorer Alexander von Humboldt. Now, with time on his hands, he began to recall that old ambition. At the ruins of "the golden city of Heliopolis," he collected leaves from a famous sycamore and some nearby flowers, which he dried and sent off to his daughter. In the cool of the evening, "we ride on donkeys," he wrote to his wife, "and we have quite a jolly party when we race across the desert, with the Arab guides stringing on behind. When we finally get to the cliffs, we have a nice fire and a picnic supper. And this is all by the light of the moon!"[6]

KOCH'S COMMA BACILLUS

By mid-December, Koch and two assistants had moved on to Calcutta. Over the next few months, they autopsied forty-two victims of cholera, most soon after death, before decomposition could complicate their findings. They also took samples from many living patients. In every case of cholera, they found the same suspected pathogen they had seen in Egypt. It was "almost unmixed" in the small intestine of the most severe cases. On January 7, 1884, Koch reported that the researchers had isolated this pathogen and developed a simple method for growing it in a pure culture.[7]

"It can now be taken as conclusive," he wrote in his next report, on February 2, "that the bacillus found in the intestine of cholera patients is indeed the cholera pathogen." It was comma-shaped and "best observed in a drop of nutrient solution suspended on the cover slip." There, it "can be seen to swim through the microscopic field of view in all directions at great speed." These characteristics, and the application of aniline dyes, made it easy to distinguish from other intestinal bacteria in victims of cholera and to confidently report its absence in other diseases.

Proof on the terms of Koch's own postulates remained elusive, however. The team continued to search for an animal model for the disease, in some cases injecting cholera samples directly into the intestines of potential test animals. But these attempts to reproduce the disease in experimental animals all failed. People assured him they had never seen the disease locally, except in humans.[8]

Koch turned instead to epidemiological evidence. Cholera mortality had declined dramatically even in Calcutta over the previous dozen years, a development he attributed "to the introduction of piped supplies of drinking-water." But he also noted that many areas still depended on open concrete tanks, or wells, for their communal water supply. The British public health authorities who were hosting Koch dismissed these tanks as a factor in cholera transmission. They subscribed instead to the anticontagionist thinking of Max von Pettenkofer, an influential German sanitarian. His scientific-sounding *Bodentheorie*, or "soil theory," held that some unknown agent of cholera, labeled x, had to combine with some equally vague factor in the soil, labeled y, to produce "the real cholera poison," labeled z. In their own testing of water from communal tanks, British researchers in India had identified no microbes specifically associated with cholera, nor even any abundance of normal intestinal bacteria. But that research had taken place in 1870–1871, ancient times in microbiology.[9]

When cholera broke out in Saheb-Bagan, then a small village outside Calcutta, Koch and his team investigated for themselves. Seventeen people had died, with the deaths clustered suspiciously around a communal water tank. Local residents relied on this tank, Koch reported, not just for drinking water but also for bathing and doing their laundry. Open defecation on the ground nearby was common. Rain routinely washed the accumulated human wastes into the water, and samples Koch and his team collected from different parts of the tank, at different times, showed that the comma-shaped cholera bacilli abounded. Interviews eventually revealed that relatives of the first victim of the outbreak had washed his contaminated clothing in this tank. Koch called it "a kind of chance experiment in humans, which substitutes for the lack of animal experiments in this case and can serve as further confirmation of the correctness of the assumption that the specific cholera bacilli are indeed the cause of the disease."[10]

Although the two episodes were almost thirty years apart, the findings from Saheb-Bagan's contaminated water tank and London's contaminated Broad Street pump were strikingly similar. Like John Snow, Koch even presented a death map showing the location of homes around the tank, with black marks on the ones where people had died. Oddly, given his fluent English and wide reading on infectious disease, Koch made no mention of Snow's work. Koch of course now possessed the one key factor that Snow had never sought—the particular microbe responsible for waterborne transmission of cholera. This was, however, the same microbe described and named *Vibrio cholerae* almost thirty years earlier by Filippo Pacini, who also went unmentioned. One way to interpret the combined omissions is that Koch, like Pasteur, was knowingly sending things into the world as new discoveries that had long been demonstrated, if not agreed upon. But even if that were so, Koch's detailed work on anthrax and tuberculosis gave him the credibility to make the world take notice. When the German Commission arrived home in May 1884, after more than eight months abroad, Koch was once again a hero on the world stage.

Pasteur was infuriated. And then, when cholera turned up that June in southern Europe, Koch had the effrontery, the sheer German *orgeuil*, to descend on the French port of Toulon with his investigative tricks. Worse, German newspapers were gleefully reporting that the French government had requested Koch's help because of the French failure in Egypt. (In fact, the German government had dispatched Koch in the hope of preventing the disease from spreading north to its citizens.)

"Try to find out the fallacy in his story," Pasteur wrote in a desperate-seeming note to veterans of the Egyptian expedition, then also investigating in Toulon. "How do his microscopic preparations differ from yours? He must have made some sort of great error. . . . As much as possible, work by yourself. Keep your cadavers to yourself. The reports which you have received that tell you how great this Koch is are wrong. His knowledge of cholera is not that good. If your results agreed with his, he alone would get all the credit. Already, the German newspapers are crowing!"[11]

Pasteur of course had a lifetime of his own accomplishments to crow about. But it wasn't enough for that massive ambition of his. Still relentlessly seeking glory, he needed one last triumph, one achievement that would forever silence those fools who still regarded him as an outsider, an interloper, a nonphysician: he wanted to cure a great human disease.

21 A SACRED DELIRIUM

Rabies typically killed fewer than twenty-five or thirty people a year in France in the 1880s. But its infrequent, unpredictable character only made it more terrifying. So did the way it often began, with an attack by a mad dog on a child. The standard remedy was cauterization, either by having a red-hot iron jabbed into the bleeding wounds, amid the sizzle and smell of scorched flesh, or by dousing the wounds with acid. In October 1834 in Arbois, in the aftermath of an attack by a solitary deranged wolf, Louis Pasteur, then just eight years old, heard the screaming of young bite victims being treated in just this manner at the local blacksmith. The memory stuck.

Cauterization fulfilled the traditional expectation that a medical remedy should entail heroic intervention and healing pain. But like a lot of traditional remedies, it didn't necessarily work. Symptoms of rabies could still develop at any time from a week to a year after the attack, a tense waiting period in which the fearfulness of the disease grew and festered.

The first symptoms included fever, discomfort, headache, and anxiety, and were common enough that almost anything could be mistaken for the onset of rabies. But once symptoms have appeared, rabies is almost always fatal. In the classic form of the disease, with the telltale confusion, excitability, hyperactivity, and hydrophobia, death by heart or respiratory failure typically occurs within about ten days. In a less common and often misdiagnosed form, paralysis advances steadily from the wound site across the body. The victim lapses into a coma and slowly dies.

Why would Pasteur have focused on a relatively uncommon condition like rabies at the moment his great rival Robert Koch was revealing the cause of major killers like cholera and tuberculosis? "If Pasteur chose it as an object of study," Émile Roux later explained, "it was above all because . . . to everyone's mind rabies is the most frightening and dreaded malady. . . . He thought that to solve the problem of rabies would be a blessing for humanity and a brilliant triumph for his doctrines." He wanted to wow the public and also, as Pasteur himself later wrote, to force "the physicians to pay attention" to those doctrines.

A veterinarian in Lyon had recently established that rabbits were a suitable model for rabies, by injecting them with saliva from rabid dogs. Obtaining the saliva wasn't easy, however. Pasteur's son-in-law, René Vallery-Radot, described the procedure in the case of "a huge bulldog . . . howling and foaming in its cage" in the animal room of the Pasteur laboratory: "Two helpers took a cord with a slip-knot and threw it at the dog as one throws a lasso. The dog was caught and pulled to the edge of the cage. They seized it and tied its jaws together. The dog, choking with rage, its eyes bloodshot, and its body racked by furious spasms, was stretched out on a table, while M. Pasteur, bending a finger's length away over this foaming head, aspirated a few drops of slaver through a thin tube." Apart from the difficulty and danger of this procedure, the larger problem was that the saliva didn't reliably produce the disease in rabbits, and the incubation period of eighteen days was too long for efficient experimentation. Pasteur and Émile Roux soon found a ghastly but more efficient way.

A Paris physician had recently described how "the morbid agent" of rabies slowly advanced during the incubation period from the location of the bite via the nerves to the brain. There, it appeared to operate on a part of the brain stem responsible for autonomic functions like breathing, heart function, swallowing, and digestion. This led Roux to propose removing material directly from the brains of dogs killed by rabies and injecting it directly into the brains of experimental animals. One drawback was that this involved using a hand drill to make a hole in the back of the skulls of live, anesthetized test animals. Pasteur balked, until Roux showed him that dogs recovered from the surgery itself overnight. And direct injection to the brainstem always produced rabies. That gave the laboratory a more dependable way to conduct the many experiments it would require to develop a rabies vaccine. Pasteur couldn't identify the microbe responsible for rabies because science did not yet possess tools to recognize viruses. Instead, he was now using the brains of living animals in effect to grow the microbe in culture. It would make him the target of vehement attacks by the growing antivivisection movement.

Pasteur's "basic procedure," according to biographer Gerald L. Geison, was to inject a variety of species with "a wide range of cultures or substances and then watch what happened." But these experiments weren't random. Pasteur was pursuing the idea that the species or environment in which a microbe develops can alter its pathogenic character. In 1883, he and Thuillier had successfully weakened a swine flu microbe to the point of harmlessness in this fashion, by passing it repeatedly through rabbits. The result was a new vaccine to protect hogs from that disease. But with rabies, this process of serial passage through rabbits produced the opposite effect at first, making the rabies microbe even more virulent for dogs. It also further shortened the incubation period, to under ten days, which was at least advantageous for experimental purposes.

Pasteur eventually managed to weaken the rabies microbe by passing it through a series of monkeys. This attenuated microbe was no longer capable of causing rabies in dogs, even when introduced directly into their brains. Pasteur then had another of his brilliant intuitions: Rabies didn't allow him time to administer an attenuated rabies microbe and simply wait, perhaps for weeks, for the body to develop what seemed to be a learned resistance to the disease. The incubation period for rabies wasn't reliably that long, in dogs or humans. Instead, Pasteur combined the attenuated rabies microbe at the start with increasingly virulent versions of that microbe over the following days, in an attempt to kick-start that learned resistance.

In May 1884, Pasteur reported that the attenuated rabies microbe appeared to protect dogs from a somewhat more virulent strain of rabies. That strain in turn protected against a still more virulent strain, and so on, until finally the dog was "refractory"—or as we now say, *immune*—to rabies. Any notion of preventing rabies in the dog population at large would of course have been wildly impractical: there were too many dogs out there, and it would have required performing a series of injections on each of them.

But Pasteur now suggested a far more tantalizing and entirely new possibility: he believed he would soon be able to treat patients *after a bite* and still render them "resistant with certainty before the disease becomes manifest." He warned that it would require further experiments "almost ad infinitum, before human therapeutics can be so bold as to try this mode of prophylaxis on man himself."[1]

Meanwhile, he called on the French government to establish a commission to oversee an experiment like the one at Pouilly-le-Fort, with dogs that had been vaccinated, together with an unvaccinated control group, all exposed to the same virulent rabies. The government naturally complied, and two months later, in August 1884, reported that two-thirds of the unvaccinated dogs were already rabid, while the twenty-three vaccinated dogs all remained healthy, some of them even after having rabies introduced directly to the brain.

Late that September, Pasteur wrote to Pedro II, emperor of Brazil, acknowledging that human experimentation was otherwise out of the question. But if *he* were emperor, Pasteur ventured, he would make an offer to condemned prisoners on the eve of execution: accept imminent death, or choose to live, after surviving "an experiment consisting of preventive inoculations of rabies designed to make the subject refractory to rabies." This would ultimately have meant exposing the prisoner, after the series of preparatory inoculations, to street rabies. Because of the absence of an animal model for cholera, Pasteur also proposed administering the cholera pathogen to condemned prisoners, without benefit of a protective vaccine. For biographer Patrice Debré, this smacked of the experiments Nazi doctors would later perform on concentration camp prisoners. Pasteur made the proposal in Brazil, not France, and even offered to travel there to conduct these experiments himself. Pedro II did not take him up on the offer.[2]

At some point, Pasteur gave up on rabies attenuation via monkeys, probably because they were impractical for producing vaccine at volume. His laboratory had continued passing rabies from rabbit to rabbit, but this still augmented virulence instead of attenuating it. Working independently, Émile Roux came up with a solution. His independence seems to have had Pasteur's tacit approval, perhaps because it had helped saved the day at Pouilly-le-Fort. But the two were bound by personality to clash, in Geison's interpretation. Pasteur was the "sturdily built, financially secure family man with conservative political leanings." Roux was a lean, tubercular ascetic, a widower who never remarried, and "of vaguely leftist or transcendental political views." Both were "stubborn, aloof, severe, demanding of others, quick to take offense, and given to outbursts of temper."[3]

A flash point in this awkward partnership came during a visit by Pasteur to the incubation room. Adrien Loir, his nephew and assistant, was carrying trays of various cultures to leave on Pasteur's shelf at the left side of the room. But when he turned to leave, he found Pasteur staring intently to the right, at a "flask with two necks, one on the top and one at the bottom, designed to cause a draft inside the flask." Dangling by a thread in mid-flask was a piece of the spinal marrow of a rabbit that had died of rabies.

"Who put this flask here?" Pasteur demanded, after a long silence.

"It can only have been M. Roux," Loir replied. It was Roux's shelf.

Pasteur "took the flask and walked out into the hallway. Lifting it up, he looked at it in bright daylight for a long time, then he returned to his work station without breathing a word." Pasteur immediately began to tinker with this new variation, and that afternoon, in the incubation room, Roux looked left and saw three flasks, each with a strip of rabbit marrow suspended on a string.

"Who put these three flasks here?" Roux demanded of Loir, who seems to have been thrust into the unhappy role of the child through whom two married adults communicate.

"It was M. Pasteur."

"Did he go into the incubation room? Did he see the flask on my shelf?"

"Yes, he did."

At that, Loir wrote, "Roux took his hat, went down the steps and out . . . slamming the door behind him as he always did when he was angry." He returned to work only at night for a time, and Loir doubted that he and Pasteur ever discussed the new procedure. Pasteur soon tweaked the method by adding sterile cotton at the two openings, and pieces of caustic potash inside the flask to dry the air. The resulting combination of air flow, dryness, temperature, length of exposure, and thinness of the spinal marrow sample somehow combined to produce attenuation of the rabies microbe.[4]

Endless trial and error followed. The result was a system that entailed injecting a test animal with a series of shots containing an emulsified spinal cord in a sterile broth. The series began with a spinal cord dried for about fourteen days. Successive shots, administered every other day, used a spinal cord dried for a slightly shorter period, Pasteur later wrote, "until one arrives at a last and very virulent cord that has been placed into the flask only a day or two previously."

Pasteur worried that performing the necessary experiments, "if allowable on animals, is criminal in man." But he had a hankering. In March 1885, he wrote to an old schoolmate, "I have not yet dared to treat humans bitten by rabid dogs. But the time to do it may not be far off, and I would really like to begin with myself, that is, to inoculate myself with rabies and then stop its effects, for I am beginning to feel very . . . sure of my findings."

Heroic self-experimentation would not happen. But an opportunity for testing on a human arose a few weeks later, when a colleague passed along word of a sixty-year-old man being treated for rabies in a Paris hospital. Pasteur visited the patient and his doctor on May 1 and apparently secured the doctor's permission to proceed. The next morning, with the doctor oddly absent, Pasteur returned with Roux, who injected the attenuated rabies, the first of the planned series of shots. But the hospital administration quickly blocked Pasteur's attempt to continue the vaccination series.

Rabies is hard to diagnose even today, and in the emotional aftermath of a dog attack, "hysterical," or psychosomatic, cases sometimes display many of the known symptoms. That patient may have been such a case. He survived without further vaccination and soon vanished from Pasteur's laboratory notebook. A second patient, an eleven-year-old girl who had been bitten on the lip by her own dog and soon showed symptoms of rabies, received two shots of the attenuated microbe on June 22, 1885. But the following morning she died, of what turned out on autopsy to be an advanced case of rabies. Her case also vanished from the record, until rediscovered in Pasteur's laboratory notebooks in the 1990s.

Then, on July 6, a mother arrived from Alsace-Lorraine with her nine-year-old son, Joseph Meister, and the local grocer, whose dog had repeatedly bitten the boy on the arms and legs. The sudden ferocity of the attack led

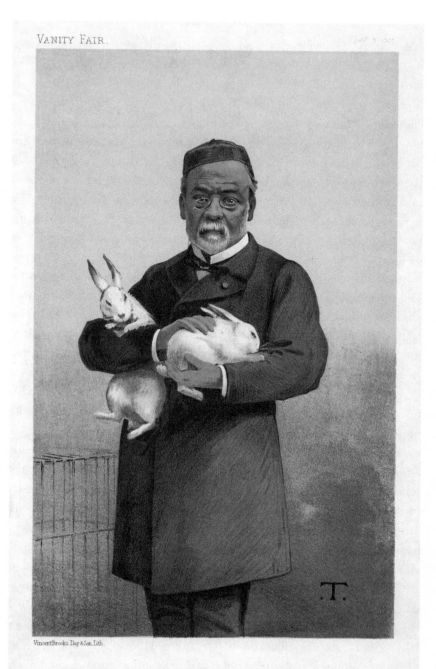

Figure 21.1

Pasteur at the time of his rabies vaccine, with some of his laboratory's experimental animals (Théobald Chartran, 1886, Wellcome Collection).

everyone to suspect rabies. An autopsy found the dog's stomach filled with hay, straw, and wood chips, also suggesting rabies. The boy's wounds were cauterized with acid. But the mother, having heard of Pasteur's research, then brought Meister by train to Paris and quickly found their way to the Pasteur laboratory. Pasteur brought in two prominent Paris physicians, both familiar with his research, to consult on the case. They agreed that the number and depth of the wounds made rabies more likely, and also that the location of the wounds on the extremities meant it might take longer for the disease to reach the brain, improving the chance for a successful intervention. That same night one of them delivered the first shot in the series. The syringe, containing the emulsified spinal cord of a rabbit that had died of rabies fifteen days earlier, went in to Meister's upper-right abdomen. Roux, who would normally have administered inoculations for Pasteur, was notably absent.

"The boy sleeps well, his appetite is good, and the inoculated matter is absorbed without leaving a trace," Pasteur wrote, six days into the treatment regimen. But he began to fret, as at Pouilly-le-Fort, and with far more reason. There, Pasteur and his assistants had vaccinated the experimental animals with attenuated anthrax microbes and waited three-and-a-half-weeks for the immune response to develop. Only then did they test the vaccine's effectiveness with fully virulent anthrax. But now Pasteur was administering steadily more virulent rabies microbes every day, and the experimental animal was a human child. Although Pasteur talked confidently of having tested his antirabies method in fifty dogs, he didn't say exactly which variation he had tested. Examination of his laboratory notebooks would later suggest that the method this time was significantly different. Roux would have been the only other person aware of how little experimental evidence in animals existed to show that the new method might potentially succeed in humans. His absence suggests that he considered it far too risky.

"If Pasteur had been a physician, if he had been made aware . . . of the danger to which he was exposing his clients," wrote Charles Nicolle, a student in whom Roux later confided, "the dreadful thought of an experimentally induced rabies would no doubt have stopped him. . . . He was possessed of that indomitable temerity that a sacred delirium imparts to genius. The scientist's conscience smothered the conscience of the man." In a letter to the doctor who actually administered the shots, Pasteur described Roux as "decidedly too timid." But that doctor in turn later reflected that "Pasteur lacked prudence in medical matters."[5]

The thirteenth and final shot in the series, containing a spinal cord from a rabbit killed by rabies just one day earlier, was due on July 16. "This will be another bad night for your father," Marie Pasteur wrote to their children. "He cannot come to terms with the idea of applying a measure of last resort to this child. And yet he now has to go through with it. The little fellow continues to feel very well." In fact, Meister seemed to thrive, and just two days after the final shot, Pasteur departed to Arbois for his summer retreat. Meister and his mother were back home in Alsace-Lorraine by the end of the month.[6]

Pasteur did not immediately shout this triumph from the rooftop. It was still possible that Meister would develop rabies, either from the original attack or, as Pasteur acknowledged, from the treatment itself. Besides, it was August, no time for major news. But on October 26, three-and-a-half months after the final shot, with Meister still in good health, Pasteur stood before the Academy of Medicine and announced the world's first successful prevention of rabies after an attack. He was already fielding other requests for treatment, sometimes several per day, he said, and the doctors with whom he worked had begun to treat a second patient just a few days earlier. That case provided additional cause for anxiety, because of a six-day lapse between the attack and treatment (with Meister, treatment had begun in less than half that time). But the new patient also came with a heroic tale, which Pasteur plainly relished.

"He's a fifteen-year-old shepherd by the name of Jean-Baptiste Jupille, of Villers-Farlay," Pasteur announced. This village near Arbois had been the scene of the rabies incident the eight-year-old Pasteur had witnessed at earshot. It was an eerie coincidence, and brought back all the old memories, though Pasteur did not mention this to the Academy. Jupille, he continued, "seeing a big, dangerous-looking dog threatening a group of six of his comrades, all younger than him, rushed forward, armed with his whip, to confront the animal. The dog grabbed Jupille by the left hand. Jupille then wrestled the dog down, and holding it under him, pried open its mouth with his right hand to release his left hand, sustaining several new bites. Then, with his whip, he bound the muzzle, and, grabbing one of his wooden shoes, he beat the dog into unconsciousness."

When Pasteur finished, one of the physicians who had approved the treatment of Meister immediately rose to declare that "rabies, this terrible disease, against which all therapeutic attempts until now have failed, has finally found its cure!" Henri Bouley, president of the Academy, added that the day would "remain forever memorable in the history of medicine and forever glorious for French science." Jupille, like Meister, soon returned home in good health.[7]

Two weeks later, the parents of Louise Pelletier, age ten, brought her to the laboratory seeking treatment for an attack that had occurred thirty-seven days earlier. It was probably too late for her. She had been bitten on the head, meaning a shorter incubation period. It was also certainly much too soon for Pasteur to take on such a risky case. But he yielded to the parents' pleading. A month later, on December 6, the girl died, with Pasteur joining the parents at her bedside. Two days after that, the headline "One of Pasteur's Patients Dies" made the front page of the *New York Times*, that paper's first mention that a means of preventing rabies existed. Critics in the Academy of Medicine muttered darkly about involuntary manslaughter or even murder, but the Pelletier girl's father wasn't among them. Decades later, with her loss still fresh in his heart, he wrote that, among all the great men he had studied, "I do not see one of them capable, as he was in the case of our dear little girl, of sacrificing long years of work, of endangering a universal reputation as a scientist and knowingly risking a painful failure, out of simple humanity." Other victims of attacks by apparently mad dogs were soon being bundled off to Paris in search of the new cure. For some—perhaps most—the vaccine merely prevented the *possibility* of rabies, sparing bite victims from the long, anxious period of uncertain waiting. For others, it was a genuine cure.[8]

The victory over rabies would be the final great research achievement of Pasteur's life, as a series of strokes steadily disabled him. It had all the hallmarks of his other great achievements—the insatiable quest for glory, the disdain for impediments of any kind, the willingness to take bold action in pursuit of what he believed to be the truth, and the unfathomable ability to get the science right and to make other people see it. The victory over rabies rendered his scientific legacy permanent. It inspired an international fundraising campaign to establish the Pasteur Institute, which remains today among the leading research centers in the fight against infectious disease.

By stopping a terrifying human disease, and seeming to snatch victims almost literally from the jaws of death, Pasteur's rabies vaccine taught the medical world that it could achieve *cures*. It was the beginning of a new era, in which those cures would proliferate. For almost the first time in the history of medical practice, physicians would have the tools to heal sick patients—or keep them from getting sick in the first place.

22 IMMUNITY AND THE STRANGLING ANGEL

One of the symptoms of the childhood disease called diphtheria is a thick, leathery, gray membrane of dead cells in the throat, which can block a child's windpipe, causing death by suffocation. Hence the disease became known as the "strangling angel." In its heyday, it used to slip through communities, dancing from child to child, on a cough or a sneeze, at schoolhouse or church service. Some parents unwittingly hastened its unholy work by having their children line up to kiss a dying brother or sister goodbye. The results are still evident in local burial grounds everywhere across New England, where a devastating eighteenth-century epidemic emptied nurseries, bedrooms, and neighborhoods.

In Lancaster, Massachusetts, for instance, mottled slate tombstones lean together, like family, over the graves of the nine children of Joseph and Rebeckah Mores. Ephraim, age seven, died first on June 15, 1740, followed by Hannah, three, on June 17, and Jacob, eleven, a day later. They shared the same grave. Cathorign, two, died on June 23, and Rebeckah, six, on June 26. The dying—five children lost in eleven days—paused long enough to leave the poor parents some thread of hope. But two months later, on August 22, Lucy, fourteen, also died. A few years after that, diphtheria or some other epidemic disease came back to collect the three remaining Mores children.

Other parents also lost all their children to that diphtheria epidemic. On a single street less than a half-mile long in Newburyport, Massachusetts, eighty-one children died over three months in 1735. The nearby town of Haverhill lost half its children, with twenty-three families left childless. The terror of dying was made more oppressive by the prospect of damnation, as a poem in the middle of the outbreak warned unruly children:

> So soon as Death, hath stopt your Breath,
> Your souls must then appear
> Before the Judge of quick and dead,
> The Sentence there to hear.
> From thence away, without delay,
> You must be Doom'd unto,
> A dreadful Hell, where Devils dwell,
> In Everlasting woe.[1]

Over the course of the nineteenth century, many other contagious diseases would become less severe, for reasons scholars still debate. But diphtheria only grew more virulent—particularly in cities, where it was a leading cause of infant mortality. By the 1880s, the United States was seeing 150,000 to 200,000 diphtheria cases a year, and a fatality rate of 50 to 60 percent was routine. Germany was losing sixty thousand children every year.[2]

BIG SCIENCE

The first Nobel Prize in Physiology or Medicine would be awarded in 1901 to honor a practical cure for diphtheria. This achievement was worthy of the honor for the countless thousands of families spared from agonizing loss. The method employed was entirely new, with eventual application to a range of other diseases. *Serum therapy*—transferring resistance to a disease from one individual to another via components in the blood—would also profoundly alter medical understanding of immunity. Unfortunately, the prize went to just one person, omitting major contributors to the discovery and ignoring the role of a surprisingly modern, international network of researchers, who fed off one another's work.

The push to defeat diphtheria got started in 1883, when the Prussian-born pathologist Edwin Klebs (1834–1913) first described the specific bacterium that causes diphtheria. But Klebs soon moved on to other topics. A year later, Friedrich Loeffler (1852–1915), an assistant in Koch's laboratory, cultured *Corynebacterium diphtheriae* and began to study its effects. This pathogen could be found only in a victim's throat. But Loeffler knew it could also cause damage at points more distant in time and in location within the body, including paralysis and heart failure. (That may be what killed fourteen-year-old Lucy Mores, seven weeks after her younger siblings.) Loeffler thought the bacteria must emit some kind of long-acting toxin to account for this damage. Preventing diphtheria, he concluded, would require finding a way to defeat this toxin. Having made this brilliant prediction, Loeffler, too, moved on to other subjects.[3]

At the Pasteur Institute, Émile Roux soon turned his attention to the disease, with his characteristic knack for devising the experiments needed to clarify any scientific question. He and an assistant grew *C. diphtheriae* in culture. Next they turned to a device designed by Pasteur's inventive assistant Charles Chamberland as a way to produce bacteria-free fluids for experiments. The Chamberland filter consisted of a metal cylinder containing a long tube of permeable porcelain, with a hollow pipe in the middle. Introducing a fluid under pressure at the top of the cylinder forced it to pass from the outside of the porcelain into the hollow pipe, leaving the bacteria behind. The purified liquid then drained out the bottom of the pipe into a sterile container. Having removed the bacteria in this fashion, Roux demonstrated in 1889 that the toxin alone could produce all the symptoms of diphtheria in experimental animals.[4]

BACTERIAL TOXINS

That research caught the interest of Emile von Behring (1854–1917), an assistant to Robert Koch in Berlin. Behring had started out as a physician and researcher in the German army focused on antiseptics, a sensible choice in the context of dressing bullet wounds and amputations. He wanted to protect the human body from infection, he declared, "as one preserves a ham against putrefactive bacteria via fumigation." Behring's thinking gradually evolved. At first, he thought that antiseptics might work not by killing bacteria, but by neutralizing their toxic products. Later, he theorized that the blood itself might function as an internal antiseptic. He suspected that the source of this apparent immunity was something in the blood serum—that is, the clear liquid portion of the blood that's left after all the cells and other solid matter have been filtered out, or coagulated.[5]

Behring began to experiment with *C. diphtheriae*. He induced the disease in guinea pigs, then attempted to do it again in the survivors. As expected, the first exposure had rendered these survivors immune to the disease. He then took blood from them and injected it into healthy guinea pigs. When he later exposed this second group to *C. diphtheriae*, they had also become immune. But he struggled to prove his suspicion that this transfer of immunity was a function of the blood serum.

At about the same time, another assistant to Koch isolated the tetanus pathogen, grew it in a pure culture for the first time, and extracted its toxin. Shibasaburo Kitasatō (1852–1931) was a physician and bacteriologist sent by the Japanese government in 1885 to train with Koch. Behring and Kitasatō soon began to collaborate, with "the advice and counsel" of Koch. The "happy situation" with tetanus, Behring wrote, was that immune rabbits produced large amounts of blood serum, to be injected into very small mice. The difference in size mattered. The donor's much greater volume of blood serum relative to the size of the recipient gave the two researchers a reliable way to make the treatment work.

On December 4, 1890, Behring and Kitasatō published their landmark study, *The Mechanism of Immunity in Animals to Diphtheria and Tetanus*. Immunity depended, they wrote, "on the ability of the cell-free blood fluid"—that is, the serum—"to render harmless the toxic substance which the tetanus bacillus produces." Blood serum from immune animals appeared to contain an "antitoxin"—a specific antidote to the toxin. The immunity transferred in this fashion seemed to persist indefinitely, at least in experimental animals, Behring and Kitasatō wrote. Even better, transferring immunity shortly after the onset of tetanus symptoms seemed to cure the disease. This was the beginning of the form of treatment called serum therapy. In a separate paper published a week later with no coauthor, Behring argued on less persuasive evidence that serum therapy also worked against diphtheria.

Behring and others attempted the first treatment of children sick with diphtheria in 1892. (By then, Kitasatō had returned to Japan and established his own research institute.) The results were unimpressive, apparently because the antitoxin in the serum was not potent enough. This was particularly embarrassing because it came soon after the heartbreaking collapse of Koch's own promised tuberculosis cure, a drug named tuberculin.[6]

THE TUBERCULIN FIASCO

That failure began at an international conference in Berlin in August 1890, just a few months before Behring and Kitasatō published their paper. Apparently under pressure from the government to deliver yet another sensational discovery, Koch had tentatively described a substance with the power "to prevent the growth of the tubercle bacteria." He had shown that guinea pigs he treated "in the late stages of disease are completely cured." Koch did not describe the treatment. But based on the care and completeness of his past work, people reacted as to "the news of the advent of Jesus of Nazareth in a Judaean village," a British publication reported. Even Pasteur telegrammed Koch with "best congratulations for his great discovery."[7]

Koch was sincere in his belief that he had found a cure. He had taken a large dose of tuberculin himself, to test its safety. It wasn't, as a critic would allege, a *tuberkulinschwindel*. But in testing on human patients, the miracle substance soon proved to be ineffective against tuberculosis. For Koch, who was simultaneously dealing with the scandal of his divorce and remarriage, this was a very public humiliation. Tuberculin was useful: the tuberculin tine test would become the most effective tool for screening large populations for tuberculosis. But the failure to save lives played into the common perception that bacteriology only pointed out causes of disease, never cures. Tuberculosis patients, their hopes raised up and dashed almost in the same painful breath, turned away bitterly to face their old terminal prognosis.

At that same moment, Behring's diphtheria cure also hovered on the brink of failure. But both French and German researchers saw a way forward in the tetanus work using rabbit serum to treat mice: choosing a serum donor significantly larger than the recipient might prove critical to obtaining diphtheria antitoxin in sufficient quantity and potency. Behring tried using cattle

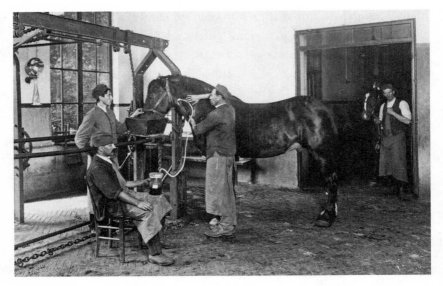

Figure 22.1
Drawing blood for diphtheria and tetanus serum therapy in the stables of the Pasteur Institute (Institut Pasteur/Musée Pasteur).

to supply serum for treating diphtheria in humans. Roux opted instead to work with immunized horses, which produced massive quantities of serum, with a much higher concentration of antitoxin. By one calculation, a bleed from a single horse could supply enough antitoxin to treat fifty patients, and the same horse could be bled at intervals throughout its life.

The Pasteur Institute began testing serum therapy in children with diphtheria in early 1894, with Behring a half step behind, now also working with horse serum. Both Behring and Roux were due to speak at a major medical conference in Budapest that September. But Behring begged off, pleading illness. It is hard now to imagine Roux stepping into the moment as a charismatic speaker. He was by nature a microbiological anchorite in the church of Louis Pasteur, and at forty, he looked the part, gaunt, bordering on cadaverous, with stark, staring eyes, a long thin beak of a nose, and a salt-and-pepper Vandyke beard. He was scrupulously fair-minded, and began his talk by crediting Behring. Then he announced his own results, which were plainly thrilling for any doctor who had ever stood by helplessly as the strangling angel carried off another child: at the Hôpital des Infants-Malades in Paris, physicians had treated 448 diphtheria patients with serum from immunized horses—and 339 had regained their health and gone home. It was as close to a cure as anyone had ever seen. The 75.5 percent survival rate compared to 50 percent at the same hospital in the recent past—and 40 percent at another Paris hospital lacking the treatment.[8]

"Hats were thrown to the ceiling," an American physician in attendance later recalled, "grave scientific men arose to their feet and shouted their applause in all the languages of the civilized world. I . . . have never seen such an ovation displayed by an audience of scientific men." The next day, in Paris, *Le Figaro* trumpeted the cure on its front page and dwelt lovingly on an "oeuvre . . . exclusivement francaise." A magazine cartoonist depicted Roux as St. George shielding a mother and child from the dragon diphtheria. When the French president named him a commander of the Legion of Honor, Roux acquiesced only on condition that Behring be honored at the same time. After the ceremony in January 1895, Behring visited the Pasteur Institute, where Roux and others warmly welcomed him. This was a new model of scientific partnership for the dawning century. Pasteur did not attend, no doubt acutely aware that Behring had been an officer in the army that had defeated France a quarter century earlier.[9]

STANDARDIZING SERUM THERAPY

Paul Ehrlich (1854–1915) would become the last of the key figures in the network of diphtheria collaborators. Born to a prosperous family in what is now Poland, Ehrlich had picked up his cousin Karl Weigert's obsession with chemical staining to reveal the nuances of microbes and cells. As a physician and chemist, he worked hard to make those nuances applicable to the care of patients. With one such application—the staining technique that enabled physicians to diagnose tuberculosis from a saliva sample—Ehrlich would later discover his own case of that disease. When he applied his blend of scientific precision and imaginative thinking to the diphtheria antitoxin, it resulted not just in a more effective treatment, but also in a bold new vision of how the immune system works.

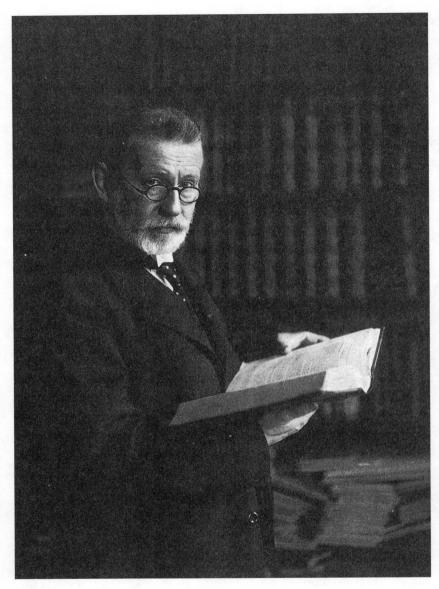

Figure 22.2
Paul Ehrlich made the diphtheria treatment effective (Wellcome Collection).

In 1891, Ehrlich's friend Robert Koch invited him to join his laboratory and put him to work with Behring sorting out the issues with the diphtheria treatment. The two became friends for a time, though they made an odd couple. Behring still had the staff officer's brusque bearing and tendency to bully, while Ehrlich, according to one biographer, was more outgoing, "overflowing and effervescing with ideas, rapidly drawing chemical formulas and diagrams on any available surface."[10]

One problem with diphtheria antiserum was that batches varied in potency. That could mean giving too weak a dose to a child already near death from diphtheria. As he sorted through the many variables in serum production, Ehrlich noticed that injecting steadily increasing amounts of diphtheria toxin into a horse—eight to eleven injections over a period of months—didn't necessarily result in a corresponding rise in antitoxin. He introduced careful testing of the blood to understand the fluctuations and find the point of maximum potency. Ehrlich soon also devised a way to sample every batch of serum for uniform effectiveness. It involved inject-ing a fixed amount of diphtheria toxin into guinea pigs, each weighing 250 grams, and then injecting a fixed amount of the serum sample to neutralize the toxin. If the guinea pigs lived six days or longer, the batch was deemed effective; if they sickened or died before then, it had to be scrapped. Later refinements would reduce the waste of animal lives. Meanwhile, the stan-dardized process developed by Ehrlich helped drive diphtheria mortality in human children down below 5 percent and eventually to less than 1 percent.

In Germany, a system of state control soon emerged for serum therapy, in part to avert another tuberculin-style failure. It entailed routine monitoring and sample testing in large-scale manufacturing facilities, with Ehrlich's work as the standard for safety and effectiveness. At that point, the partnership with Behring came to an abrupt end. The two had signed an agreement to share profits from the diphtheria treatment. But before any profits could appear, Behring made a secret agreement with a drug manufacturer to cut his former collaborator out of the deal. As a result, just in the first year of commercial production, Behring pocketed 350,000 marks, a fortune. (His annual salary as an assistant to Koch had been just 1,200 marks.) He moved his family into an Italianate mansion suited to a prince of science in Marburg, where he became a university professor, and he also acquired a villa in Capri.

Along with the profits, Behring claimed the glory. When the first Nobel Prize in Physiology or Medicine was awarded in 1901, it made no mention of Edwin Klebs, Friedrich Loeffler, Shibasaburo Kitasatō, Émile Roux, Paul Ehrlich, or others in the diphtheria network. Their research had in fact turned serum therapy from another tragic failure into what the prize statement called "a victorious weapon against illness and deaths." But the prize honored only Behring.

Behring's later career was largely undistinguished, perhaps in part because after a certain point, no one wanted to work with him. His posthumous reputation has also suffered by association. In 1940, on the fiftieth anniversary of his diphtheria paper, Nazi officials and scientists fervently celebrated Behring as "the savior of children." It was a useful distraction, according to biographer Derek S. Linton, from the Nazi program then already murdering thousands of children deemed eugenically unfit. Those celebrations simultaneously treated Ehrlich, a Jew, as a nonperson.[11]

THE PUZZLE OF IMMUNITY

The great unresolved question of serum therapy and vaccination alike was how they worked—that is, how immunity worked. The then-accepted explanation came from Rudolf Virchow (1821–1902), who described various diseases as the result of physical or chemical changes that caused a body's cells to malfunction. Likewise, he thought, various undefined modifications of the cells enabled the body to protect itself from certain other diseases. But this cell-mediated, or cellular, immunity was unsatisfyingly vague.

In the 1880s, Elie Metchnikoff (1845–1916) took up the question of immunity from an outsider's perspective. He was a striking figure of Russian and Ukrainian background, with a shock of uncombed hair pushed back from his forehead. In his youth, by his own description, he was hypersensitive, prone to depression, and briefly addicted to morphine. Twice in his life, he attempted suicide. But he was also prone to imaginative scientific insights. His deep-set eyes lit up with the excitement of new ideas, which he could defend against the fiercest critics. He was so passionate about science that, when he later worked at the Pasteur Institute, he asked in his will to be cremated in the same furnace researchers used to destroy the remains of experimental animals. (His ashes now rest in an urn in the Pasteur Institute's former library.)[12]

Metchnikoff was a zoologist with no medical training. His early research focused on comb jellies and other gelatinous creatures, which generally lack organized digestive tracts. Instead, tiny, cell-like structures roam through their digestive cavity gobbling up intruders, along with the host's own discarded tissue. Metchnikoff became obsessed with these cell-like structures, and especially with the way they sometimes bunched up around a new food source. Influenced by evolutionary thinking about the connectedness of all life, he wondered if their digestive behavior might shed light on biological processes in vertebrates. In 1882, shortly before a research trip to Sicily, Metchnikoff took a course in general pathology. He came away thinking about inflammation in humans and the way certain white blood cells migrate through the capillary walls to flood the site of an injury.[13]

In Sicily, he set up his laboratory to study the transparent, jelly-like larva of a starfish species. There, as he later recounted it, two ideas merged: Maybe the invertebrate feeding cells bunching up on food and the vertebrate white blood cells flooding an injury were different forms of the same behavior? To test the idea, he took a thorn from a rose bush in the garden and used it to prick some of the starfish larvae. "And the next morning, at a very early hour," after what he said was a night sleepless with anticipation, "I observed with immense joy that the experiment was a perfect success!" The feeding cells flooded the site of the injury in the same fashion as did white blood cells in vertebrates. Metchnikoff went on to demonstrate that both are capable of engulfing and destroying pathogens. He named these cells *phagocytes*, from the Greek, meaning "cells that devour." With the help of aniline dyes, he described the largest of them and named them *macrophages*, or "big eaters." It was an entirely new view of the immune system, but also just a beginning.[14]

The next great contribution to the immune question came from Paul Ehrlich in the mid-1890s. His work with staining had shown him the importance of *side chains*, chemical structures on any given molecule that determine its characteristics and reactivity. He later described how certain living cells also depend on side chains to take up the specific nutrients they need. Another Berlin chemist, Emil Fischer, then expanded this idea to explain how specific structures on an enzyme's side chains enable it to bind with corresponding structures on a target molecule, in lock-and-key fashion, to speed up a chemical reaction.

As he worked on diphtheria, Ehrlich began to think the combination of side-chain and lock-and-key theory might also explain how substances in the bloodstream identify and latch onto specific intruders, including the diphtheria toxin and various microbes. Each intruder carried an identifying molecular structure, a sort of key, which he later called an *antigen*. The antigen caused the body to produce a flood of antibodies with corresponding structures to lock onto the intruder. Later, he added the idea that the antibodies also bind with "complement" factors in the blood serum, which aided in the destruction and removal of intruders. Ehrlich couldn't actually see antibodies, antitoxins, or the complement system. But he sketched out his concept of a Y-shaped antibody, with the two arms representing the side chains. He also illustrated examples of how antibodies attach to intruder antigens, and how the complement system then aided in the destruction of these intruders. It was a display of extraordinary visual imagination—not just to see what was invisible, but to map it out on paper for others to understand.

As he developed his hypothesis, Ehrlich inevitably got some details wrong. But he also wrote with astonishing foresight about antibodies being passed on in breast milk to build immunity in young children, and about the "horror autotoxicus," or autoimmunity. His ideas led to fierce debate about the existence of antibodies, and also about whether the correct understanding of the immune response was Ehrlich's side-chain theory, or Metchnikoff's phagocytes roaming around like Pac-Men gobbling up intruders.[15]

The resolution of this apparent conflict came early in the new century, in research by British bacteriologist Almroth Wright. He and a coauthor took finger-prick samples of their own blood, then tested how various samples handled invasion by *Staphylococcus* bacteria. After briefly incubating a sample at body temperature, they measured the sample's "phagocytic power" by counting how many of the white blood cells had consumed bacteria. When they tried this with blood plasma (the liquid portion of the blood including clotting factors) and blood serum (the liquid portion minus the clotting factors), the count of white blood cells happily fattened on bacteria was roughly identical. But when they tried the same experiment using serum heated at a high enough temperature to impair its biological effectiveness, Metchnikoff's phagocytes lost their ability to gobble up intruders. They needed Ehrlich's antibodies and complement system, which also needed Metchnikoff's phagocytes, to accomplish the critical business of devouring and removing threats to human health.

"We have here conclusive proof," the researchers wrote, in a 1904 paper, "that the blood fluids modify the bacteria in a manner which renders them a ready prey to the phagocytes." They called the elements in the blood that identified substances for attack by phagocytes *opsonins*, from the Latin *opsono*, meaning "I prepare the meal." Or as Wright's friend George Bernard Shaw later put it in a medical drama, "Opsonin is what you butter the disease germs with to make your white blood corpuscles eat them."[16]

As further research confirmed and expanded these results, it became clear that Metchnikoff and Ehrlich hadn't after all presented rival concepts of immunity. Instead, they had described two interdependent aspects of the same system. In 1908, the Nobel Prize in Physiology or Medicine honored both men as founders of the science of immunology. It was a long way from looking at starfish larvae, or at a disease that had until then kept the world's graveyards stocked with the fresh corpses of unfortunate children. But by following their idiosyncratic paths, Metchnikoff and Ehrlich had produced the first useful road map of the body's complex system for defending itself from a vast and constantly shifting array of enemies.

23 DEADLY CARRIERS

Patrick Manson (1844–1922), a Scottish surgeon and physician, set out at twenty-two to make his fortune in the colonies. He had completed the medical course at the University of Aberdeen—but for the next twenty-three years, in southeastern China, he learned mainly by paying close attention to the symptoms of his patients, among them the grotesque swellings of the lower body caused by elephantiasis.

Manson called himself "a good carpenter but an indifferent surgeon," but he was actually deft and innovative with a scalpel. The standard British practice then for one effect of elephantiasis, massive enlargement of the scrotum, was to constrict arteries to the affected area and cut off the genitals. The peculiar heartlessness of this procedure may have been influenced by the far higher incidence of the disease among the colonized than the colonizers. Manson instead devised the method of elevating the scrotum on a board above the body to drain the blood before surgery. This reduced bleeding during the operation and made it clear which tissue needed to be removed, allowing him to alleviate the problem while keeping the patient largely intact.[1]

In the coastal port of Amoy (now Xiamen), where he was based, the likelihood of elephantiasis built up over a lifetime and afflicted one elder in three. That, plus the unrelenting misery of the disease, led Manson to study elephantiasis more carefully. During a year-long leave in Britain in 1875, he married, but also spent long hours researching tropical diseases in the library of the British Museum. There he stumbled upon the work of another colonial physician, who had identified filarial worms in patients with chyluria, a symptom Manson had often seen in patients who also had elephantiasis. He returned to Amoy in 1876 with his wife, and with a new microscope to search for these worms in blood samples from elephantiasis patients.

In fact, the microfilaria consistently appeared in elephantiasis patients, and sometimes in patients who had yet to show any symptoms of the disease. Manson was aware of the recent discovery that parasites can pass through one or more intermediate host species in their life cycle. He reasoned that a blood-sucking species was the likeliest culprit for delivering microfilaria into the human bloodstream. Mosquitoes happened to coincide in their distribution with incidence of elephantiasis, and he soon found microfilaria in their abdomens.

Manson next induced an elephantiasis patient named Hin-Lo, who was also his servant, to spend the night in a "mosquito house" he had set up, with mosquito netting all around. The idea was to leave the door open long enough to let the mosquitoes inside, then shut them up with Hin-Lo overnight. In the morning, mosquitoes belly-fattened with Hin-Lo's blood clung to the sides of the hut. An assistant then trapped each of them beneath a wine glass, immobilized it with a breath of tobacco smoke, and placed it in a small, screened container with some water in which to lay its eggs. A microscope slide containing the blood from one of these mosquitoes typically contained about twenty or thirty microfilaria. The individual worm was a "long snake-like" animal with "a perfectly transparent structureless body," shortening and extending itself within a sort of sheath. It soon wriggled out of the sheath and transformed into a "sausage-like" creature with a "pursed up" mouth, Manson wrote, then developed into what he took to be its final stage, with a "boring-apparatus," like a hole saw, at one end. He thought this was for "escaping from the mosquito" and "penetrating the tissues of man."[2]

In 1878, Manson sent a paper to the Linnean Society in London describing the mosquito as the carrier of elephantiasis. A critic supposedly mocked it as "either the work of a genius or more likely the emanations of a drunken Scots doctor in far-off China." A year later, Manson filed a second report, which must also have elicited incredulity. He employed two hospital assistants to count the number of microfilaria in the blood of elephantiasis patients. One worked by day, the other in the evening, and they reported strikingly different results: the worms were almost totally absent from the blood in the morning, but "invariably begin to appear in the circulation at sunset" and increase in number until about midnight. "For the meaning of it I think we have not far to look," Manson concluded. The filarial worms had adapted to appear in the blood just when mosquitoes, their intermediate host, would be feeding. It was a reversal of the Biblical paradigm: Instead of other species in service to humanity, the human body was a habitat in the service of other species.[3]

Manson's work persuaded some researchers. But two major flaws prevented a complete triumph for the idea of insects as agents of disease: Manson assumed that mosquitoes bite only once to get the blood meal needed for egg laying. So he completely missed the mosquito's role in direct transmission of elephantiasis from person to person. Instead, he thought the filaria escaped into the water where the mosquito died. They found their way back to a human host, he wrote, by "piercing the integuments" of someone wading in that water, or, "what is more probable, being swallowed" in drinking water.

THE MALARIA PARASITE

Manson didn't at first extend his mosquito transmission hypothesis to malaria. But his work influenced others. One of them was Charles Alphonse Laveran (1845–1922), a French military physician in Algeria. Laveran's microscope was rudimentary. But he possessed excellent vision and the patience to use it carefully. In October 1880, while examining fresh blood from a malaria patient, he noticed "elements that seemed to [him] to be parasites" because of their rapidly moving appendages, called *flagella*. He found them only in patients suffering from malaria, or those who had died of the disease. But they vanished from the blood of patients cured with quinine. He published a brief account of the parasite and the phases of its development, concluding, "The presence of these parasites in the blood is probably the principal cause of malaria." Laveran didn't, however, link the parasites to mosquitoes.[4]

Others were prepared to attribute malaria to mosquitoes even without new evidence. "Viewed in the light of our modern 'germ theory' of disease,"

Albert King, an obstetrician, told an audience in 1882, mosquitoes "deserve consideration, as the probable means by which bacteria and other germs may be inoculated into human bodies, so as to infect the blood and give rise to specific fevers." King also suggested protecting the malaria-riddled city of Washington, DC, by surrounding it with a mosquito-proof screen the height of the Washington Monument, then nearing completion as the world's tallest building. This may have nudged the mosquito transmission idea back to fringe theory.[5]

Laveran continued to advance his research, reporting in 1884 that he had found the malaria parasite in 432 cases—and never in cases that didn't involve malaria. Italian researchers also recognized the role of the parasite, which they identified as a protozoan belonging to a new genus, *Plasmodium*. They reported that different species of *Plasmodium* occur in different bird species. They also identified the species responsible for two different forms of human malaria. By 1890, the parasite theory had become the accepted understanding of malaria. This was a momentous achievement, given that malaria (literally "bad air") had the miasma theory embedded in its very name. But it didn't prove that mosquitoes played any part in malaria.

Laveran leaned on Manson's elephantiasis work when he wondered in 1884, and again in 1891, if "mosquitos play a role in the pathogenesis of malaria as they do in filariasis?" But he remained tentative, and he made no effort to test the idea. At about the same time, Cuban epidemiologist Carlos Finlay (1833–1915) proposed mosquito transmission in far more specific terms. Unlike Manson, he recognized that the same mosquito can bite more than one person over the course of its short life. He also understood the anatomy of the mosquito's proboscis, and how it could pick up the germ of a disease with one bite and pass it, with another, to the next victim. Finlay's concern was yellow fever, which swept across Havana in deadly seasonal waves. The disease gets its name from the yellow skin color caused by liver damage in severe cases. Other symptoms include high fever, bleeding from mouth, ears, and nose, and bloody vomiting resembling coffee grounds, leading to death in up to half such cases.

Finlay didn't merely implicate the mosquito. He actually tested the idea, and at the 1881 International Sanitary Conference in Washington, DC, he reported five cases in which he had mosquitoes bite yellow fever victims and then bite healthy volunteers, transmitting the disease. Soon after, he correctly identified *Aedes aegypti* mosquitoes as the culprit in yellow fever. But most physicians were still struggling to come to terms with germ theory, and the notion of a deadly pathogen transmitted by a creature as trivial as the mosquito apparently required too great an intellectual leap. Finlay's theory went unheeded for another twenty years. Meanwhile, powerful evidence linking insects and other arthropods to disease came instead from cattle.[6]

TEXAS FEVER

Late in the era of cattle drives from Texas to urban markets in the north, Wilbur E. Campbell, a rancher in Kiowa, Kansas, got wind of a huge herd due to pass near his ranch on the trail to Dodge City. Campbell, who had been a cattle driver himself, rode out to meet the drivers while they were still ten miles off and warned them to stay well clear of his land. What worried him was "Texas fever," sometimes called "red water" fever for the dark urine of afflicted animals. This disease made cattle listless, unwilling to eat, with trembling limbs and sad eyes. Their weight plummeted and within days entire herds lay dead.

Ranchers knew that Texas fever tended to hit after a cattle drive passed through—much as eighteenth-century Italian farmers had connected rinderpest to newly arrived oxen. The herd could ramble along "without remaining for any length of time on any portion of the ground they traverse" and yet "leave behind sufficient poison to destroy all or nearly all" the local cattle, a British veterinarian hired by the US Department of Agriculture reported in 1871. Infuriatingly, the infected southern cattle themselves remained healthy, apparently having adapted to the sickness over time.

Campbell found himself in a standoff. The furious drivers shouted that they would "go through if they had to wade blood up to their chins." Overnight, Campbell rounded up enough ranchers armed with revolvers and carbines to make this a real possibility. The herd prudently swung away, heading instead for Abilene. Confrontations like that finally put an end to cattle drives in the late 1880s. By then, though, Texas fever was killing cattle from California to Maine.

Ranchers blamed the disease on the ticks with which southern cattle were often afflicted. But the same British veterinarian dismissed this as "an absurdity," presumably because ticks were too trivial to take down entire herds. No one else paid much attention until 1889, when a physician in the US Department of Agriculture set out to test the tick idea.[7]

Theobald Smith (1859–1934) devised a painstaking series of experiments at a research farm in Arlington, Virginia. (It's now part of Arlington National Cemetery.) In one field, he and a colleague put disease-free cattle together with cattle from North Carolina carrying the usual load of ticks. All but a few of the healthy cattle soon came down with Texas fever. Separately, the researchers removed all the ticks from three other Carolina cattle. (To put this in perspective, imagine the effort to pick all the ticks off a fifty-pound feral dog, then extrapolate to a one-thousand-pound steer—times three.) They put the picked-clean cattle together in a field with disease-free cattle to see if disease transmission occurred in the absence of ticks. It didn't.[8]

That was suggestive evidence for the tick theory. But Smith, born Schmitt to German immigrant parents in upstate New York, had taught himself bacteriology by reading Koch and Ehrlich in the original German. He was a modest, soft-spoken man, with a wife and three children. His amusements included home repairs and calculus. He was also a thorough researcher. So he repeated the cattle experiments, adding useful variations. A field infected with ticks from southern cattle, but minus the actual cattle, also sickened healthy animals. So did the offspring of ticks from southern cattle, reared in the laboratory. He identified a parasite now called *Babesia bigemina* in both the ticks and the blood of infected animals. That blood, injected into healthy animals, transmitted the sickness, too. These experiments, conducted over four years and finally published in 1893, established beyond refute that ticks were the agents of Texas fever. Spraying or dipping cattle to kill the ticks quickly became standard—and continues in the United States today to prevent outbreaks that would cost $1.2 billion or more annually.[9]

The Texas fever research was the first time anyone had proved conclusively that arthropods, meaning insects, arachnids, and other creeping things, don't merely drive people mad with their buzzing, biting, and itching.

They are also *vectors* (from the Latin word meaning "carriers") of some of the deadliest diseases known.

MOSQUITO MANSON

In 1889, Patrick Manson left China for good, to return with his family to Britain. He set up practice in London, where he became the leading expert on the tropical diseases being encountered in the British Empire's many colonies. He also made a name for his stubborn insistence on the medical importance of mosquitoes, and in certain circles he was derided as "Mosquito" Manson. The idea of malaria transmission by mosquitoes was so well grounded, he thought, that if circumstances permitted, he would himself "approach its experimental demonstration with confidence." He was already fifty years old, though, and no longer up to the hardships of tropical research. His applied for funding to undertake a study in the West Indies, but unsuccessfully. He commended his hypothesis, however, "to the attention of medical men in India and elsewhere, where malarial patients and suctorial insects abound."[10]

In fact, just such a medical man had literally come knocking at his door earlier that year. Ronald Ross would shortly be on his way back to India to begin the necessary experiments under "Mosquito" Manson's careful, long-distance direction.

For much of his life until 1894, Ronald Ross (1857–1932) was a typically undistinguished product of the colonial system. He had been born in a Himalayan hill town, the first of ten children of a general in the British Indian Army. His parents packed him off to England for his schooling at age eight, a common practice among such families then. For young Ross, it seems to have instilled a sense of being treated unfairly that would stay with him for life. But he also flourished. Living at first with an aunt and uncle, he developed a passion for music, poetry, and other genres, as well as for mathematics. He yearned to attend a good university and establish himself as a writer.

Instead, his father pushed him into medicine. Ross responded by performing poorly in medical school and idling his way into a third-tier medical posting back in India. There, he hunted, fished, played golf, scribbled, and failed to advance in his assigned career. During an 1888 furlough in England, Ross began, at thirty-one, an effort to make something of himself. He took a course in public health and also learned bacteriology. Like Manson at the same age, he acquired a wife and a microscope before returning to his colonial posting. There, he tried and failed to identify *Plasmodium* in the blood of malaria patients. In the process, however, he published articles in the *Indian Medical Gazette* correcting other workers who had mistaken normal blood forms for the malaria parasite.

The turning point for his career came on another furlough back in England in 1894. Ross had been spending time in the British Museum reading malaria research that was unavailable in India. Another physician directed him to Manson as the acknowledged expert on the disease. On April 9, Ross knocked on the front door of Manson's home in London to express his interest in working on mosquitoes. Manson was not in, but immediately wrote to express regret. He had read Ross's papers in the *Indian Medical Gazette*, he added, and admired "the minuteness and accuracy" of his microscopic observations.[1]

On April 10, Ross returned for the first of many visits with Manson, who quickly taught him how to find *Plasmodium* in a blood sample. The process of tutoring had begun. Along with the essential education he provided, Manson may also have represented the sort of medical father figure Ross needed. For Manson, Ross was a younger, healthier alter ego, who could carry out his research program in the tropics. It would become one of the most productive partnerships in the history of medicine, though with seeds of its destruction built in from the start.

THE COLLABORATION

One afternoon in November 1894, Manson and Ross were walking together on Oxford Street when the older man outlined the idea he was about to publish in the *British Medical Journal*. He had decided to focus on mosquitoes as the agent of malaria transmission, for reasons far more nuanced than the analogy with filarial worms in elephantiasis. Since Laveran's discovery of the malaria parasite, other researchers had sorted out at least some of the stages of its development. Camillo Golgi (1843–1926), a pathologist at the University of Pavia, had described how *Plasmodium* colonizes the red blood cells, develops there, and then divides. In the process, it ruptures the cell, spills a new generation into the bloodstream, and sets off the characteristic malaria fever.[2]

This led to a general assumption that the parasite's reproduction was entirely asexual, by division. But no one understood why two other stages in the development of *Plasmodium* seemed to appear only after that, in blood samples taken from a malaria patient. One stage was crescent-shaped; the other, which emerged from the crescents, was spherical, sometimes with wriggling flagella, which eventually separated from the spheroid and moved independently. To some researchers, this wriggling had "the appearance of agony" and represented the dying struggles of the parasite on being moved into the hostile environment of a microscope slide.

Another researcher suggested, however, that the flagella represented the beginning of the parasite's new life outside the body of the malaria victim. That idea, together with his own experience with mosquitoes, led Manson to a hypothesis: Maybe these puzzling forms of the *Plasmodium* parasite showed up in the laboratory only after blood was drawn because that was how they showed up in nature. But instead of a finger prick, nature's way of drawing blood was with the bite of a mosquito. And the mosquito's body was also where the next stage of the parasite's life was meant to take place.[3]

Ross soon departed for India, "wild with excitement" to carry out the experiments to test Manson's hypothesis. He was so eager to get his hands on malaria that he even solicited finger-prick blood samples from likely cases among his fellow passengers on the ship from Malta. Over the next four years, Ross and Manson would exchange about two hundred letters, the vast majority from Ross ("Dear Dr. Manson") recounting his struggles and seeking direction, with Manson ("My Dear Ross") sending back praise, updates on malaria developments elsewhere, and recommendations at every stage on what Ross should try next.[4]

In India, Ross soon found the parasite in the blood of malaria patients who had not yet been treated with quinine. The mosquitoes he caught with the intent of having them bite these patients were at first "obstinate as mules" in their refusal to do so, making it difficult to find out what happens next. But he soon succeeded not only at making mosquitoes bite, but also at dissecting them and observing the living parasite within the mosquito. Manson wrote back in evident delight: "The mere fact that the parasite is not digested is enough to prove to my mind that it is in its proper habitat."

To prove it to other minds, however, Manson needed further experiments and a detailed description of how the parasite developed. He urged Ross to look on the work as a quest for the "Holy Grail and yourself as Sir Galahad and never give up the search for be assured you are on the right track." Ross badly needed this encouragement. First, he had to make himself

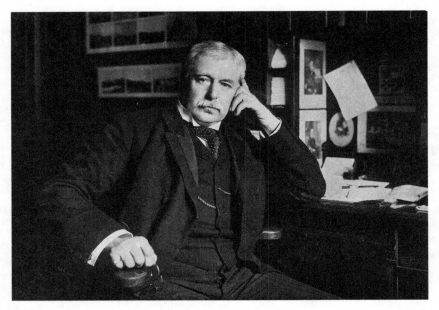

Figure 24.1

At a distance of five thousand miles, "Mosquito" Manson directed research to pin down the origin of malaria (Wellcome Collection).

an expert in mosquito anatomy and learn to dissect its minute body parts properly. He also had to make sense of different *Plasmodium* species, each passing through multiple developmental forms in a complicated life cycle. And he had to sort out various mosquito species, with no entomology text other than an angler's guide to insects. This was in addition to Ross's regular military duties, which in one case took him away for six months on a cholera outbreak in Bangalore.[5]

Ross achieved his next important success on August 20, 1897. The characteristic pigmentation seen in *Plasmodium* from malaria patients turned up that day in the cellular lining of the intestines of certain mosquito species fed on malaria patients. It was the first tantalizing evidence that the human malaria parasite developed in mosquitoes, and Ross celebrated the date thereafter as "Mosquito Day." The *British Medical Journal* made Ross's account its lead article, together with an endorsement from Manson, who wrote, "I am inclined to think that Ross may have found the extracorporeal phase of malaria. If this be the case, then he has made a discovery of the first importance."[6]

In fact, another account of that "extracorporeal phase" had appeared a month earlier in the *Lancet*. On summer break, William MacCallum (1874–1944), a student at Johns Hopkins Medical School, was working in a "makeshift laboratory in a woodshed" at his family home in rural Ontario. As he was examining blood of a mosquito that had fed on an infected crow, he described two forms of sphere, one producing flagella, which swarmed around the other "quiet spherical forms." One of the flagella eventually "plunges its head into the sphere and finally wriggles its whole body into that organism." This somehow blocked out the others, which circled around "vainly beating their heads against the organism." The interior of the sphere became "churned up" by the flagellum. Then it began to grow and divide.

The parasite was reproducing not just asexually, as Golgi had described, but also sexually, with the flagellum equivalent to a sperm, the sphere to an egg, and the combination to a zygote (now called an *oocyst*). MacCallum found this pattern repeated soon after in a case of human malaria. Ross confessed years later that he had previously noticed a flagellum entering a sphere and lashing about frantically. But "I thought it was *trying to get out!*" He had "felt disgraced as a man of science ever since"—and plainly blamed Manson for the idea that the parasite needed to escape the mosquito into a body of water.[7]

In fact, though, it was Manson who had alerted Ross to the *Lancet* article and pushed him to test the conclusion with his own research. It was Manson who worked his political connections in London to free Ross from other military distractions, ultimately winning him a six-month leave at the beginning of 1898 for his malaria research. When human malaria cases then proved scarce in Calcutta, where Ross had relocated for access to a good laboratory, it was Manson who urged him to continue the malaria work in birds. It was Manson, finally, who served as Ross's voice in the scientific world, arranging publication under Ross's name and promoting the work in medical meetings. Ross was, in fact, completely dependent on Manson's guidance.[8]

The next breakthrough came in mid-1898. As he dissected mosquitoes at various stages after they had fed on infected birds, Ross observed the zygote, or oocyst, begin to develop and then, to his surprise, burst open and spill forth numerous rod-like bodies. At first, he thought these *germinal rods*, as he called them, might be spores, or spore-like. "Nature probably makes some extraordinary effort here in order to complete the life cycle," he wrote to Manson, adding, "What the dickens she is going to do next I cannot imagine at all." Manson urged him on: "You are like Captain Cook now—sailing into unknown seas which may reveal wonders unconceived."

In July, Ross wrote Manson again, saying, "My last letter left me face to face with the astonishing fact that the germinal rods were to be found in the thorax as well as in the abdomen." In fact, they were "far more numerous" there, and they weren't tough and spore-like at all, but "a multitude of delicate little threads" apparently circulating in the insect's blood. Next, he found them in the mosquito's head, and he searched "until [he] was blind and half silly with fatigue" for some place where they might accumulate and continue their development. On July 4, he discovered a long duct-like gland at the juncture between thorax and head. The rods were "swarming here and were even *pouring out* from somewhere in streams."

After dissecting several other mosquitoes, he found that "the duct led straight into the headpiece, probably into the mouth. In other words it is a thousand to one, it is a *salivary gland*." Ross thought he was "*almost* entitled to lay down the law" on malaria transmission: "Malaria is conveyed from a diseased person or bird to a healthy one by the proper species of mosquito, & it is inoculated by its bite," with the rods "poured out in vast numbers under the skin of man or bird," to be swept away by the blood and "develop into malaria parasites." Soon after, Ross wrote to Manson, "Hence I think I may now say Q.E.D., and congratulate you on the mosquito theory indeed." Student, like master, could be adept at deploying flattery to advance his cause. But he added, in an ominous foreshadowing, "The door is unlocked, and I am walking in & collecting the treasures."[9]

Manson published an account of Ross's latest work in the *British Medical Journal*. He wanted to put Ross's claim to the discovery on the record and also redeem his own reputation. Skeptics had "stigmatized" him, he wrote, as "a sort of pathological Jules Verne . . . governed by 'speculative considerations' and . . . 'guided by the divining rod of preconceived idea.'" Now his mosquito-malaria theory was vindicated. Laveran contributed a testimonial endorsing "the very great importance" of Ross's discoveries.[10]

At the British Medical Association meeting on July 28, Manson delivered an impressive account of this work, waiting to the end to reveal a telegram he had just received from Ross detailing his final triumph: He had fed laboratory-reared mosquitoes on infected birds. When he then fed these mosquitoes on healthy birds, those birds also came down with malaria. A friend later wrote to Ross to recall "the profound sensation produced when Sir Patrick read out the telegram." It "created quite a furore," according to another friend, leading to unanimous approval of a resolution congratulating Ross on "your great and epoch making discovery." At the end of February 1899, Ross boarded a ship to return to Britain and collect the treasures due him as a freshly minted great man of science. "Well, I have left many things undone which I ought to have done," he wrote Manson, "but congratulate myself that the task you imposed on me is finished. You must cease *rubbing the lamp* for a little, at all events."[11]

THE ANOPHELES CONNECTION

In fact, Ross had left two critical parts of the malaria question unresolved: He had demonstrated transmission only in birds, not humans. And because he was not a naturalist, he had not bothered to pin down exactly which species transmitted the disease. They were merely "dapple-winged" mosquitoes, a useless description for anyone setting out to control the disease. The full epoch-making work fell to Italian physician and zoologist Giovanni Battista Grassi (1854–1925). In November 1898, he fed captive-bred mosquitoes on malaria patients and used the bite of those mosquitoes to produce malaria in a human volunteer with no prior history of the disease. Grassi and his coauthors identified mosquitoes of the genus *Anopheles* as the specific agents of malaria transmission, and they also delivered a complete account of the life cycle of *Plasmodium falciparum*, a form of the malaria parasite often fatal to humans.[12]

What has become known as *Grassi's law*—"There is no malaria without *Anopheles*"—remains the one essential fact making malaria control possible:

to rid people of the disease, you must first rid them of *Anopheles*. Ross had missed it, and this may have deepened his outrage when he felt the Italians were not giving him the credit he deserved. He fired off a note to Manson: "It is a mistake to allow this sort of thing to take hold for a moment. I shall strike back at once with full force. The theory belongs to you & Laveran absolutely"— though in truth, neither of those two names much concerned him.[13]

CREDIT

Ross would spend the rest of his life seeking sole credit for solving the mosquito question. This campaign started even before he returned to Britain in 1899, when he began quietly shifting his intellectual paternity to Laveran and nudging Manson out of the family tree. In a paper read to the French Academy of Medicine, Ross praised Laveran for having originated the mosquito hypothesis. Manson he credited merely with "guessing" the reproductive role of the flagella and thus adding "an important argument to those already advanced by Laveran."[14]

Fictionalizing the origin of the mosquito hypothesis probably appealed to Ross for several reasons. The familiar feelings of injury, and even abandonment, were there after Manson secured him a position as a lecturer at the Liverpool School of Tropical Medicine, rather than at the London School of Tropical Medicine, which Manson was then founding at the center of the British Empire. Those feelings intensified when Ross learned that Manson was collaborating with Grassi. After Ross left India with the work unfinished, it was simply the quickest way to confirm that mosquitoes transmit malaria to humans. Using infected mosquitoes supplied by the Italians, Manson replicated their work on transmission to a human volunteer—his own twenty-three-year old son, Thurburn, a medical student—as a dramatic way to convince the public of the importance of mosquito control. (Manson began his son's treatment with quinine immediately after witnesses confirmed the appearance of malaria parasites in his blood. One Oedipal drama at a time was perhaps sufficient.)[15]

Ross may have seen minimizing Manson as a way to maximize his own importance, according to medical historian Jeanne Guilleman: Manson had shaped Ross's research with such "decisive, timely directions" that an honest account of the story might have led people to question "Ross's research autonomy." Laveran was an "almost ideal" substitute. "As the discoverer of the malaria plasmodium, he had prestige, yet he posed no competitive threat to Ross's claim to originality. Unlike Manson, he had published no prior research on the mosquito's role in disease . . . and he took no later initiative to prove the mosquito-vector theory for humans. As a foreigner, Laveran was in no position to judge Ross's teaching or clinical performance," while Manson clearly was.[16]

Of his Italian rivals, Ross wrote in a way a casual reader could at first mistake for respect, using generalized praise ("great brilliance and success") to lead into specific diminishment: Grassi's proof that an *Anopheles* mosquito could transmit malaria to a human test subject was merely "the first confirmation with human malaria of my previous inoculation experiments with the malaria of birds."[17]

When the malaria work began to be talked about as a candidate for the Nobel Prize in Physiology or Medicine, Ross was dismayed to hear Manson and Grassi's names mentioned, not just his own, as likely candidates. He persuaded Robert Koch to lobby the Nobel jury on his behalf. And even after winning the 1902 prize, Ross still felt compelled in his Nobel Prize acceptance speech to belittle Grassi and make Manson merely one of four intellectual forebears. (The others were Laveran, Koch, and Albert King, proponent of the mosquito net as tall as the Washington Monument.) That speech also didn't bother pretending that the colonized people who were most vulnerable to malaria would get much benefit from his discovery. On the contrary, controlling malaria was about access to "the fertile, well-watered, and luxuriant tracts" where the disease "strikes down, not only the indigenous barbaric population, but, with greater certainty, the pioneers of civilization, the planter, the trader, the missionary, and the soldier."[18]

Ross's rage at his own imagined mistreatment only burned brighter with time. In 1923, a quarter century after his triumph in India, Ross published his *Memoirs*, with an entire chapter attacking Italian researchers as "rascals," who perpetrated "impudent scientific frauds" and "piracy." It was an endless victory dirge of bitter feelings and self-pity—bitter perhaps because

greatness, having briefly found him, cast him aside again when his partnership with Manson ended. "Enthusiasm is a tender plant," he moaned, "and
I fear that the events of 1898, followed by those of 1900, murdered mine
for medical research. . . . So the Great Passion died."[19]

MANSON'S LEGACY

Manson remained gracious throughout, merely thanking Ross for being
included in his accounts of the discovery. What mattered to him was the science, and it mattered in ways he could never have imagined when he began
his elephantiasis research in the 1870s. That work, together with Theobald Smith's irrefutable implication of ticks in Texas fever and the sensation
attending the success of Ross and Grassi against malaria, persuaded others
to look more closely at the creeping, flying, biting, and stinging creatures
of the world.

Beginning in 1898, infectious disease researchers would demonstrate
that arthropods transmit bubonic plague (vectored by fleas), African sleeping sickness (by tsetse flies), yellow fever (by mosquitoes), and epidemic
typhus (by body lice). The endlessly expanding list of vector-borne diseases
would eventually also include dengue fever, Chikungunya virus, Zika virus,
and various forms of filariasis and encephalitis (all mosquito-borne); Rocky
Mountain spotted fever, Crimean-Congo hemorrhagic fever, Lyme disease,
ehrlichiosis, babesiosis, and tularemia (all tick-borne); Chagas disease (from
the kissing bug); river blindness (from a black fly); leishmaniasis (from a
sandfly); and schistosomiasis (from a snail), among others. Discovery of
vector-borne diseases would lead to massive control programs, which continue to prevent hundreds of millions of deaths and untold misery every
year. It is an unfinished story: climate change and the political inclination to
underfund prevention sometimes allow vector-borne diseases to reemerge.

Even so, it is a legacy—better than any Nobel Prize—that "Mosquito"
Manson would relish.

25 FIT FOR DUTY

On September 6, 1914, after retreating for two weeks as the German Army drove deep into France, Allied forces began their counterattack northeast of Paris. French and British troops poured into the area around Meaux by train, truck, and a midnight caravan of six hundred taxicabs—the last quickly becoming a symbol of unity in the face of the enemy. For three bloody days, the First Battle of the Marne raged across farm fields awaiting their harvest. In the wake of battle, wounded soldiers were gradually picked up, if they were lucky, and carried back to hospitals in Paris.

At the Hôpital Val-de-Grâce, hundreds of them came in, some gunshot, others with deep, jagged wounds from shrapnel, all covered in filth. Along with improved antiseptics, most of the wounded received injections of antitoxin against tetanus. As a result, a physician there could boast of treating 135 French wounded without a single case of tetanus. At a hospital in Mary-sur-Marne, on the other hand, a German medical officer attending a dozen wounded German prisoners was said to have refused the enemy's antitoxin—and lost half his soldiers to tetanus.[1]

As the Great War dragged on for the next four bloody years, it would become the harsh proving ground not just for tetanus antitoxin, but for all the infectious disease research of the past half-century. It would be the first war not just of modern weapons, but of modern remedies.

LOCKJAW

Tetanus must have seemed like an unlikely candidate to become the war's first great medical triumph. The anaerobic bacteria first described by Kitasatō in 1889 and now called *Clostridium tetani* routinely occur in the guts of livestock and other animals. Even before the fighting, farm fields were heavily manured with their wastes. Eight to ten million horses served in the war and further enriched the soil, as did the wastes of the soldiers themselves. Trench warfare kept soldiers "literally covered from head to foot with clay and earth and mud," largely of fecal origin, and unable to change their clothes for months at a time.

What was on the surface entered the wound, according to British abdominal surgeon Berkeley Moynihan, who delivered a devastatingly clinical account of the impact of a heavy German bullet moving at high velocity: "When the bullet impinges upon any substance, even the soft clothing or the flesh, the infinitely brief arrest in the point which strikes first allows the base, which is, of course, much heavier, to overtake the apex, and the bullet then lies sideways, or begins to turn over and over as it ploughs its way through the soft parts." Within the damaged tissues, tetanus bacteria and other microorganisms "grow apace." The incubation period for tetanus varies from six to sixteen days. Symptoms begin with abdominal rigidity, followed by uncontrollable, agonizingly painful muscle spasms and contractures. This leads to the lockjaw that gives tetanus a common name and to death from asphyxiation or cardiac arrhythmia. Military hospitals reported death rates from 58 to 100 percent.[2]

The immediate success of tetanus antitoxin against such odds was so impressive that, at the end of that first September, the French Academy of Medicine urged preventive injections of tetanus serum "in all wounds, and especially those soiled by earth or clothing." British and German authorities made similar recommendations soon after. Demand outstripped supply. At Val-de-Grâce after the First Battle of the Marne, a physician was so short-stocked, or perhaps just so hostile to an enemy invading his country, that he attempted a sort of controlled experiment: He gave the tetanus antitoxin to one hundred wounded German prisoners but withheld it from one hundred others. In the first group, only one patient died, the day after being admitted. In the second group, eighteen patients came down with tetanus.[3]

Horses were not just contributors to the tetanus problem, but also the solution, as providers of antitoxin serum. The Pasteur Institute rapidly expanded from three hundred horses to nearly 1,500, producing a wartime total of eight million doses for Allied troops. British and American suppliers added to this total, and a similar effort took place on the German side. As a result, the warring armies were able to drive down the incidence of tetanus in the first months of the war from nine cases per thousand soldiers treated in hospitals to just two per thousand thereafter, with mortality cut almost to zero.

Tetanus antitoxin was still relatively crude and could cause side-effects. Hence the lines in a Canadian soldiers' song, "Then he painted it with iodine to keep the germs away; He injected anti-tetanus that hurts me to this day." The worst of these side effects, anaphylactic shock, undoubtedly killed some patients. Recent historians of World War I have concluded that "tens to hundreds of men on both sides of the conflict" may have died due to hyper-allergic reaction to antitetanus serum. But the serum therapy saved several hundred thousand others. Kitasatō's discovery, which had seemed so much less important at the time than Behring's work on diphtheria, saved whole armies of fathers and sons to return home to their families—or at least to go back to the trenches to fight again.[4]

MAGIC BULLETS

Medical discoveries also reduced the wartime hazard of venereal disease. Three German innovations made the difference: identification of the cause of syphilis, a pale, spiral rod now called *Treponema pallidum*; development of a blood test, the Wasserman reaction, to detect these spirochetes; and the introduction of a drug to destroy them.

The drug came from the laboratory of Paul Ehrlich. He experimented early in the new century with aniline dyes as a potential treatment for sleeping sickness, then shifted to an arsenic preparation called atoxyl after other researchers showed that it killed the trypanosomes responsible for that disease. Finding a way to protect people and livestock from sleeping sickness was a colonial rather than a humanitarian priority: Germany considered Uganda and the Congo basin, then suffering an epidemic of the disease, valuable areas for economic expansion. On a 1906 expedition in East Africa,

Robert Koch attempted to use atoxyl to cure sleeping sickness. When it left some of his unwitting patients permanently blind, and few, if any, actually cured, he recommended forced isolation of the sick in "concentration camps." (Apart from the devastating effect on test subjects, this callous experimentation has further damaged Koch's modern reputation.)[5]

At his laboratory in Frankfurt, Ehrlich assigned an assistant to synthesize and test atoxyl derivatives, with the aim of reducing toxicity. Each derivative required multiple experiments to assess its value, and the careless assistant found the 606th derivative, arsphenamin, to be ineffective against various pathogens, like most of its 605 predecessors. But in 1909, Ehrlich's old colleague Kitasatō sent Sahachirō Hata (1873–1938) to train in Ehrlich's laboratory, noting that he had worked with syphilis in experimental rabbits. Ehrlich started him off retesting his repertoire of atoxyl derivatives against various pathogens. One of them was syphilis, which produces telltale eye inflammation in rabbits. Hata soon reported that Compound 606 appeared to correct this symptom, restoring cloudy, inflamed eyes to normal health. A second test also suggested effectiveness against syphilis. The two men shook hands excitedly over these results, both of them repeating Ehrlich's gleeful denunciation of his previous assistant as "der ungeschickte Taperkerl!" (literally, "the clumsy teakettle").

Ehrlich then ordered an extensive series of tests in various experimental animals, and later in human patients. In 1910, he announced the discovery of a drug "whose value and activity in all stages of syphilis are now beyond doubt." The manufacturer Hoechst quickly released it under the name Salvarsan, a neologism meaning "the arsenic that saves." It was the first good alternative to treatment with mercury in the four hundred years since the arrival of syphilis in Europe, and demand was massive and immediate. Ehrlich had previously described serum therapies, or *serotherapy*, as "magic bullets" for diphtheria, tetanus, and other pathogens. Now he coined the parallel term *chemotherapy*, with Salvarsan as the first chemical magic bullet. The magic came with nausea, vomiting, and a few cases of damaged hearing. But Ehrlich soon produced an improved version, reducing the arsenic and thus the side effects.[6]

There were complications. Some patients took the first signs of improvement as a cure and did not bother returning for the full series of injections. British Army researchers soon also found that completely eradicating spirochetes from the blood was rarely possible. Adding a small amount of the dreaded old mercury seemed to help. From a military perspective, the key conclusion was that Salvarsan cases spent less time in hospital—just fifteen days, compared with the previous average of forty-two days followed by two years of mercurial injections. Soldiers treated with Salvarsan also "enjoyed a much greater interval of freedom between the first and any further manifestations of the disease"—freedom, that is, to return to the trenches. About one hundred thousand British soldiers received syphilis treatment during the war, and their quick reclassification as "fit for Active Service" represented a major improvement in manpower on the front lines. The same of course was also true on the German side.[7]

WAR FEVERS

The medical fight against two other diseases, typhus and typhoid, was a mixed success. The filth and chaos of wartime had always produced what was called *ship fever* or *camp fever*, as circumstances dictated, or sometimes just *war fever*. It routinely killed more soldiers than died in combat. But in the decades before the war, researchers sorted out the very different origins of typhus and typhoid and developed methods of prevention specific to each disease.[8]

In 1909, Charles Nicolle, Émile Roux's former student, was working at the Pasteur Institute in Tunisia when he described a eureka moment: he saw typhus victims in their filthy rags outside the hospital entrance transformed, on being admitted to the hospital, into freshly washed and laundered hospital patients. Hospital staff who handled the patients' discarded clothing, on the other hand, tended to become infected with the disease. In a flash, he realized that the body lice crawling along the seams of the discarded clothing were the carriers of typhus. It was a good story—and an instance of the common tendency of storytellers to "improve" their narrative.

In fact, Nicolle and his colleagues had been studying typhus since 1903. Well before the hospital epiphany, both epidemiological evidence and laboratory experiments had implicated lice as the culprit. Nicole then proved it in 1909 by using lice to produce the disease in experimental primates and later in guinea pigs. The discovery was considered important enough to earn him the Nobel Prize in Physiology or Medicine for 1928.[9]

Wartime measures to prevent the disease could be simplistic. Both Allied and German armies instigated "delousing" measures, including intermittent bathing in facilities set up in former breweries and specialized laundries to delouse soldiers' underclothes. Soldiers devoted free time to picking "cooties" from their clothing, or sometimes burning them out by running a lighted candle along the seams. None of this was completely effective. Washing inner but not outer garments could mean rapid recolonization of the former from the latter. And neither washing nor picking removed the louse's nits, its eggs. A study found the average soldier in the trenches played unwilling host to about twenty lice, though a count of one hundred or more was common.

On the eastern front, typhus quickly became epidemic, crippling the forces fighting there for Germany and the other Central powers. It also killed an estimated three million Allied soldiers and civilians in Russia. And yet on the western front, typhus remained mysteriously absent. One possible explanation for the difference is that the typhus pathogen carried by the lice was already endemic among the impoverished peasantry on the eastern front. It may have been less common, or absent altogether, in the more prosperous conditions of northern France and Belgium. On the western front, soldiers suffered instead from a new, less severe louse-borne disease called *trench fever*.[10]

If infected lice had been imported to the western front, Nicolle argued in his Nobel Prize speech, the war would have ended not in a "bloody victory" but "in an unparalleled catastrophe. . . . Men would have perished in millions, as unfortunately occurred in Russia." This was at least an arguable proposition, given the extraordinary concentration of soldiers and civilians along the four-hundred-mile western front. But luck—and Nicolle's warning about the danger of lice—deserves some of the credit.[11]

TYPHOID

The wartime victory over typhoid fever was more complete, and almost entirely the result of vaccination. In the final decades of the nineteenth century, German researchers had identified the bacterial subspecies responsible for the disease. British bacteriologist Almroth Wright then experimented with a heat-killed version of this bacteria and in 1896 developed the first vaccine against typhoid. The methodology wasn't new, but typhoid was a worthy target. It often required hospitalization, and commonly killed 10 to 20 percent of victims.

Unlike typhus, typhoid was all too familiar in the cities and suburbs of Western Europe and North America. It spread through fecal contamination of water or food. The 1907 case of "Typhoid Mary" Mallon, a cook with asymptomatic typhoid, served as a notorious reminder of the everyday risk of infection. Mallon, who acknowledged that she almost never washed her hands, was implicated in spreading the infection to seven of the eight New York City–area families for whom she cooked, resulting in at least three deaths. Later, after being released from isolation, she returned to cooking under a false name, again spreading the disease through the hotels and restaurants where she worked.

Recent events had also painfully alerted the military to the threat of typhoid from poor sanitation: the Spanish-American War lasted less than four months in 1898, but one-fifth of US troops were put out of action by typhoid fever and 1,500 died—many times more than in combat. The disease proved equally devastating for British troops in South Africa during the Boer War, from 1899 to 1902. Wright, a professor at the Royal Army Medical College, won permission from the British Army to offer his new vaccine on a voluntary basis to soldiers heading off to that war, and his disciples worked hard to win recruits to the procedure. "The doctors lecture in the saloon," wrote Winston Churchill, a reporter aboard a troop ship bound for South Africa. "Wonderful statistics are quoted in support of the experiment. Nearly everyone is convinced. The operations take place forthwith, and the next day sees haggard forms crawling about the deck in extreme discomfort and high fever." The vaccine was still relatively crude, and severe reactions were common. "The day after, however, all have recovered and rise gloriously immune." Churchill held back, but joked that he would happily submit to "a system of inoculation against bullet wounds."[12]

In fact, immunity against typhoid proved elusive at first. Most of the 8,022 British soldiers who died of typhoid over the course of the war were unvaccinated. But some who had completed the two-course vaccination nonetheless also came down with what appeared to be typhoid fever, and some died of it. Part of the problem was that Wright's vaccine at that point protected only against typhoid. But an equally dreadful cousin, paratyphoid, was also present in South Africa. Some vaccine lots may also have been produced at too high a temperature, or been stored improperly, rendering them ineffective.

Wright's record-keeping was too careless to make a convincing case that his vaccine had done much to reduce the loss. His abrasive personality also hurt the cause. In public, he was "erratic and disputatious," according to medical historian Anne Hardy, "known and disliked for (among other things) his attitude to women and his opposition to women's suffrage." To adversaries, he became "Sir Almost Right."[13]

Other physicians in Britain and the United States soon improved his vaccine, reducing its toxicity and adding protection against paratyphoid. They conducted careful studies to demonstrate safety and effectiveness. The United States Army, badly stung by the disease in 1898, made typhoid vaccination mandatory in 1911, and it documented a dramatic decline in peacetime incidence of the disease. When the war began, one eminent British physician wrote that sending soldiers to the front without the typhoid vaccination was "little short of murder." Even so, the British military made typhoid vaccination voluntary for soldiers going overseas.

Britain had just reversed its policy of compulsory smallpox vaccination of infants, under pressure from antivaccination protesters. That controversy may have influenced the Army's decision. But after sharp early losses to typhoid, almost all British troops in France had rolled up their sleeves for the vaccine by 1915. Over the entire war, the British Expeditionary Force counted just 1,191 deaths from typhoid or paratyphoid disease, a fraction of the 8,022 killed by these diseases in the Boer War—though ten times as many soldiers were in the field, in far worse conditions.[14]

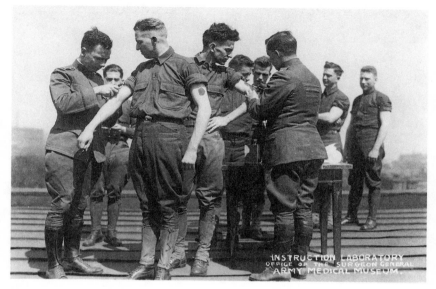

Figure 25.1
American soldiers take part in a vaccination exercise (National Museum of Health and Medicine).

The wartime success against typhoid would have a dramatic effect in peacetime: soldiers who survived to return home would spread the word about new medical treatments and help ease public acceptance of other vaccines, beginning in 1921 with the first vaccine against diphtheria and continuing with vaccines against whooping cough, polio, and a steadily expanding list of other deadly infectious diseases.

Whether these new treatments shaped the outcome of the war is, however, debatable. Medical advances "meant that the time-honored link between war and epidemic disease was broken in 1914," according to historian Jay Winter. It stayed broken through 1917, freeing soldiers from the old, random mortality by clotted lungs and open bowels, instead keeping them alive for the more purposeful business of killing and being killed by mustard gas, machine gun, and cannon fire. The great epoch of medical discoveries may thus have inadvertently made the misery of the trenches more bearable and the brutality of modern warfare more sustainable.[15]

26 A PATHOGEN TOO FAR

In 1918, epidemic disease and war once again embraced with all their old passion. The deadly pandemic begun that year became known as the Spanish flu because Spain was a neutral country, and its press was the first to report the devastating outbreak. The warring countries meanwhile suppressed the news, leaving their citizens unprepared. This flu was particularly terrifying because it spread so easily and because it concentrated its venom on the young. (Their elders may have acquired immunity from exposure to a previous flu outbreak.) It filled up its victims' lungs with fluid, and the desperate hunger for air turned their skin blue as they suffocated.

The first of three waves hit soldiers in France early in 1918. But the flu soon spread from there, in two subsequent and far more virulent waves, to sicken soldiers and civilians almost everywhere. Over the course of two years, it infected an estimated five hundred million people worldwide, a quarter to a third of the human population, and killed fifty million of them, with most of the dead between twenty and forty years of age. (By comparison, the COVID-19 pandemic has infected about six hundred twenty million people at this writing—well under 10 percent of the current human population.)

In most fatal cases, the immediate cause of death was pneumonia, marked by an abundance of *Streptococcus*, *Staphylococcus*, and other bacteria. But something else seemed to be preparing the way for these common microbes to proliferate. As a later physician put it, "The specific virus ploughs the land and the secondary bacteria germinate in the furrows."[1]

A half century of germ theory and triumphant bacteriology led almost everyone to suspect a bacterial, not a viral, pathogen. In fact, they suspected one specific bacterial pathogen. *Haemophilus influenzae* was also known as Pfeiffer's bacillus, for Richard Pfeiffer, a researcher at the Robert Koch Institute, who had identified it as the cause of an 1889–1890 influenza pandemic. Pfeiffer's indictment of this bacillus went largely unquestioned for a quarter century, until the bodies started to pile up in 1918. Researchers around the world then searched desperately for *H. influenzae* in victims of the new pandemic, with little success. Pfeiffer himself admitted that he could find it in only about half of flu victims. Other scientists found it but couldn't get it to produce flu even when sprayed as a pure culture into the respiratory tracts of monkeys and human test subjects.

GOING VIRAL

The failure of Pfeiffer's bacillus—the failure of bacteriology—led some researchers to think back twenty years to a different and still relatively obscure line of microbial research. In 1898, a Dutch microbiologist named Martinus Beijerinck (1851–1931) was studying a disease of tobacco plants. Beijerinck took an extract from plants infected with tobacco mosaic and put it through a Chamberland filter to screen out bacteria and other contaminants. With the filtered extract, he infected other plants, then took filtered extracts from those plants and infected still other plants, and so on in a series. Unlike the diphtheria toxin that Roux had extracted with a Chamberland filter, this "contagium" could reproduce itself, but only within the tissue of living organisms. Beijerinck thought the contagium consisted of nothing more than dissolved molecules. So how to explain its reproductive capabilities? He concluded that it "must be incorporated into the living protoplasm of the cell, into whose reproduction it is, in a manner of speaking, passively drawn." This must have seemed to his contemporaries like a wildly improbable speculation. In fact, though, it fits remarkably well with the modern understanding of how a virus reproduces. What may also seem wildly improbable was that Beijerinck developed this first good description of a virus within a short walk of where Antoni van Leeuwenhoek had seen and described the first known bacteria. Thus Delft secured its place, over a distance of more than two hundred years, as the cradle of microbiology.[2]

That same year, a German team led by Friedrich Loeffler, who had previously discovered the bacterial agent of diphtheria, used filtration to identify the first animal virus, for foot-and-mouth disease. And in 1901 in Cuba, Americans James Carroll (1854–1907) and Walter Reed (1851–1902) demonstrated that the agent of yellow fever remained infectious after passing through a bacteria-proof filter, making it the first known human disease caused by a virus. (This was a footnote to their previous work demonstrating that yellow fever, like malaria, was a mosquito-borne disease.) By 1906, at least eighteen such pathogens affecting plants, animals, or humans were known. Contemporaries called them *filter-passing*, or *filterable*, *pathogens*, or increasingly just *viruses*. But it would be years before anybody could see one or describe one morphologically or chemically. Virology meantime remained clouded in confusion and doubt.[3]

The 1918 pandemic pushed researchers to look more closely and think much harder about this new science. Different research groups began to apply their Chamberland filters to samples from flu victims. Charles Nicolle and Charles Lebailly at the Pasteur Institute in Tunisia were the first to report success, in October 1918, after using filtered sputum from a flu victim to pass the disease to two volunteer test subjects. In Germany, two researchers tested a filtrate from a flu victim on themselves, with unknown results; and in Flanders, a British researcher died while experimenting with a filtrate. In Japan, researchers exposed twenty-four volunteers—"our friends, doctors and nurses"—to the flu, some with an emulsion of fluids straight from victims of the pandemic, others with a filtered extract. Six who had recovered from the flu showed no signs of a recurrence. The other eighteen, who were new to the disease, all came down with flu, in some cases with "very severe" symptoms. The filtered extract was equal to the emulsion as a source of contagion.[4]

Skepticism persisted, however, with some critics still arguing well after the war that "the invisible virus concept" was little more than a ruse to absolve "the discoverers from the necessity of producing evidence of a characteristic microbe." When a few researchers attempted to develop a flu vaccine in 1918, they worked instead with attenuated bacteria. Older defensive measures—quarantine and closures of schools, churches, movie theaters, and restaurants—proved more effective in bringing the pandemic to a close. That, and what may be the oldest measure: by 1920, almost all potential victims had acquired immunity by surviving the flu—or dying.[5]

The pandemic launched medical thinking in a dramatically new direction over the next decade and, indeed, for the remainder of the twentieth century. Having been routed by influenza, medical researchers now regrouped to address the puzzle of filter-passing viruses. "There could hardly be a set of problems whose solution has more potential importance for the community than this," the secretary of the British Medical Research Council declared in 1922, noting that "in a few months in 1918–1919 [flu] killed more persons in India than had died from the plague there during the previous twenty years." It was the beginning of a major initiative to apply "new technical methods of investigation" to viruses.[6]

Other developed nations also pursued viral research, and by 1927, a Rockefeller Institute researcher could list close to one hundred diseases thought to be viral, though he allowed plenty of room for subtractions from this list, on the reasonable assumption that some would later turn out to be caused by very small bacteria or protozoa. Among those affecting humans, the list correctly included smallpox, chicken pox, herpes, encephalitis, yellow fever, dengue, polio, rabies, mumps, measles, rubella, the common cold, and influenza.

The questions about viruses that were still outstanding seem like the ones we would ask on encountering a featureless but disturbingly forceful presence from some distant planet: What does it look like? Can it mutate? Is it alive? And always the one the pandemic had put in the front of peoples' minds: Will it kill us? Getting the answers would be difficult. Viruses were obligate parasites—that is, totally dependent on living cells. Researchers trying to study them struggled with the challenge of keeping them alive outside a host species.[7]

The British effort focused on canine distemper as an animal model for influenza, using dogs and later ferrets as experimental animals. By 1927, they were testing a distemper vaccine in a two-shot sequence, first with the killed virus, then with the live virus. By 1931 it was available commercially—for dogs. "Is it too much to ask," the *Times* (London) wondered, peevishly, "that

work on similar lines should be undertaken on the cause of influenza? . . .
Has not the time arrived to launch a campaign and to come to grips with
the enemy?"[8]

In fact, researchers were already doing just that. In 1933, at Britain's
National Institute of Medical Research, workers filtered throat washings
from flu patients, used the filtrate to infect ferrets, and identified the culprit
as the influenza A virus. Soon after, a researcher at the Rockefeller Institute
in New York used the same technique to identify a second potential culprit,
influenza B. At Vanderbilt University, researchers devised a way to grow
viruses apart from their normal host species, using fertilized chicken eggs.
Max Theiler (1899–1972), a South African–born researcher at the Rockefeller Foundation in New York, soon put this technique to work developing
an effective live attenuated vaccine against yellow fever. Other researchers
used it to develop and improve the first flu vaccines. Having risen up and
become strong on the bones of the tens of millions lost to the 1918 pandemic, the science of viruses would go on to save hundreds of millions from
premature death in the decades just ahead.

27 MIDNIGHT WORK

On a windy November evening in 1932, two women set out at the end of their normal working day into the streets of Grand Rapids, Michigan. The Great Depression was entering its fourth year. Banks had shut down, and the city's dominant furniture industry had collapsed. Pearl Kendrick and Grace Eldering, biologists for a state laboratory, were putting their free time to use identifying victims during an outbreak of a potentially deadly childhood disease.

"We learned about the disease and the Depression at the same time," Eldering later recalled. "We listened to sad stories told by desperate fathers who could find no work. We collected specimens by the light of kerosene lamps, from whooping, vomiting, strangling children. We saw what the disease could do."[1]

It could seem at first like nothing, a runny nose and a mild cough. A missed diagnosis is common even now: "just a cold, nothing to worry about." After a week or two, though, the coughing can come in violent spasms, too fast for breathing, until the sharp, strangled bark breaks through of the child desperately gasping to get air down her throat. That sound makes the diagnosis unmistakable.

"It's awful, it's awful," says a modern researcher who has seen whooping cough, also known as pertussis. "You wonder how they can survive the crisis. I mean, they're suffocating. They're choking. They become completely blue. They cannot overcome the cough, and you have the impression that the child is dying in your hands." It can go on like that for weeks, or months, and there is nothing much medicine can do to help.[2]

Until the mid-twentieth century, there was also nothing anyone could do to prevent the disease. It was so contagious that one child with whooping cough was likely to infect half his classmates and all his siblings at home. In the 1930s, it killed four thousand Americans on average every year, most of them still infants. Survivors could suffer permanent physical and cognitive impairment.[3]

All that changed because of Kendrick and Eldering, now largely forgotten. Their day job was to conduct routine testing of medical and environmental samples. But whooping cough became their obsession. They worked on it late into the night, without funding at first, but supported by the state laboratory's research team, which was remarkably diverse for that era in race, gender, and even sexual orientation. They also enlisted the trust and enthusiasm of their community.

Medical men with better credentials were deeply skeptical. But where other researchers had failed repeatedly over the previous thirty years, Kendrick, Eldering, and their team succeeded in developing the first reliably effective whooping cough vaccine. Childhood deaths from whooping cough soon plummeted in the United States, and then the world.

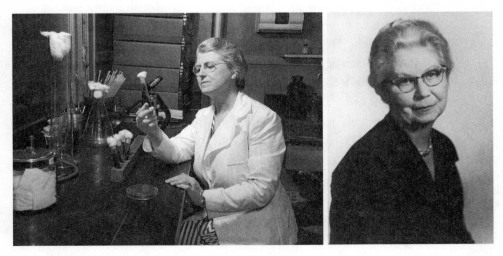

Figure 27.1
Pearl Kendrick (left) and Grace Eldering (right) were among the early recruits as public health laboratories began hiring women researchers. They soon devised a vaccine to stop a disease that killed thousands of children every year (Grand Rapids Public Library).

COUGH PLATES

Pearl Kendrick (1890–1980), raised in upstate New York, went on to earn her degree in science from Syracuse University. Educational opportunities for women had been expanding for decades, but job opportunities did not necessarily follow. For a time, Kendrick became a schoolteacher and principal in upstate New York, the expected career path for an educated woman then, preferably leading to marriage. The conventional attitude, as one medical educator put it in 1922, was that "education enhances womanly charm, attractiveness and fitness for domestic happiness."[4]

Public health was one of the few scientific areas that had begun to seek out educated women. The success of infectious disease control in World War I had opened minds to the possibilities for improving public health at home. Much of the new work fell to state departments of health. Their laboratories needed staff to bring new diagnostic tests, vaccines, and other preventive measures into routine use. Men with public health training gravitated to the prestige and higher pay of jobs in universities or research institutions. State laboratories, offering lower wages, less status, and mostly repetitious work, needed women.

Kendrick spent the summer of 1917 studying bacteriology at Columbia University. She worked briefly as a laboratory assistant in New York. Then Michigan's enterprising director of state laboratories recruited her, promising to "make it interesting" and "with every chance for advancement." He was true to his word. When the Michigan Department of Health opened a laboratory in Grand Rapids in 1926, Kendrick became its first director. In 1932, on leave from her job, Kendrick completed her doctorate in science from Johns Hopkins University. She returned to Grand Rapids determined to study a single disease. When Kendrick asked her male boss for permission to work after closing time on the city's whooping cough outbreak, he replied, "Go ahead and do all you can with pertussis, if it amuses you."[5]

Grace Eldering (1900–1988) had graduated from the University of Montana, and then worked as a schoolteacher in Hysham, Montana, the ranching and farming community where she grew up. Teaching did not hold her interest. Instead, in 1928 she became a volunteer and then a paid employee at the Michigan state laboratory in Lansing, later transferring to

Grand Rapids to work on pertussis. There, she and Kendrick became lifelong partners, at work and at home.

In the beginning, the main goal of their research was to diagnose pertussis faster and more accurately so that contagious patients could be isolated as early as possible, and safely returned to school or work when the contagious stage ended. Their weapon of choice was the *cough plate*, basically a petri dish with the culture medium painted on the bottom. Doctors, nurses—and Kendrick and Eldering, too, after working hours—held up the open dish a few inches away while the patient coughed into it. The dish, covered with a lid, then went into an incubator, to grow the bacteria into colonies suitable for analysis.

On November 28, 1932, Kendrick and Eldering identified their first *Bordetella pertussis* specimen. The bacterium that causes whooping cough had been known since Belgian researchers first described it in 1906, but no one in the laboratory had seen it before. They had to compare the ones on their cough plate against published accounts. The bacterial colonies, they reported, "appear smooth, raised, glistening, pearly, and almost transparent," encircled by a pale halo where the bacteria had eaten into the blood in the culture medium.

Kendrick and Eldering devised a series of improvements to grow bacterial colonies quickly and in quantity. Instead of using human blood in the culture medium, as other scientists had done for much smaller studies, they turned to sheep blood because it was less expensive and more readily available in the volumes they needed. They soon expanded their study into an ambitious citywide cough plate service for monitoring and controlling whooping cough.

MIDNIGHT WORK

Developing a vaccine for any disease was still a rudimentary, cooking-without-recipes enterprise. It meant experimenting with a long list of variables, leading to a killed or weakened pathogen that was safe enough to inject into human patients and yet strong enough to elicit lasting immune resistance to the disease. Adverse effects, from sore arms to anaphylactic shock, were common. But people accepted the risks because they still had vivid experience of how much deadlier it was to experience the actual disease. In 1931, however, the American Medical Association declined to endorse any of the existing pertussis vaccines, concluding that they had "absolutely no influence" on prevention and were "useless" as remedies after onset of the disease.

In January 1933, just seven weeks after their first glimpse of the pathogen, Kendrick and Eldering produced their first experimental pertussis vaccine. It consisted of whole-cell *Bordetella* bacteria killed with a common antiseptic, purified, sterilized, and suspended in a saline solution. Others who had developed similar vaccines before them often neglected to provide critical information on preparation, dosage, and other considerations, with the result that one batch could vary wildly from the next. Kendrick and Eldering took a far more systematic approach, at every step, from collecting the bacteria to delivering the vaccine. They learned as they went—for instance, that bacteria collected at a certain stage in the illness were more likely to elicit a strong immune response—and they tested various versions of the vaccine for safety by injecting them into experimental animals, and themselves.

They had no prior experience with clinical trials, which were practically a new science then. But testing whether their vaccine protected children would require a large-scale, controlled field study—comparing a group of vaccinated test subjects against a similar, but untreated, control group. The trial would have to be part of what Kendrick called "our midnight work," after business hours.

Grand Rapids then was a leader in putting medical advances to work saving lives. The city government and private donors stepped forward to cover the clinical trial's cost of $1,250 over the first two years. Doctors, nurses, and ordinary city residents rallied to help. Mothers volunteered not just their time, but also their children's well-being as experimental subjects.

After a vaccination clinic, the two researchers waited in dread for a call about a bad reaction, beyond the usual mild fever. "I felt scared to death most of the time," Kendrick later admitted. But that call seems never to have come. In the first round of the field study, 1,600 children took part, 712 of them vaccinated, and 880 as untreated controls. In the untreated group, there were sixty-three cases of whooping cough, all but ten of them serious. Among the vaccinated children, only four cases occurred, all of them mild.

The medical establishment didn't believe it. James Doull, an epidemiologist at Case Western University in Cleveland, had completed a similar study using a different vaccine and had shown no real benefit from vaccination. When public health leaders asked Johns Hopkins epidemiologist Wade Hampton Frost to review the conflicting results and make a recommendation, he seemed interested at first mainly in avoiding a trip to Michigan. "I very strongly suspect that Miss Kendrick's field studies are not set up in such a way as to give a really good control," he wrote. Getting it right was hard even for specialists in clinical testing, and "the odds are strongly against Miss Kendrick's experiment being sound."[6]

Frost ended up visiting Grand Rapids despite himself. There, he soon came to appreciate Kendrick and Eldering's commitment to careful science. He recommended improvements in the design of their clinical trial, and the two women went back to work. Their new study would require a larger staff to follow patients over a period of years. This time they enlisted the help of First Lady Eleanor Roosevelt, who visited the laboratory on a busy 1936 tour of Grand Rapids. She was one of the few outsiders who seemed to understand what they were doing, Kendrick said, and funding soon followed from the federal Works Progress Administration. The new study attracted 4,200 test subjects, and the vaccinated group again experienced whooping cough at a dramatically lower rate than their unvaccinated counterparts. The same protective effect showed up in an independent clinical trial of the vaccine in New York State.

In 1944, the American Medical Association added Kendrick and Eldering's vaccine to its list of recommended immunizations. As a result, incidence of the disease in the United States fell by more than half just in that decade. Deaths dropped from 7,518 in 1934, the peak year for pertussis, to just ten a year by the early 1970s. Other countries, from Mexico to Russia, introduced the vaccine with similar success.[7]

To minimize the "pincushion effect" of giving so many shots in the early years of a child's life, Kendrick and Eldering worked on a combined diphtheria, tetanus, and pertussis vaccine, a forerunner of the DTaP/Tdap vaccine that now routinely protects 85 percent of the world's children. They also developed what has become the required method for testing the effectiveness of every batch of whole-cell pertussis vaccine worldwide. In place of the hodgepodge, cooking-without-recipes past, these women made whooping cough prevention standardized, reliable, and reproducible—in a word, scientific.

"What did Kendrick and Eldering really do?" asks Michael Decker, a pertussis specialist at Vanderbilt University Medical Center. "They persevered in their belief that a successful vaccine could be made. They figured out how to make it. They engineered a clinical trial using novel techniques to prove their point. And in the face of intense criticism from people of high standing, they showed that their results were correct. They basically laid the pathway for modern pertussis vaccination."

MODESTY

It may seem surprising that such monumental achievements did not make Kendrick and Eldering famous. But they never meant the work to be about them, according to Carolyn Shapiro-Shapin, a historian at Grand Valley State University, who began researching the two women in the 1990s. Their vaccine was the product of "a whole community working together," in her phrase, and they liked it that way.

One part of that community was an African-American woman named Loney Clinton Gordon. She had come to Grand Rapids in the early 1940s seeking work at a local hospital as an experienced dietitian. It didn't go well, she recalled in a 1998 interview with Shapiro-Shapin. Prospective employers praised her credentials, but then added, "we just don't think chefs would want to take orders from you." Word reached Kendrick, who phoned to offer a job.

Gordon was soon at work sorting through "piles of cultures" every morning. One pertussis strain could be up to ten thousand times more virulent than another, and finding the right strain was crucial to improving the vaccine. "Every day I worked so hard. Millions of plates. It's a wonder I still have eyes." One day, she went in and "started looking, and all of a sudden here was a plate. My God, it was so big and so clear," she recalled, describing the halo where the bacteria had eaten into the blood in the surrounding culture medium. "It just talked to me. 'Here I am.'" Gordon took the plate to Kendrick and Eldering, who put it through "all of these processes, repeated and repeated and repeated," to see if it met their criteria for a better vaccine, "and, *bingo*, there it was." No other record of Gordon's contribution exists. But like others who remembered working in the lab, she mainly expressed gratitude at having been part of the work of saving lives.[8]

"All these medical breakthroughs are a result of the work of many persons," Eldering later told a reporter, who wondered why their vaccine hadn't become known as the Kendrick-Eldering vaccine, on the model of the Salk vaccine for polio. "We disapproved of that notion because there were just too many people involved and we didn't want the sole credit. You'd have to put a whole string of names on the vaccine." They also preferred to remain private. In the 1970s, when the feminist movement was shining a light on women's overlooked contributions, an invitation arrived for Kendrick and Eldering to appear on NBC's *Today* show. They politely declined.[9]

Given the gender politics of their era, modesty may have seemed obligatory. In college, Kendrick once told a reporter, she had gotten male science faculty to take her seriously and provide the instruction she needed by acting "as humble as I could be." Managing feelings and emotional displays in this fashion could easily become a career strategy. When a student once asked, "Were you discriminated against?" as a woman in a male-dominated medical world, Kendrick answered, "If so, I didn't recognize it." Focusing on the work at hand, she explained, "kept me from worrying if I was getting [paid] as much as my friend John, say, who was working beside me—though I knew very well I wasn't."

With Kendrick, though, the determination also showed through. "I never thought there was anything I couldn't do," she once told a reporter. She was talking about a time in college when she had to organize meal service for seventy-five fellow students during a two-week Christmas break. The point was that she was single-minded about whatever she took on. That determination also showed up outside of work. Shirley Redland, Eldering's niece, recalls visiting the two women as a child and sitting in the back seat of the car, wide-eyed, when Kendrick was at the wheel: she had a "heavy foot, and people better get out of her way."[10]

From the 1930s on, Kendrick and Eldering shared a comfortable four-bedroom house in an old apple orchard, on a hilltop overlooking the city. It was common for single working women to live together then, to eke out systematically meagre salaries, and the arrangement raised no eyebrows in Grand Rapids. They shared the same outside interests, in reading, gardening, and bird-watching. They kept cats and dogs. They owned a summer cabin on Lake Michigan, often traveled together, and clearly cared for each other. After Eldering lost a finger while attempting to repair an air conditioner at work, it was Kendrick who stitched down that finger on her gloves. "They had a wonderful life together," Redland recalls. "I don't think there was ever a harsh word."

Were they more than devoted friends? At one point in her research, Shapiro-Shapin was interviewing a chemist named Lucile Portwood, who had worked in the laboratory in the 1940s. She asked about the relationship, and Portwood, who was then eighty and near-deaf, "yelled into my tape recorder, 'I'm a lesbian and I would have known if those gals were up to something.'" In any case, Kendrick and Eldering would have considered it nobody's business but their own.[11]

THE PREVENTION PARADOX

There is another reason history has largely ignored two such important medical pioneers. It has to do with the paradoxical nature of prevention: When a vaccine or some other healthcare measure largely eliminates a disease from people's lives, the vaccine itself can become a target because real or imagined adverse effects may now seem worse than the forgotten disease. That happened to Kendrick and Eldering's whole-cell pertussis vaccine in the 1970s. It caused fever and injection site reactions, and in rare cases temporary neurological problems. Anti-vaxxers also accused it of more serious adverse effects, though a scientific review debunked most of these accusations. The vaccine was steadily improved over time and was always infinitely safer than risking the disease. But public confidence in it was shaken.

A stripped-down *acellular vaccine*—basically just three or four of the original three thousand or so antigens—soon replaced the whole-cell vaccine in the United States and some other developed nations. The acellular vaccine has, however, recently turned out to provide strong protection for only a few years. Together with increasing vaccine hesitancy, that shorter period of effectiveness has contributed to a whooping cough resurgence in the United States. Undervaccination in poorer countries has also allowed whooping cough to persist there, killing an estimated 160,000 people each year, mostly children. The death toll is likely to get worse: in 2020, an estimated twenty-three million children missed out on their pertussis vaccinations, largely due to disruptions caused by the COVID-19 pandemic.

An answer to these problems may soon be available. Molecular biologist Camille Locht, a devoted admirer of Kendrick and Eldering at the Pasteur Institute in Lille, France, has developed a new whole-cell vaccine. It will of course be different from theirs—made with live bacteria that are genetically altered to render them harmless, and not injected in the arm, but sprayed into the nose. In addition to being easier to administer and avoiding needle fear, it needs no refrigeration, all advantages in remote and impoverished areas. If all goes well, it could become available by 2025.

Meanwhile, the current descendant of Kendrick and Eldering's vaccine continues to save lives in countries around the world. After Kendrick's death in 1980, a colleague estimated that the vaccine had prevented hundreds of thousands of premature deaths in the United States alone. It is probably in the tens of millions by now worldwide. "Who are the men and women living today who would be dead from whooping cough had it not been for Pearl Kendrick's vaccine?" he wondered in a memorial note. "Name one. You can't do it and neither can I. . . . The accomplishments of disease prevention are statistical and epidemiological. Where's the news value, the human interest in that?"

News value of course had little meaning for Kendrick and Eldering. They wanted only to save children's lives. Having accomplished that, they were content to be forgotten. But we should remember.

28 THE ANTIBACTERIAL REVOLUTION

In December 1943, British Prime Minister Winston Churchill was homeward bound across North Africa after a series of meetings with world leaders in the Middle East. He was sixty-nine years old, tired, overweight, an avid drinker and smoker with a bad heart. Now, as his Avro York transport landed in Tunisia, he had a nasty case of pneumonia. His heart went into fibrillation. Doctors were unsure they could save him.[1]

Churchill was hardly an ideal patient. He agreed to lay off cigars but continued to see visitors and do business. What followed, despite the patient, was a triumph of modern medicine—and also propaganda. British newspapers enshrined the new wonder drug penicillin as the prime minister's savior, and their reports grew into legend: When Churchill was a boy, the story went, a man had saved him from drowning, prompting Churchill's grateful father to pay for the man's son to attend medical school. That son, Alexander Fleming, had in turn discovered the penicillin that supposedly saved Churchill's life.[2]

In fact, Churchill had experienced no near drowning in his youth. The Churchills and Flemings were not acquainted. And what cured the prime minister's pneumonia wasn't even penicillin. Instead, as he publicly declared soon after, he was saved by "this admirable M & B"—a sulfa (or sulfonamide) drug manufactured in England by May & Baker Ltd. The mythmaking about penicillin was perhaps understandable. The new wonder drug was a British innovation (with considerable American help), while sulfa drugs had originated in Germany. But sulfa drugs were in fact the first great breakthrough of the twentieth-century revolution in antibacterial medicine.[3]

The real story began with Paul Ehrlich's fascination with the way different dyes selectively stain different biological structures. It led him to think that the dyes themselves might have therapeutic value against specific pathogens. Alternatively, it might be possible to attach a toxic substance for the dye to carry to the pathogen. This hadn't worked with his drug against sleeping sickness, and the success of Salvarsan had distracted him from further attempts at turning dyes into drugs. But Ehrlich's thinking strongly influenced his many followers in the German pharmaceutical industry.

In the late 1920s, researchers at a facility in Elberfeld, Germany, began to explore the therapeutic possibilities of azo dyes, synthetic compounds that had become important colorants in the textile industry. The researchers' employer was a conglomerate of major chemical companies joined together under the unwieldy name Interessengemeinschaft Farbenindustrie Aktiengesellschaft (roughly translated as the Dye Industry Syndicate, Inc.). But it was far better known by a name that would become notorious in the aftermath of World War II: IG Farben.

In the 1920s and early 1930s, IG Farben was widely envied for its highly productive system of pharmaceutical invention. Heinrich Hörlein, a skilled chemist, oversaw a carefully integrated network of seven research laboratories in the conglomerate's Bayer division. He functioned as a sort of military strategist surveying "the field where chemistry and medicine joined battle against disease," according to historian John E. Lesch in his 2007 book *The First Miracle Drugs*. "He could spot the points where the enemy's line was broken, and the reverse salients in his own"—that is, the areas where research and development lagged behind the general line of advance. He knew how to marshal his resources accordingly. One such "reverse salient" was the failure to produce safe and effective chemical therapies against bacterial infections. Ehrlich's chemotherapy had succeeded thus far mainly against diseases caused by protozoa, with new drugs for malaria, trypanosomes, and kala-azar, an often-fatal form of leishmaniasis. But doctors were still helpless against major bacterial killers like pneumonia, tuberculosis, dysentery, and childbed fever.[4]

Hörlein set out in the late 1920s to change that. IG Farben had already succeeded in synthesizing the first successful means, other than quinine, of preventing and treating malaria in humans. Atabrine, as it became known, was based on yellow acridine dyes, helping to fuel optimism that azo (or azobenzene) dyes might be next to yield powerful new therapies, this time against bacterial pathogens. Other researchers had already detected signs that these dyes might have some effect on bacteria. The challenge was to make the effect powerful and precise enough, without also amplifying toxicity.[5]

Chemist Josef Klarer (1898–1953) did much of the work devising novel compounds around the basic azo dye molecule. This was a like working on a bicycle frame, according to writer Thomas Hager: "A chemist as talented as Klarer could easily change the wheels and gears, customize the handlebars and seat, add a cart in back or a basket in front, make a thousand variations on the core structure." Klarer spun out so many compounds in this fashion that he had a rubber stamp made for the core azo structure, then sketched in the variations for each new compound by hand. Chemist Fritz Mietzsch (1896–1958) sat at a neighboring laboratory bench and the two regularly shared their thinking about different compounds. Gerhard Domagk (1895–1964), a pathologist, tested their new compounds against bacteria. His laboratory notebooks were, however, largely a chronicle of failure, recording tests of different compounds by different means against different targets, usually followed by the words *ohne Wirkung*, or just *oW*, meaning "without effect."[6]

COLOR BLINDED

The breakthrough came in September 1932, when Hörlein or one of the others thought back almost a quarter century to research at Bayer that made azo dye coloring in textiles more durable by attaching sulfur side-chains. Why not try the same variation against bacteria? Really, it's a wonder the idea had not occurred sooner: Hörlein himself had been lead author of that 1909 study, on his first assignment at Bayer. As a result, Mietzsch and Klarer soon sent the sulfonamide azo compound KL695 to Domagk, who tested it against *Streptococcus* bacteria from a human patient with sepsis.

In vitro testing produced the usual *ohne Wirkung*, without effect. But when Domagk went on to in vivo testing in mice, KL695 proved strikingly successful against streptococcal infection. On Christmas Day, 1932, IG Farben applied for a patent on KL695. While researchers elsewhere remained mired in the "general atmosphere of caution and resignation" about antibacterial chemotherapy, Lesch wrote, the Bayer/IG Farben system of "industrialized invention" and its "robust optimism" about turning dyes into drugs had triumphed. The company would eventually market the first sulfa drug under the trade name Prontosil.[7]

But not quite yet. Over the next two years and three months, the researchers cranked out a thousand variations on KL695, by Hörlein's estimate, and performed "tens of thousands of experiments" on different bacterial infections. Clinical testing also began, though by modern standards it was haphazard. The results suggested considerable success against a broad range of streptococcal infections, particularly using a variation called KL730. On February 15, 1935, an article by Domagk announced the discovery of a drug with "the best chemotherapeutic effect in streptococcus infections in animals that we have ever seen." Experimental mice given ten times the streptococcal dose needed to kill them within twenty-four hours and then promptly treated with an oral dose of Prontosil showed no signs of illness. Bayer began selling its new drug for treatment in humans a few months later.[8]

There was one hitch, from the perspective of Bayer/IG Farben profits: Tipped off about the new drug by publication of the company's French patent in 1934, researchers at the Pasteur Institute had quickly gone to work. In November 1935, they published their startling analysis. It was the sulfa side-chain, not the azo dye, that made Prontosil effective. To prove it, the Pasteur team stripped away the azo framework and achieved cures in animal experiments using the sulfa compound alone. Bayer also held the patent on the sulfa compound, but it was now expired, freeing anyone to produce sulfa drugs without payment. Moreover, the raw materials were cheap, and sulfa drugs were easy to manufacture.[9]

The reason Prontosil had failed during in vitro testing but succeeded in vivo, the Pasteur team explained, was simple: in the guts of humans and other animals, digestion flushed away the useless azo dye framework and liberated the sulfa to do its antibacterial work. Paul Ehrlich's great dream—the "myth and fascination of color"—had given the German researchers confidence to achieve a great cure for bacterial infections. But along the way, it had also kept them from understanding what it was they were achieving. Decades later, a chemist who had participated in the Pasteur analysis confessed continuing astonishment that research "based on an erroneous hypothesis" could have yielded such "technically impeccable results." It was the conundrum at the heart of a massively beneficial transformation in human health.[10]

BRINGING HOME THE BENEFITS

For Gerhard Domagk, the success with Prontosil soon unexpectedly turned personal. On December 4, 1935, his six-year-old daughter Hildegard fell while coming downstairs to bring her mother a sewing needle for some Christmas handicrafts. The needle penetrated her hand, eye-end first, and broke off in her wrist. After surgery, the entire length of her arm became swollen. Dizziness and fever indicated systemic infection. The surgeon thought the only hope was to amputate her arm. But Domagk determined that the infection was streptococcal and asked for permission to begin administering Prontosil. The child's fever began to abate that same night, and Hildegard soon returned home with her arm intact.[11]

The world beyond Elberfeld did not at first recognize that a great revolution in infectious disease treatment had begun. But in June 1936, the *Lancet* published an account of experiments with Prontosil at Queen Charlotte's Maternity Hospital in London. Bacteriologist Leonard Colebrook and obstetrician Méave Kenny had administered the drug to thirty-eight maternity patients with severe puerperal fever caused by the same pathogen Domagk had used in his experimental mice. The researchers couched their first report in cautious terms, but also marveled at "the spectacular remission of fever and symptoms observed in so many of the cases."

Only three of the women died, a fatality rate of eight percent—compared with a 26.3 percent death rate in the thirty-eight women treated at the same hospital immediately before arrival of the new drug. By the time the authors had treated sixty-four patients with Prontosil, the death rate was down to

4.7 percent. In one memorable case, a Mrs. S. was admitted three days after delivering her first child, "very gravely ill" and with a high fever. Her blood sample cultured *Streptococcus* bacteria at a rate of five thousand colonies per cubic centimeter—that is, in a volume roughly equal to a small sugar cube. In her entire blood stream, this translated to about thirty million bacterial colonies. But on the fourth day of treatment with Prontosil, her temperature fell back to normal and a blood sample was entirely free of infection. Given that such an intense bacterial load had "never previously been observed by us except in the terminal stages of a fatal infection," Colebrook and Kenny wrote, "this patient's prompt recovery was astonishing." After dutifully listing the caveats, they confessed, "We find it difficult to resist the conclusion that the treatment has profoundly modified the course of the infection" in the most severe cases of childbed fever. The salvation that had eluded so many young mothers seemed finally to have arrived. Three weeks after admission, Mrs. S. went home to her family.[12]

In the United States, the general public, and many physicians, first became aware of the new drugs when the president's son, Franklin Delano Roosevelt Jr., a senior at Harvard, spent Thanksgiving 1936 in Massachusetts General Hospital with a sinus infection. The infection spread to his throat, and he began to cough up blood. On December 17, the case made the front page of the *New York Times*, under the headline, "Young Roosevelt Saved by New Drug." The *Times* reported that he had "faced death" until his doctor administered an oral form of "the new chemo-therapeutic agent to ameliorate the streptococcus infection." The patient was now responding "beautifully," according to the report, and the American distributor of Prontylin, an oral form of the sulfa drug, was already being "besieged" by patients demanding the new "cure." Young Roosevelt then faded from the news, after a reassuring note in late January about his recuperation in Florida, with his fiancée by his side as he landed a forty-pound tarpon after a "20-minute struggle." It was a touching tableau of resilient American manhood and the power of modern medicine.[13]

Demand for sulfa drugs surged in the aftermath, with production for the US market climbing from 350,000 pounds in 1937 to fourteen million pounds in 1942. The effect on public health was dramatic. Sulfa drugs caused deaths in childbirth and from pneumonia to decline by perhaps a third, and from scarlet fever by almost two-thirds, according to a modern comparison of the periods before and after 1937. But the trend in deaths from tuberculosis, which was untreatable with sulfa drugs, remained unchanged over the same period. Overall life expectancy at birth for Americans increased by almost five years from 1936 to 1943, with sulfa drugs as a major contributor to the gain.[14]

THE MESSY AFTERMATH

This astonishing change was taking place across the developed world, and the judges at Sweden's Karolinska Institute were quick to acknowledge it. In October 1939, they awarded the Nobel Prize in Physiology or Medicine to Gerhard Domagk, the lone physician among the discoverers, characteristically omitting any mention of chemists Klarer, Mietzsch, and Hörlein. The prize put Domagk at odds with Adolf Hitler.

Hitler had demonstrated hostility to drug companies from the start. He considered them havens for Jewish scientists, and he thought their discoveries mainly benefited Germany's enemies. He also opposed the animal experimentation on which pharmaceutical development depended. Early on, the chairman of the executive board of IG Farben had visited Hitler and warned him that his virulent anti-Semitism would damage German science and trade. Hitler threw him out in a rage, saying Germany could get by for "one hundred years without physics and chemistry." Hitler also hated the Nobel Prize because the Peace Prize in 1936 had gone to a pacifist writer imprisoned in one of his concentration camps. Thereafter, Germans were forbidden to accept a Nobel. Domagk made the mistake of seeking a way around this ban, and in mid-November Gestapo agents raided his home and carried him off to jail. He was released after a week, arrested again, and finally released after signing what amounted to surrender. It would be 1947 before he was finally able to claim his prize.[15]

For Hörlein, the aftermath of World War II was more complicated. As Hitler secured his hold on the government through the 1930s, IG Farben's opposition had collapsed. It purged its Jewish staff and became a massively profitable contributor to the war effort, employing concentration camp prisoners as slave labor. A subsidiary supplied the concentration camps with Zyklon B, a cyanide gas originally marketed in the 1920s for delousing clothing, ships, trains, and barracks. From 1942 on, Germany used Zyklon B in gas chambers for the mass murder of Jews. Hörlein thus became one of the IG Farben executives tried at Nuremberg as a war criminal, for his role as a member of an administrative committee overseeing a subsidiary that produced Zyklon B, and for having authorized use of slave labor in company factories and criminal experimentation on concentration camp prisoners. Hörlein's lawyers presented evidence that he was not directly aware of the poison gas program. Hörlein himself pointed to the many lives saved by his work, particularly with sulfa drugs and atabrine. He was acquitted, though with one judge dissenting. Hörlein went on to finish his career as a member of the board of directors at Bayer. Heinrich Hörlein Strasse in Leverkusen, where the company is headquartered, now honors him.[16]

One other aftermath of the development of sulfa drugs bears mentioning. These drugs seemed so miraculous in their power to cure diseases that people used them indiscriminately at first—for instance, as a "lightning cure" for gonorrhea. But overuse only served to knock out susceptible pathogens, clearing the field for resistant ones to flourish. Resistant gonorrhea soon became a common problem. The battlefield accomplishments with sulfa drugs were also underwhelming, though the scene of a soldier or medic tearing open a sulfa packet and sprinkling it on a wound would be immortalized in countless World War II films. Reporting on combat use by American soldiers, Colonel Elliott Cutler, the army's chief surgical consultant in the European theater, could not say with confidence that sulfa drugs had actually saved lives. Cutler acknowledged that soldiers themselves had absolute faith in their magic powder. But he also knew that wounded soldiers deserved the psychological and physiological benefits in a single drug.[17]

That drug was already on the way, though with resistant bacteria trailing close behind.

29 PENICILLIN

The antibiotic revolution began with a combination of bad housekeeping and good luck, in the laboratory of Alexander Fleming (1881–1955), a physician and microbiologist at St. Mary's Hospital in London. But the founding event wasn't his accidental 1928 discovery of penicillin, for which he would become famous. Instead, it was a foreshadowing that happened seven years earlier, by the same haphazard means.

Fleming was then about forty years old, "small, with blue eyes, a large head, a bent nose and a broad Ayrshire accent" from his childhood on a farm in the Scottish Lowlands. He led "a comparatively blameless and contented existence," wrote bacteriologist Ronald Hare, who worked with Fleming in the 1920s. He spent weekdays with his wife and one child in a Chelsea flat, and weekends gardening at a country house a few hours northeast of London. "The nearest he got to excitement," Hare wrote, "was a visit to the Chelsea Art Club on the way from the laboratory, before going home to dinner. . . . He was not lazy, but he was never in a hurry. He arrived every morning on the stroke of nine and departed punctually at five. Although taciturn, he liked company. If there was a party to go to, he went and enjoyed himself."[1]

His one arguably unfortunate trait was a tendency to be untidy. He left laboratory dishes painted with various bacterial cultures and bodily fluids to pile up for weeks before he got around to cleaning them. Fleming was otherwise an agreeable workmate, and careful not to offend. At the time of the discovery, he was sharing his office, a turret room twelve feet across, with V. D. Allison, a young bacteriologist.

During one of his irregular bouts of housekeeping, in November 1921, Fleming turned to Allison and remarked, "This is interesting." He held out a plate, Allison recalled, "covered with golden yellow colonies of bacteria," except in one area where they were entirely absent, encircled by a halo where something had made the bacteria "translucent, glassy and lifeless in appearance." In a 1922 paper, Fleming explained that he had prepared the plate during "investigations made on a patient suffering from acute coryza."

Allison put it more plainly: Fleming was studying a "blob of nasal mucus," his own, while suffering from a bad head cold. He had deposited this sample on the lab plate and set it aside. Bacteria of unknown origin had drifted in and proliferated—except around the blob. "Obviously something had diffused from the nasal mucus to prevent the germs from growing near to the mucus," Allison wrote, "and beyond this zone to kill and dissolve bacteria which had already grown."

Fleming called this unknown something a *lysozyme*, a combination of *lysis*, meaning loosening or dissolving, and *enzyme*, meaning a protein that speeds up (or catalyzes) a chemical reaction. Soon after, Fleming prepared a glass with "an opaque yellow suspension" of bacteria and, on introducing fresh nasal mucus, turned the liquid "clear as water." He then repeated this little miracle,

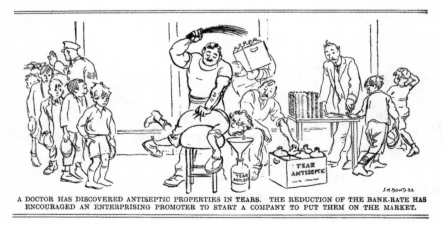

A DOCTOR HAS DISCOVERED ANTISEPTIC PROPERTIES IN TEARS. THE REDUCTION OF THE BANK-RATE HAS ENCOURAGED AN ENTERPRISING PROMOTER TO START A COMPANY TO PUT THEM ON THE MARKET.

Figure 29.1
A 1922 *Punch* cartoon on Alexander Fleming's antibacterial research (Punch Cartoon Library).

but this time, Allison wrote, "A single drop of tears dissolved the germs in less than a minute—it was an astonishing and thrilling moment." Contrary to the common belief that tears, saliva, and other secretions "rid the body of microbes by mechanically washing them away," Fleming wrote, they "have the property of destroying microbes to a very high degree." The immediate response from medical colleagues was indifference. *Punch*, however, took note, publishing a cartoon of boys lining up to be caned, for a small fee, with their tears collected in jars for sale by a "Tear Antiseptic" entrepreneur.[2]

Fleming later discovered penicillin in much the same way. It involved a neglected petri dish full of staphylococci, a chance introduction of a *Penicillium* mold with a highly unusual antibacterial effect, and a resulting zone of inhibited growth in the bacteria. It took an extraordinary series of lucky breaks to make the penicillin discovery happen, including the precise temperature fluctuations needed to give the *Penicillium* a leg up on the bacteria. Despite being "keenly interested" in the discovery, Fleming's "enthusiasm for developing it was minimal," according to chemist and science historian Trevor I. Williams. This may have been due partly to skepticism among British scientists about the potential of chemotherapy against bacteria in those years before the arrival of sulfa drugs.

Fleming may also have been discouraged by the scientific challenge of working with penicillin, which proved highly unstable and difficult to produce in useful quantities or to extract from the mold juice in which it grew. He made a few tentative experiments with topical infections, but failed to pursue the results even when his assistants produced more promising research. "After 1931," Williams wrote, "Fleming's own interest in penicillin lapsed almost entirely; he did nothing, he promoted nothing, he published nothing, and he made no public mention of it." While IG Farben was assiduously turning its misguided pursuit of azo dyes into a miracle cure, Fleming was squandering two of the luckiest breaks in the history of science.[3]

THE BLOODY AUSTRALIAN

The turning point for penicillin came years later, when a terse, plain-talking Australian immigrant named Howard Florey (1898–1968) took note.

Where Fleming was inoffensive, Florey was blunt. It's one thing to "call a spade a spade," a colleague later remarked, but Florey was more likely to call it "a bloody shovel," and the British Medical Association was "that pack of bloody trade unionists." In place of Fleming's contented family life, Florey endured an unhappy marriage. He and his wife Ethel, also a physician, found reason to spend more time at work than at home. But Florey was a thorough scientist, a skillful and at times diplomatic administrator of his department, and, above all, not the sort to squander opportunities.

Florey's own dyspepsia led him to lysozymes. He suffered from abdominal troubles, said to result from his stomach's overproduction of mucus. The functioning of natural products like mucus then became an important part of his research as a pathology professor at Oxford University. In 1938, he hired biochemist Ernst Chain (1906–1979), a Jewish refugee from Nazi Germany, and began a broad study of natural products antagonistic to microbes. They were merely looking to understand how lysozymes and antibacterial inhibition worked, with no expectation of clinical results.[4]

Chain undertook a preliminary literature search and, by good luck, ran across the obscure 1929 paper in which Fleming reported that a *Penicillium* mold produced a bacteria-inhibiting substance he named *penicillin*. Chain thought Fleming had discovered "a sort of mould lysozyme" capable of inhibiting a surprising range of bacteria. He located a specimen of Fleming's *Penicillium* mold at Oxford, left behind by another researcher. Penicillin thus became one of three representative antibacterial substances chosen for detailed study. It would be necessary to extract and purify the penicillin, Chain wrote, "but I did not foresee any undue difficulties with this task."[5]

The job of researchers then as now required what Florey called "shaking a hat in all possible directions" for financial support. He applied for a grant from the government's Medical Research Council, which came through in September 1939 with the grand sum of £25, roughly a quarter of a coal miner's annual wage then. But a Rockefeller Foundation commitment of $5,000 per year for five years was in hand by March 1940. It was the beginning of a gradual shift in the focus of penicillin development—and infectious disease research more generally—to North America.[6]

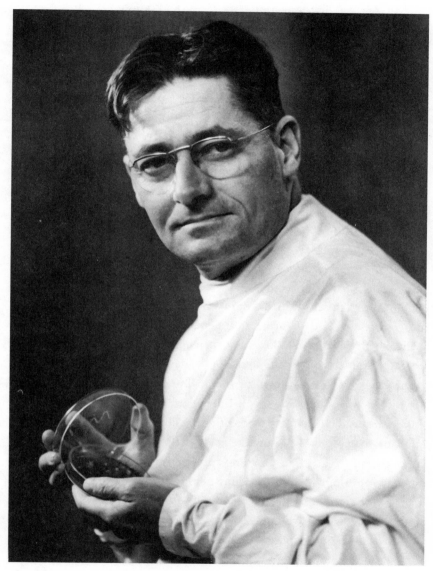

Figure 29.2

The plain-talking Australian Howard Florey turned penicillin from a scientific curiosity into a life-saving antibiotic (University of Adelaide Library, Rare Books and Manuscripts).

Growing the *Penicillium* mold in a liquid medium called *mold juice* and extracting the penicillin proved more difficult than anticipated. Norman Heatley (1911–2004), Florey's research assistant, contributed key breakthroughs. He was a skilled biochemist, with a genius for making fixes with whatever materials happened to lie at hand. To test penicillin samples for effectiveness against various bacteria samples, for instance, Heatley devised the cylinder-plate method, which became standard. It required six or eight tiny glass cylinders standing in a petri dish in which a bacterial sample was growing. A drop of penicillin went into each cylinder, and after incubation Heatley measured how far the zone of bacterial inhibition had spread out around each cylinder. This device enabled the researchers to develop the standard measure of penicillin effectiveness, the Oxford unit.[7]

On Saturday, May 25, 1940, as Hitler's Blitzkrieg was trapping British troops at Dunkirk, Florey was conducting an experiment that must have seemed utterly disconnected from the war effort. At 11:00 a.m., he injected eight white mice with a lethal dose of *Streptococcus* bacteria. Four of the mice, the controls, received no further treatment. Florey injected half the other four with a single dose of ten milligrams of penicillin, and half with a smaller dose repeated at intervals over the course of the day. By 10:00 p.m., when Florey went home, the four control mice were all ill and struggling to breathe. Heatley took up the watch, and by the time he left at 3:30 a.m., all four control mice were dead. The mice treated with penicillin remained healthy. Heatley, jubilant, rode his blacked-out bike home in the dark, singing so loudly that a policeman flagged him down on suspicion of public drunkenness. On Sunday morning, at about the time a hodgepodge flotilla in the English Channel was beginning to evacuate troops from Dunkirk, Florey, Heatley, and Chain returned to the lab. Seeing that the four mice given penicillin had all survived, Chain "danced with excitement." Even Florey acknowledged, "It looks quite promising."[8]

Florey tempered their enthusiasm, however, noting that a man weighs three thousand times more than a mouse. It also became apparent, when the treated mice also began to die after a few weeks, that stopping an infection even in mice was no easy matter and would require an extended course of penicillin treatment. Heatley set out to produce much larger quantities of the drug. Because *Penicillium* requires oxygen, the mold grew only a few millimeters thick, in a felt-like mat on the surface of a fluid nutrient medium. To maximize the area of oxygen exposure, he haunted rubbish dumps and experimented with salvaged containers. Enameled bedpans from the nearby Radcliffe Infirmary worked best, with a lid for keeping out contaminants and a spout for drawing off raw penicillin. Soon after, Florey commissioned a Staffordshire pottery to produce ceramic pans designed by Heatley, rectangular this time to avoid wasted space in the incubator. The first publication reporting results ("Penicillin as a Chemotherapeutic Agent") appeared in the *Lancet* on August 24, 1940, with the Battle of Britain then raging in the skies overhead. The Oxford researchers were so concerned about an imminent German invasion, with tanks "rolling down Headington Hill," as Heatley put it, that they rubbed *Penicillium* spores into the fabric of their coats. If forced to destroy their work and evacuate, they would at least have raw material to start up again wherever they landed.[9]

Early in the new year, the researchers had enough of the drug on hand to try penicillin in humans. A fifty-year-old woman with terminal breast cancer, Elva Akers, proudly volunteered as a test subject for toxicity. When she spiked a fever and began to shiver, the researchers quickly worked to weed out impurities. Akers volunteered again, and when she experienced no further reaction, the researchers moved on to test the drug's effectiveness.[10]

A middle-aged police officer named Albert Alexander had arrived at the Radcliffe Infirmary desperately ill with systemic infection. It had started with a thorn scratch to his face as he tended his rose garden, or, as other evidence suggests, with a minor injury suffered in a German bombing raid. The infected wound had developed into an abscess and cost him an eye. He was oozing pus all over. Sulfa drugs had not helped. But his condition began to improve within twenty-four hours after injection of two hundred units of penicillin on February 12, 1941. By the fourth day of treatment, he was well enough to leave his bed to take lunch.[11]

Because the drug was still scarce, hospital staff had to collect Alexander's urine—bedpans again—and carry it by bicycle back to Florey's laboratory, which recovered the excreted penicillin for reinjection. On the fifth day, the penicillin ran out and treatment ended, with the patient seemingly recovering. But Alexander's infection soon returned, and in mid-March, he died. The researchers shifted their focus to children, who would require smaller amounts of penicillin. Four of the next five patients recovered.

British pharmaceutical companies were under intense pressure to meet other wartime needs, and in continual danger from German bombing raids. Taking on the highly speculative project of manufacturing penicillin had little appeal. Instead, the Rockefeller Foundation wangled scarce plane seats for Florey and Heatley to travel to the United States, to encourage production there. It was a dangerous trip in wartime, Bristol via Lisbon, the Azores, and Bermuda to New York. An intriguing double date the two had gone on a few months earlier made it more anxious: Howard and Ethel Florey, joined by Heatley and Margaret Jennings, a histologist in the laboratory, had gone to see Alfred Hitchcock's *Foreign Correspondent*. Jennings was Howard Florey's mistress. More to the point, the movie included Hitchcock's vivid imagining of a mid-Atlantic crash of a Pan Am Clipper, the exact plane on the precise route they were about to travel. It was, they agreed, "Rather a bad thing to see."[12]

Hitchcock notwithstanding, they arrived safely at the beginning of July 1941. A friend of Florey's connected them to a US Department of Agriculture administrator with an interest in mold fermentation. He opened doors for them at the newly established Northern Regional Research Laboratory in Peoria, Illinois, which had the latest fermentation equipment. In an offhand note in a telegram ("I know it will occur to you"), the administrator suggested researchers there attempt submerged fermentation, producing penicillin not in a thin layer on the surface of shallow pans, but in huge vats.[13]

Some British writers later bemoaned having "given away" penicillin to the Americans. Bacteriologist Ronald Hare, who worked on penicillin production in Toronto during the war, depicted the United States as a land of corn pone, cowboys, and maverick manufacturing operations. But that would turn out to be just what penicillin needed. Because Peoria was in the corn belt, fermentation researchers there were trying to find uses for corn steep liquor, a watery by-product from the process of turning corn into cornstarch. It quickly proved superior to yeast extract as a growth medium for the *Penicillium* mold, and a series of tweaks rapidly boosted penicillin production.[14]

Heatley stayed on in Peoria for five months to work with the research team there. They were soon growing *Penicillium* mold with corn steep liquor in vats like oversized milkshake machines, with an agitator shaft in the middle to keep the mixture oxygenated. A higher-quality strain of *Penicillium* found on a rotten cantaloupe at a local market provided a further boost. By November 1941, the Peoria team had already boosted penicillin production tenfold, with exponentially greater progress still to come. It's a measure of Heatley's adaptability that he managed to work on friendly terms with a microbiologist he described as "the most violently anti-British man I have ever come across." He seemed not to hold a grudge even afterward, when he learned that the American, Andrew J. Moyer, had deleted Heatley's name from a paper they coauthored and also brazenly taken out *British* patents on parts of the manufacturing process. (Historians have ensured that, whatever else Moyer may have gotten from those patents, he earned a bad name.)[15]

Florey meanwhile headed off on a "carpetbagging" tour to interest drug companies, university researchers, and government officials in penicillin manufacturing. His listeners were eager to hear more, but also daunted by the limited experience with penicillin's therapeutic potential and by the expensive and uncertain challenge of producing the drug in quantity. As if to answer their questions, Florey and his team published a twelve-page report that August in the *Lancet*. It detailed their early success with human patients, and also proposed methods for large-scale manufacturing. It turned out, moreover, that the Florey team's original 1940 article had already been enough to rouse the interest of a few alert researchers. Merck, Squibb, and Pfizer were already on the case, and in August, Lederle Laboratories announced that the company was committing $40,000 to penicillin development. At Columbia University Medical School in New York that autumn of 1941, researchers had flasks of penicillin growing on every laboratory bench, and under the seats of a two-story amphitheater. They had even attempted treatment in a patient four months before Florey's group. But their patient also died when the penicillin ran out. (His name was Aaron

Allston. Together with Albert Alexander and Elva Akers, it was as if penicillin was at the starting line, preparing to run the human alphabet.)[16]

Florey headed home in late September, disappointed that the Americans hadn't already cranked out enough penicillin for him to carry home five million units—a kilo's worth in powder form, or about five hundred doses—for further human testing. But his succinct sales pitch had launched a multinational crusade. It would grow to the scale of the Manhattan Project, with an effect on the shape of the modern world that would be at least as large, and far more beneficial.

At the beginning of October 1941, two months before the United States entered the war, authorities suspended antitrust rules to allow drug companies to pool information on penicillin production. The entire penicillin effort came under the thumb of a "'Dictator of Penicillin' in Washington" who "had to approve of everything we did or required. We were, for a time, mortally afraid of him," Ronald Hare recalled of his time working in Toronto. But again, a dictator was just what the penicillin effort needed, to manage the far-flung efforts of research laboratories, universities, Allied governments, and pharmaceutical companies on both sides of the Atlantic. Hare implied as much, almost on the same page. When the American ordered a martini at a lunch meeting, he did the same "and we had quite a jolly party," leading him to wonder "how many Canadian soldiers owe their lives to the mollifying influence of gin in Washington."[17]

Governments at first reserved all penicillin for the war effort. But on March 14, 1942, Anne Miller, a nurse married to the Yale athletic director, became the first patient in the United States successfully treated with penicillin, for childbed fever. (She would live to be ninety.) Another batch of penicillin went to Boston that November to treat victims of the catastrophic Cocoanut Grove nightclub fire. By February 1943, the record of a hundred or so such cases had built enough confidence in penicillin for the US government to commit $7.6 million to construction of manufacturing plants by a half-dozen pharmaceutical companies. The companies themselves tripled that amount. John L. Smith, a vice president at Charles Pfizer & Co., then a little-known chemical manufacturer, had previously balked at a proposal to manufacture the new drug. The penicillin mold, he warned, was "as temperamental as an opera singer, the yields are low, the isolation is difficult, the extraction is murder, the purification invites disaster and the assay is unsatisfactory." But Smith was soon gambling his career, and possibly the company, on deep fermentation of penicillin.[18]

Microbiologist Gladys L. Hobby, who had moved from Columbia University to Pfizer, later attributed this change not to government pressure for the war effort, but to a New York City two-year-old named Patricia Malone. She had sepsis, and on August 11, 1943, her doctor gave her just hours to live. Hearing about the case, an editor at the *New York Journal-American* got on the phone to Washington to plead for immediate release of penicillin for treatment. That same evening, a police motorcycle escort raced the drug into the city, sirens wailing, and the story became nationwide news. "This child aroused the interest of many of us," Hobby recalled, "but particularly of John L. Smith whose sixteen-year-old daughter had succumbed to an infection prior to the development of penicillin." The widely reported happy ending was that penicillin saved Patricia Malone's life. In September, around the time she went home from the hospital, Pfizer purchased an old ice factory in Brooklyn for conversion to penicillin production.[19]

Penicillin was just undergoing its first field trial in North Africa and Sicily, to treat Allied soldiers for combat injuries. Writing in the *Lancet*, a military physician who witnessed the results predicted "the greatest revolution in treatment" of wounded soldiers, adding that "sepsis as we know it might almost disappear." The highly public tale of rescuing Baby Malone amplified this message, as a congressman made clear in a tribute that October: "The people of America owe a great debt to the *Journal-American* for the part it played in educating the public at large to the benefits of penicillin, the powerful germ killer." Keeping up wartime morale may have played a part in the final episode in the Baby Malone story. That December, when the child died during surgery for a congenital heart condition, it went unreported in the press.[20]

Hobby was witness to another key event in penicillin history that autumn. At a crowded meeting of the American Public Health Association in New York City, a US Public Health Service researcher took the lectern to report a recent penicillin trial. He did not strive for drama, and "loudspeakers and projection equipment were not as sophisticated then as now," Hobby wrote. "Everyone strained to hear what was said." What he was describing was the treatment of four men with early stage syphilis.

"The impact was electrifying," Hobby wrote. After intramuscular injection with penicillin over eight days, the patients appeared to be cured. "By then much had been written on the activity of penicillin, but no one had expected that an antibacterial agent would be active against spirochetes as well," Hobby wrote. One giddy physician in the audience rose to declare it "probably the most significant paper ever presented in the medical field." The researcher cautioned that it would require a longer study on a larger test group. But that same month, a US official was touting penicillin in a meeting with British and Canadian counterparts as "the beginning of a revolution in the treatment of syphilis."[21]

By March 1944, just seven months after the Malone episode, the Pfizer factory in Brooklyn was manufacturing penicillin in fourteen fermenters, each with a capacity of 7,500 gallons. The overall penicillin effort turned out 684 billion units in the first half of the year, and on June 6, Allied soldiers carried penicillin with them onto the beaches at Normandy. It was a lifesaver for the hundred thousand or so soldiers who benefited from penicillin treatment in the European theater between D-Day and the final German surrender. The same was true for their counterparts in the Pacific.[22]

THE WRONG DICTATOR

The surprising thing is that Germany did not match the Allied effort, especially as they had access to publications by Florey and others detailing their work with penicillin. The BBC also broadcast news about penicillin in several languages across Europe. That helped inspire clandestine penicillin manufacturing in occupied Denmark, France, and the Netherlands, where researchers at a liquor factory dubbed their secret version of the drug Bacinol, to discourage German interest. (Fortunately, their German watchdog liked Jenever gin, "so [they] made sure he got a lot. He slept most afternoons.")[23]

One explanation for the German failure to produce its own penicillin is that it had lost so many scientists into exile, like Ernst Chain, or to the death camps. But Germany's pharmaceutical companies were still world leaders in developing chemotherapies. In the occupied Netherlands, they had access to the world's most complete collection of microbial specimens, including many *Penicillium* cultures. Perhaps their own sulfa drugs seemed like miracle enough? The consolidation of dye companies into IG Farben had also perpetuated the German emphasis on synthesizing new drugs. This required expertise in chemical engineering, not fermentation. But the larger problem, historians have argued, was that Germany never created "a coordinating force or body to draw together knowledge and experience of penicillin and to plan production." That is, it had no dictator of penicillin to match the highly coordinated Allied campaign.[24]

It had only one dictator. On July 20, 1944, Adolf Hitler suffered burns and abrasions when a bomb planted by one of his own officers exploded in a room where he was meeting with staff. A spattering of wood splinters posed a threat that infection would lead to sepsis. Hitler's personal physician, Theodor Morell, recalled what had happened to Reinhard Heydrich, "the Butcher of Prague" and one of Hitler's personal favorites. Heydrich survived the immediate effects of a 1942 explosive attack by resistance fighters, only to develop a bacterial infection from the leather and horsehairs blasted into his body from his car's upholstery. In the absence of penicillin, Heydrich succumbed to blood poisoning.

Morell not only knew about penicillin by 1944, he had taken out a patent in his own name for manufacturing rights in Germany. He had also obtained a quantity of it, either from captured Allied soldiers or from Germany's own faltering attempts to manufacture the drug. There wasn't enough to administer this precious horde to General Rudolf Schmundt, Hitler's adjutant, who later died of injuries in the bombing. Instead, Morell gave it to Hitler, who lived.[25]

Thanks in part, however, to the lifesaving effects of penicillin on Allied troops pushing east from Normandy, he would not live for long.

PANACEA

As antibiotics and vaccines became commonplace in the decade after the war, it could seem to people in the developed world as if a golden age of endless health was unfolding at their feet. "The bringing of each disease under control was in itself a separate miracle," a New York physician recalled, years later. "These were thrilling events. . . . Therapeutic triumphs coming rapidly one after another imprinted the physicians with almost too great a readiness to believe. Faced with the tale of some new remedy an impulse to seek proof would arise from the science-based portion of their education, only to be met by the internal rejoinder, 'why not believe?'"[26]

Drug companies scrambled to bring streptomycin, aureomycin, erythromycin, tetracycline, and other new antibiotics into an eager medical marketplace. They were no longer just magic bullets, but a panacea, overused against almost any imaginable problem. The goal, one microbiologist wrote, "is simply *to live in a world without menacing microbes*, to have all disease-producing microbes rendered harmless and domesticated; to see infectious diseases vanish from the earth. . . . All the evidence supports the contention that sooner or later we will no longer need to fear disease-producing germs."[27]

A few early observers worried that the apparent reprieve might be temporary. In 1947, shortly after penicillin became available to British civilians, a bacteriologist reported that *Staphylococcus* bacteria resistant to penicillin were already widespread among patients at a London hospital. It was enough to raise a shadow of technological foreboding.

"Those deadly staphylococci . . . are not pirates or privateers accidentally encountered, they are detachments of an army. They are also portents," a London physician warned. Medicine risked blindly transforming the human landscape, he thought, the way modern agriculture was transforming the British countryside. "We plough the fields and scatter insecticides and selective weed-killers on the land and we find we have killed birds, bees and flowers who minister in various ways to our health and happiness and with whom we have no quarrel. . . . We should study the balance of Nature in field and hedgerow, nose, throat and gut before we seriously disturb it. Again, we may come to the end of antibiotics. We may run clean out of effective ammunition and *then* how the bacteria and moulds will lord it."

He was a voice crying in the opposite of a wilderness.[28]

30 RACE TO THE VACCINE

As other infectious diseases seemed to fade away in the mid-twentieth century, one terrifying exception mysteriously grew more severe and more frequent. Summers were made over as "polio season," shutting down swimming pools and movie theaters, locking children indoors, and leaving parents to whisper among themselves about the latest victims. The dead were at least out of sight. But paralyzed children in their wheelchairs and braces kept the peril fresh in mind. So did the news of strangely mechanized lives confined in iron lung machines, which breathed with a leathery bellows sound for victims no longer able to breathe on their own.

"I couldn't take it, that's all," writer Wilfred Sheed recalled thinking, as a fourteen-year-old in one such summer. "I'd go crazy if I got polio and had to give up baseball, and of course, football—and *walking*, which I'd almost forgotten about. And I'm sure that if someone had chosen that moment to show me a picture of myself as I would look a year or two hence, crawling spindle-shanked . . . over an ice-cold floor to get to the bathroom in the middle of the night, I'd have gone crazy on the spot."[1]

In the United States, people turned to the National Foundation for Infantile Paralysis, founded by President Franklin Delano Roosevelt, to put a hopeful face on this nightmare. More than that, they had its March of Dimes, a mass movement to raise funds for polio education, rehabilitation, research, and, ultimately, a vaccine.

CELLS MADE SICK

Attempts to grow poliovirus in chicken eggs had failed. The only other way to study it outside a living host was to grow it in a tissue culture. "Bits of tissue" from a human or some other organism "were stuck to the wall of a test tube with fibrin and nutrient fluid added" to keep the tissue alive, one researcher explained. In an incubator, "cells grew out from the fragments on the wall of the test tube and could be observed directly with a low-power microscope." This was cheaper, more efficient, and more humane than testing in an experimental animal. It also enabled researchers to see exactly how a virus affected individual cells, though the virus itself remained invisible.[2]

One tissue culture study, however, had thrown up a roadblock to progress toward a polio vaccine. In 1936, researchers used the technique to grow a poliovirus strain in tissue samples taken from a human embryo. They succeeded, but only in samples from the brain or spinal cord. That was a major problem. It would take lots of tissue cultures for large-scale vaccine production—and the tissue was going to have to come from monkeys, which were also susceptible to polio. But painful experience ruled out using monkey neural tissue to make a human vaccine: in 1935, two scientists had produced separate polio vaccines that way—and nine children died. That disaster, and the lack of an alternative, stymied polio vaccine development for the next thirteen years.[3]

The breakthrough, for polio and a host of later vaccines, came from John Enders (1897–1985) at Boston Children's Hospital. Enders was the son of a wealthy Connecticut banker, and he looked the part, in his three-piece suit and fob watch, with bow tie askew. As a virologist, he made a reputation for careful research, working mainly on mumps, chicken pox, and measles. In March 1948, Enders and his associates, Frederick Robbins (1916–2003) and Thomas Weller (1915–2008), were working to grow different viruses in tissue samples from a human fetus.

"One day when Fred and I were preparing new sets of cultures," Robbins wrote, "Dr. Enders suggested that, since we had some poliovirus stored in the freezer, we might inoculate some of the cultures with this material, which we did." The two younger scientists didn't expect much: the cultures included

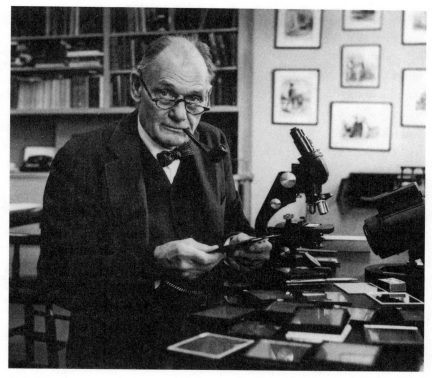

Figure 30.1

On a hunch, John Enders removed a major roadblock to the polio vaccine (Irene Shwachman, 1954).

tissue samples from skin, muscle, and intestines, when everyone knew that poliovirus grew only in neural tissue. But Enders was thinking about how polio victims commonly shed the virus in their feces—one way the disease spreads to new victims, especially in areas with poor sanitation. "It was in the back of my mind," he later explained, "that, if so much poliovirus could be found in the gastrointestinal tract, then it must grow somewhere besides nervous tissue."[4]

When the test tubes with their tissue samples were capped to contain the nutrient fluids, they went into slots in a wooden roller drum. The drum held them in a horizontal position as it slowly rotated inside an incubator. Every third or four day, the researchers replaced the nutrient fluid in the test tubes. The idea was to replicate conditions in the human body. After twelve to twenty days, they took samples of the tissue cultures, injected them into mice and monkeys, and waited. To their surprise, poliovirus cultured in nonneural tissue caused paralysis in the test animals. Enders then examined samples of the tissue cultures under his microscope. The poliovirus had left the cells visibly swollen and damaged. He looked up at his two colleagues and uttered a mouthful of a word he coined on the spot: "Cytopathogenicity." Literally: cells made sick.[5]

"Much to our amazement," Robbins wrote, "the virus grew, not only in brain tissue but in skin, muscle, kidney, and intestine." In some of the cultures, the poliovirus multiplied a trillion or more times over a few weeks. The study that had created the thirteen-year roadblock, it turned out, had tested only a single poliovirus strain, and it happened to be the one strain that grows only in neural tissue. The Enders group published their findings in *Science* in January 1949, clearing the way for vaccine development by almost any other strain. It was, said one scientist, "like hearing a cannon go off."[6]

WILLING TO SHOOT THE WORKS

Jonas Salk (1914–1995) had started out helping perfect the flu vaccine in the laboratory of Thomas Francis Jr. at the University of Michigan. He made a reputation for being an adept and innovative scientist—and also for routinely lobbying to put his own name first on the papers they coauthored. "Everyone knows who *you* are," Salk told his boss. "It doesn't matter whether your name is first or last." Salk moved on in 1947 to the University of Pittsburgh School of Medicine, where he started out in two rooms in the basement of the Municipal Hospital, and soon launched a campaign for more space. "A closet this week, an extra office next week," a friend recalled, "the auditorium next year." Salk was equally enterprising in seeking financial support to expand his work into that new space.

The great need in polio research then was for someone to sort through the many polio strains and organize them by type. It mattered because an individual immune to one type could still be susceptible to another. No established scientist was likely to undertake this work because it promised to be so dull. "The solution necessitated the monotonous repetition of exactly the same technical procedures on virus after virus, seven days a week, fifty-two weeks a year, for three solid years," the research director for the National Foundation for Infantile Paralysis acknowledged.

But the funding, $200,000 a year, was enormous for that time, and the experience could prove critical for a scientist just starting out. "Whoever did the work," Richard Carter wrote in *Breakthrough: The Saga of Jonas Salk*, "would develop the kind of laboratory team, the kind of laboratory space, the kind of familiarity with poliovirus, and therefore, the kind of running start that might, on completion of the drudgery, find the drudges ready to scoot home free with experimental polio vaccines." In 1948, the National Foundation selected Salk to be one of four such drudges, each heading his own laboratory at sites around the country. It was a logical choice: he was young, and experienced with both viruses and vaccines, and he was willing. Many established polio scientists then preferred small-scale, fundamental research to vaccine development, which one of them called "essentially an industrial process." Salk, by contrast, "wanted lots of space, was perfectly comfortable with the idea of using hundreds of monkeys, and running dozens of experiments at a time," said the research director for the National Foundation approvingly. "He always wanted to expand his program so that it would encompass as much of the subject as possible. . . . His willingness to shoot the works was made to order for us. Furthermore, he was entirely without fear of the concept of vaccination." His elders were still traumatized by the failed polio vaccines of 1935. "You cannot imagine how gingerly these ideas had to be broached in those days." Salk was soon tinkering with the possibilities of producing a killed (or inactivated) vaccine.[7]

What must have been hardest for Salk was acting the part of the junior scientist. In his laboratory, members of his team were obliged to address him as Dr. Salk. But to the senior scientists who supervised the work of typing different polio strains, he was a glorified menial. This was particularly true for Albert Sabin, who was then developing a live polio vaccine at Cincinnati Children's Hospital. At one meeting, Salk asked a question intended as gently as possible to suggest that the panel was too focused on the infectivity of different strains. However he phrased his question, it didn't have the intended effect. Sabin, who was notoriously abrasive, "turned to me and said, 'Now, Dr. Salk, you should know better than to ask a question like that,'" Salk later recalled. "It was like being kicked in the teeth. I had offered an oblique challenge to one of the assumptions, you see, and now I was being put in my place." His wounded pride felt "the resistance and the hostility" every time he appeared at these meetings. It was the beginning of a bitter rivalry with Sabin.[8]

STARS ALIGNING

By the early 1950s, circumstances made a polio vaccine more likely. The known poliovirus strains were now categorized into just three types. The Enders tissue culture technique made it possible, as Salk put it, to do the same work with two hundred test tubes that had required two hundred monkeys a few months before. The course of poliovirus within the body was also becoming clearer. Years earlier, Sabin had demonstrated that it enters the body through the mouth, not the nose, as formerly believed. But how it got from the alimentary tract to the nervous system remained a puzzle.[9]

Researchers rarely found poliovirus in the blood of paralyzed victims, and they tended to dismiss the exceptions as accidental spillovers from the nervous system. Because polio was a nerve disease, they also thought immunity must depend on some obscure factor in the nerve tissue itself. That put it beyond the scope of known science. And yet the demand for a vaccine was rapidly becoming more insistent. In 1952, the disease paralyzed 21,300 Americans. The iron lung machines filled converted gymnasiums, lined up in rows, as if in a machine shop, with the disembodied head of a polio victim visible at one end of each machine.[10]

On March 1 that year, Dorothy Horstmann, a pediatrician and virologist at Yale, published the results of experiments closely tracking the course of polio in monkeys and chimpanzees. She proved that the virus enters the blood in the early days of the disease. The normal immune response then produces antibodies to eradicate it—but not soon enough in some cases to keep the disease from entering the nervous system and causing damage. "Everyone was relieved," John Enders recalled, "to find that poliomyelitis was not an exceptionally bizarre disease, but similar to others." A vaccine might work, as it had for other viral diseases.[11]

HAVING TO CHOOSE

In a different world, the prize for developing the first effective polio vaccine might have gone to another woman. Isabel Morgan (1911–1996), the daughter of two pioneering geneticists, started her career as a virologist at the Rockefeller Institute, where "it didn't take her long," Thomas M. Rivers, the institute's director, recalled, "to demonstrate that she was a crackajack experimenter," so good he "could never understand" why her former doctoral supervisor hadn't hung onto her. But after six years, the Rockefeller Institute couldn't hang onto her either.

"I watched Isabel Morgan very carefully during her years at the Rockefeller Institute," Rivers said, admitting more than he perhaps realized. "Hell, I watched anyone at the Institute who worked with viruses carefully, and it was apparent from the very beginning that, girl or not—and by the way she was a very handsome looking girl—Isabel knew which way was up." Then he added, as if talking of circumstances outside his influence as director of the institute, "It's just that I don't think that she could have advanced very far at the Institute. As I said before, few Ph.D. ladies ever had much of a chance for advancement at the Institute during the early days."[12]

Morgan moved on to a leading polio group at Johns Hopkins University. There, she soon developed a killed (inactivated) poliovirus using formalin, a formaldehyde solution, and proceeded to experiment with its ability to elicit an antibody response. In a series of papers beginning in 1947, she announced the successful immunization of experimental monkeys. "By 1951," Rivers said, "Morgan had demonstrated beyond a shadow of a doubt that she had been able to immunize rhesus monkeys with formalin-inactivated viruses of all three basic immunologic types to a point where it was impossible to bring down such animals by the most sensitive routes"—that is, by injecting wild poliovirus directly into their brains. "Up until the time she did her work, most virologists believed that you couldn't immunize against poliomyelitis

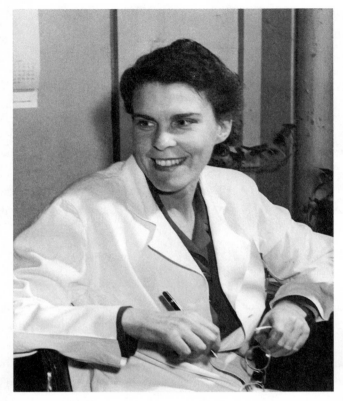

Figure 30.2
Isabel Morgan developed a critical forerunner of the first polio vaccine (March of Dimes).

with a formalin-inactivated poliovirus" and that only a live vaccine would work. "She converted us and that was quite a feat."

She went no further, however. In 1949, at thirty-eight, she married and left Johns Hopkins for minimally demanding work at a county laboratory in the suburbs north of New York City, where she also devoted herself to a stepson with a learning disability. Polio histories tend to say merely that she married a "data processor," implying boredom and security. But Joseph D. Mountain, her husband, had trained as a biplane pilot with the US Army Air Service and later worked as a pilot and aerial photographer in the desert kingdom of Arabia. A 1935 photo shows him bearded and in full Arab headgear and robe. He had had a life. The difference for Morgan was that she had to *choose* a life, either as an ambitious scientist or as a wife. "It was a different time," a friend later explained. "A woman like Ibby had a hard choice to make, and she made it."[13]

"Would Morgan have beaten Salk to the polio vaccine had she remained at Johns Hopkins?" asked historian David M. Oshinsky, in his book *Polio: An American Story*. "It's certainly possible since Salk had barely entered the starting gate by 1949. The Hopkins lab was first rate in every way. Morgan had the knowledge, the technique, and the funding to move forward quickly on her killed-virus vaccine." She later told friends that she lacked the confidence to move on to human testing. "In truth," Oshinsky wrote, "she never got the chance."

WORKING OVERTIME

Salk's ability to think big and pursue multiple lines of research soon came to the fore, along with his undeniable courage. From an early interest in a live attenuated polio vaccine, he had moved on to a formalin-inactivated vaccine like the one Morgan had developed. By the winter of 1951–1952, he was being pressed by the polio research community to answer a multitude of questions about the vaccine, all requiring a multitude of experiments: Which poliovirus strain to work with? How much formalin to eliminate infectiousness but also maximize immune response? How many days to reach inactivation? How to test batches of the vaccine for safety? His laboratory operation was "like a factory," according to one worker there, "but those of us who knew how unusual that kind of speed-up was in a university lab did not mind, because we felt we were part of a closely knit team engaged in a great effort." Salk was continuously absorbed in his thoughts, and increasingly demanding of his team, "but we attributed that to the strain of the work. The bravery he was showing in going ahead so rapidly toward human experiments was also terribly admirable, we felt."[14]

Salk's fellow polio researchers cross-examined him with their habitual ferocity at a meeting in December 1951 and sent him back to Pittsburgh with more questions in need of urgent experimentation. By May 1952, he felt ready. At the D. T. Watson Home for Crippled Children outside

Pittsburgh, he explained the importance of the work he hoped to accomplish there, and the need to keep it secret. The first step was to identify the type and amount of antibodies left in the children's blood by the polio that had crippled them. In July, he injected them with vaccine of the same type and found, as he had hoped, that it significantly increased the level of those antibodies. Next, he went to the Polk State School, north of the city, to test a *trivalent vaccine*— that is, one containing inactivated poliovirus of all three types.

The mentally handicapped children to be tested had never been exposed to polio, making this experiment far riskier. But the vaccine produced no ill effects. (Testing on the disabled was common then, though by modern standards, another polio researcher who did the same thing later acknowledged, he "would be in jail and the company would be sued" for it.) After a waiting period for immunity to develop, Salk took blood samples from the Polk children back to the laboratory. Testing revealed a high level of all three antibody types. A few drops of that blood added to a tissue culture infected with poliovirus destroyed the virus but allowed the tissue culture to continuing growing. Salk sat down at a microscope to see the results for himself. "It was the thrill of my life," he later recalled. Compared to that moment, "everything that followed was anticlimactic." The Polk State School children had become the first people successfully protected from polio by the Salk vaccine.[15]

GOING PUBLIC

Salk faced another grilling by fellow polio researchers at a meeting in Hershey, Pennsylvania, in January 1953. Acutely aware of the thousands killed or paralyzed by polio the previous summer, some pushed for a quick move to large-scale field testing. Others urged caution. "I would suggest more experimentation along the same lines that he is doing so admirably at the moment," said Enders, with characteristic tact, "and not enter into a large experiment which will inevitably be connected with a lot of publicity and may jeopardize the entire program."[16]

Enders was right about the publicity. Salk would be publishing his early results at the end of March 1953. But gossip columnist Earl Wilson broke the story in January, and newspapers ran lead stories next day. "Officials raise guarded hopes," said the *Cincinnati Enquirer*, "that this spells the death knell of polio as a crippler and killer." *Time* magazine followed up, with a photo of Salk captioned, "Ready for the big attack."[17]

The National Foundation for Infantile Paralysis introduced Salk more formally in late February 1953 to a meeting of invited medical and other dignitaries at New York's Waldorf-Astoria hotel. The Rockefeller Institute's Tom Rivers, who chaired the foundation's vaccine advisory committee, reviewed the history of the 161 people tested so far and the back and forth among polio researchers about how to proceed with the vaccine. Salk, momentarily cautious, questioned the use of that word: "I don't know that we even have a vaccine yet. . . . We have preparations which have induced antibody formation in human subjects."

"I think you have a vaccine, Jonas," Rivers gently advised.

At his own suggestion, Salk went on the radio, with CBS providing fifteen minutes of airtime at 10:45 p.m. on a Thursday for a coast-to-coast broadcast from a studio in Manhattan. ("Jonas went on the air that night to take a bow and become a public hero," one envious scientist complained. "And that's what he became.") A spokesman for the National Foundation began by reminding the American people that their donations had made them "active partners—stockholders, if you will—in this cooperative enterprise which seeks to attain better health for all the peoples of the world." Then Salk led listeners through an account of recent polio research, with results that "provide justification for optimism." No vaccine would be widely available for the 1953 polio season, he said, but "we are now faced with facts and not merely with theories. With this new enlightenment we can now move forward more rapidly and with more confidence."[18]

As soon as the On Air light blinked off, Salk headed for the overnight train back to Pittsburgh, where he continued straight to the lab. The new vaccine was front-page news everywhere, and the laboratory was now a factory in overtime. Details of all sorts still needed to be resolved, from the effect of potential adjuvants—additives to improve immune response—to the optimal interval between first injection and booster shots. The National Foundation worked to set safety protocols for a large field trial and to negotiate procedures with drug makers and independent testing labs. Thomas Francis Jr., Salk's old boss at the University of Michigan, agreed to supervise the field trial, making additional stipulations about proper double-blind procedures and his own independence in assessing the results.

Weeks before the field trial was to begin, gossip columnist Walter Winchell went on the air to warn that the new vaccine "may be a killer!" In recent testing, seven of ten batches "contained live (not dead) polio virus," he said, which had "killed several monkeys." The National Foundation replied that those batches had been found and eliminated by rigorous safety testing, which also identified and corrected deviations from the manufacturing protocol. Worried parents pulled 150,000 children from the field trial.[19]

A NATIONAL EXPERIMENT

On April 25, 1954, the US Public Health Service endorsed a nationwide field trial of the Salk vaccine. Next day, schoolchildren with signed parental consent forms lined up for their shots. In all, more than six hundred thousand children received either the vaccine or a placebo injection that spring, with local doctors, nurses, schoolteachers, mothers, and other volunteers doing most of the legwork and record-keeping, and the evaluation center at the University of Michigan compiling the data.[20]

Salk and his staff were shut out to avoid biasing the results, but they still worked furiously to improve the vaccine, assuming a successful outcome would lead to a rapid nationwide launch. In these tense circumstances, Salk committed a blunder that jeopardized working relationships in his laboratory. Two of his top researchers had given him the only copy of a paper they had written describing a valuable new technique for measuring the level of poliovirus in tissue cultures. Salk took it with him on a trip and afterward claimed to have lost it. A few days later, he presented a recognizably similar manuscript with the data tables intact, supposedly based on his notes—and with his own well-known name as first author. One of the actual authors mustered the nerve to challenge Salk, who replied that he deserved to be first author because he had gone to the trouble of reconstructing their research. His subordinates seethed helplessly and went back to work.[21]

The National Foundation for Infantile Paralysis was also shut out of the field trial, which was costing its donors $7.5 million, in addition to the millions being spent on its regular research program. At the same time, it needed to prepare for public demand ahead of the 1955 polio season. In the event of a successful result, millions of doses would need to be quickly distributed. The foundation had little choice but to bet on success. That meant paying a half-dozen drug companies $9 million to manufacture and stockpile enough vaccine to treat nine million American schoolchildren.

In the middle of the field trials, the National Foundation got at least one bit of good news: The 1954 Nobel Prize in Physiology or Medicine went to John Enders and, at his insistence, to his associates Weller and Robbins, for their tissue culture technique. It was work developed, the *New York Times* noted, with grants made "from coins that were collected in the 'March of Dimes.'" In an interview with Edward R. Murrow for his television show *See It Now* soon after, Salk gracefully acknowledged the importance of the tissue culture work to his own vaccine, saying, "Enders threw a long forward pass and we happened to be at the place where the ball could be caught."[22]

In early March 1955, Francis phoned from Ann Arbor to let the National Foundation know he was nearing completion of his analysis. He would deliver the results at the University of Michigan on April 12, the tenth anniversary of the death of the March of Dimes founder, President Franklin D. Roosevelt.

SPREADING THE WORD

That morning, 150 or so journalists were corralled in an upstairs press area. When the doors of an elevator finally opened to reveal messengers carrying information packets, the crowd of reporters surged forward. "Appalled, the messengers backed off, pitching packets into the crowd like oceanarium keepers throwing fish to leaping porpoises," in one writer's account. The ones who got the packets raced off to their typewriters and telephones.[23]

At 10:20, as scheduled, Thomas Francis, "a short, chunky man with a close-cropped mustache," in a black suit and horn-rimmed eyeglasses, appeared on stage and delivered his report "in a slow, conversational tone," the *New*

York Times reported. He talked for ninety-eight minutes. The gist of it was that the vaccine was 60 to 70 percent effective against Type I poliovirus, by far the most common type, and 90 percent or better against Types II and III.[24]

Reporters had agreed to hold their stories until Francis finished speaking, but an NBC reporter had already glanced at the first few sentences of the press release and phoned in a news flash. The *Today* show immediately broadcast word that Salk's polio vaccine was good to go. "By the time Francis spoke, there were church bells ringing in some towns," the Associated Press reported. "One courtroom observed a moment of silence. Department stores delivered the news over their public-address systems. In whitewash paint, a shop keeper daubed on his window: THANK YOU, DR. SALK. Parents and teachers wept." It was the beginning of Salk's elevation to sainthood in the public mind.[25]

Late that afternoon in Washington, DC, a federal official authorized production of the vaccine. The plan was to start with the most vulnerable population, children in first and second grades, and move on from there as supplies allowed. But right at the start, a pharmaceutical disaster almost ended the program. Sloppy manufacturing at Cutter Laboratories in California resulted in injection of 120,000 defective vaccine doses, containing live virus. Of the children vaccinated, fifty-one developed severe paralytic polio, five of them fatally. They infected others in turn, leading to 113 additional cases of paralysis and five deaths. Public health officials pulled the Cutter product off the market and conducted emergency testing of other manufacturers. They resisted calls to stop all polio vaccinations, however. No one was willing to risk another polio summer. Vaccinations went forward without further incident, and US polio cases plummeted over the next few years, from fifteen thousand cases in 1956 to fewer than a thousand in 1961.[26]

GOING LIVE

Much of the credit for the elimination of polio thereafter belongs not to Salk but to Albert Sabin, who had continued to develop and improve his live vaccine throughout. Sabin was a thorough, demanding scientist. But he played the street fighter to Salk's saint—making the front page of the

New York Times in June 1955, for instance, with Congressional testimony demanding an immediate halt to use of the Salk vaccine to prevent another Cutter incident. "Coming from Sabin this is old stuff," a spokesman for the National Foundation replied, managing to sound like a schoolteacher with a bright but unruly child. Sabin, he added, said much the same thing "on every possible occasion to stop the use of the Salk vaccine."[27]

Sabin had reason to believe his own vaccine was better. He tested it first on monkeys and chimpanzees, then on himself, as was the custom. In the winter of 1954–1955, he conducted his first human field trial on thirty inmates at a federal prison in Chillicothe, Ohio, eliciting immunity in all of them. The National Foundation continued to fund this work, but Sabin felt that it was focusing resources on the Salk field trials at the expense of progress on his live vaccine. At one point in 1955, Sabin said, an exasperated Tom Rivers even told him to take his live vaccine and dump it "into a suitable sewer." But in 1956, even Rivers acknowledged that Sabin had achieved the vaccine characteristics he needed. This didn't mean the National Foundation would endorse, much less fund, another costly field trial. That would risk disrupting the Salk program, which had in any case already immunized much of the vulnerable population in the United States.

Instead, other countries came to Sabin for the materials to conduct field trials of their own. This helped establish a pattern that would shape the subsequent campaign to eradicate polio worldwide: individual nations would provide their own medical expertise and healthcare teams to make new technologies work with local economic, cultural, and religious realities, though they could call on international support or training as needed. With permission from the US State Department, Soviet scientists visited Sabin, and he visited the Soviet Union in turn to lobby for his vaccine. The field trial there in 1959 protected ten million people. The Health Ministry then expanded the program to a total of seventy-seven million Soviet citizens.[28]

Sabin's live vaccine was significantly less expensive than the Salk vaccine. It was also easier for community healthcare workers to administer with relatively little training. And children naturally preferred a vaccine on a sugar cube to an injection. Precisely because it was live, it was also better at inducing and maintaining immunity in the mucus lining of the intestines. That meant secondary immunizations could occur by "contact immunity"—as a consequence of inadequate hand washing, or via drinking water contaminated with fecal matter, in areas with poor sanitation. This ability to protect people who had not been vaccinated would prove critical to the rapid elimination of wild poliovirus from communities, and ultimately entire continents.

In August 1960, the US Surgeon General licensed the Sabin vaccine, which quickly supplanted the Salk vaccine in the United States, for the same reasons it was being adopted abroad. It was soon everywhere in American life. One day in 1963, a Hollywood songwriter struggling to revise a song for the movie "Mary Poppins," came home to learn that his child had gotten the polio vaccine. "Did it hurt?" he asked. "No," the child replied, "they just put it on a cube of sugar and we swallowed it down." Next day, that became a song hook, "A spoonful of sugar helps the medicine go down," a sideways homage to Albert Sabin, one of the least saccharine men in the history of medicine.

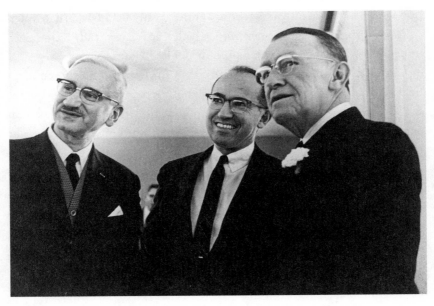

Figure 30.3
Rival polio vaccine developers Albert Sabin and Jonas Salk in 1961, with March of Dimes president Basil O'Connor (March of Dimes).

THE TRADE-OFF

Sabin's vaccine had one major drawback. Because the attenuated virus remained alive in the intestines, it could evolve there and revert to its original virulence. By mid-1964, when more than one hundred million doses had been distributed in the United States, a study in the *Journal of the American Medical Association* found that it had already caused fifty-seven cases of paralytic polio. The authors also noted the benefits of the vaccine: from a record low of 691 cases in the United States in 1962, paralytic polio had dropped to 331 cases in 1963, and appeared to be dropping by half again through June of 1964. "Epidemics of poliomyelitis as previously known have disappeared; outbreaks have become infrequent and localized," they noted.

It was a trade-off: risk of vaccine-derived paralytic polio was about one per million immunizations, much lower than the risk of going unimmunized. The study recommended pushing on. By 1979, as a result, wild poliovirus was gone from the United States. But six to eight people a year paid the price in some form of paralysis, until the nation switched back to a higher-potency Salk vaccine in 2000. Other wealthy nations now also rely on the Salk vaccine. Most developing nations, however, still mainly use the Sabin oral vaccine, based on a similar risk analysis and the need for secondary immunizations. As a result, combined with lack of immunization in many poor areas, three hundred cases of vaccine-derived poliovirus were detected worldwide in 2019. In 2020, that spiked to one thousand cases after a COVID-19-induced suspension in routine polio vaccination. The best hope to end this problem is a new Sabin vaccine genetically modified to block it from becoming virulent. Distribution began in March 2021, under an emergency authorization by the World Health Organization (WHO).[29]

The other side of the ledger suggests the trade-off was worth it. In 1988, when the Rotary Club and other organizations launched a campaign to eradicate the disease, roughly 350,000 people were becoming paralyzed by polio every year worldwide. In 2019, that was down to just 112 people. The WHO has certified continent after continent free of wild poliovirus— most recently Africa in 2020. Wild poliovirus Types II and III have been eradicated everywhere. Type I survives in only two countries, Afghanistan and Pakistan, and in 2021, Pakistan reported just a single case of wild polio-virus. (It's back up to twenty cases as of mid-October 2022.)

Eradication of all forms of polio, forever, is now achingly close. When it comes—if it comes—it will be thanks to both Salk and Sabin, neither of whom profited from the vaccines they developed, and to those who donated their dimes to make polio vaccines possible. That victory will also belong to countless unnamed community healthcare workers, often women, who still carry polio vaccine into the most remote and difficult corners of the world, risking their lives to protect their neighbors.

31 ZERO POX

By the mid-1950s, North America and Europe had eliminated smallpox. But 160 years since Edward Jenner's bold prediction that his vaccine would lead to "annihilation of the small pox," the disease still raged across the developing world, killing or maiming ten to fifteen million people a year. Much as in Jenner's time, the impediment to smallpox vaccination campaigns was still the failure of vaccine to remain viable over long distances and in harsh climates.

A breakthrough came in the early 1950s, in the form of a freeze-dried vaccine. It remained stable for months, without refrigeration. But member states of the newly formed WHO voted down a proposed smallpox eradication campaign in 1953. A Soviet proposal in 1958 won approval, but with almost no budget or staff. The sheer audacity of trying to eradicate a major infectious disease wasn't what held them back. On the contrary, WHO had already overcommitted to another eradication campaign, against malaria. Proponents of smallpox eradication argued that it would be an easier target. Where malaria required repeated application of insecticides and prophylactic drugs, smallpox required only a single dose of vaccine. And where malaria had countless host species, smallpox had only humans.[1]

WARMEST THANKSGIVING GREETINGS

By a roundabout route, John Enders's "long forward pass" not only sped up development of the polio vaccine, but also played a part in getting smallpox eradication started. In the aftermath of the Salk vaccine, Enders had applied his laboratory's cell culture technique to develop the first effective measles vaccine, licensed for use in the United States in 1963. A pilot study with this vaccine soon dramatically reduced measles incidence in the West African nation of Upper Volta (now Burkina Faso), where the disease routinely killed up to 25 percent of infected children.[2]

The US Agency for International Development (USAID) proposed following up with a measles vaccination campaign in eighteen West African nations. It sought help from the US Communicable Disease Center, as the CDC was then known. It badly needed that help. In a preliminary USAID effort, planners had assumed that vaccinating children in equal quadrants of a country over four years would result in 100 percent coverage. They did not grasp that other children would be born and become susceptible every year along the way.[3]

USAID was also planning to drop out of the new measles program after the fourth year. Donald A. Henderson (1928–2016), a young CDC infectious disease specialist, pointed out that poor nations would be unable to continue on their own because the measles vaccine cost $1.75 a dose. On the other hand, the USAID program *might just work* if it focused instead on smallpox. That vaccine—Jenner's vaccine—cost only a penny or two a dose.

The unexpected, momentarily horrifying result came at Thanksgiving 1965, when President Lyndon Johnson announced a five-year plan to vaccinate one hundred million West African children against *both* diseases, with USAID and the CDC collaborating on the program with the WHO and the participating nations. "Neither the CDC nor I had any experience in managing a program in a foreign country," Henderson wrote, a little plaintively, and his longtime boss and mentor threw him out of his office in a rage. To further complicate things, the US program, with its budget of $36.5 million, helped convince member nations to commit the WHO in 1966 to global eradication of smallpox—with the unwritten goal of getting there in just ten years.[4]

The WHO's director-general was already saddled with the embarrassing failure of malaria eradication, as mosquitoes became resistant to DDT and other insecticides. Now he was "displeased," according to Henderson, that the Americans were foisting this new obligation on him. His answer was to put an American in charge of the eradication program so that the inevitable failure would land where it belonged. That American, he stipulated, would be D. A. Henderson.

Henderson, then just thirty-eight years old, was tall, with a voice that could command a room, combined with a penchant for "ebullient hospitality and kindness." He was inexperienced by the standard of WHO senior program managers. But he would turn out to be a better choice than anyone expected. As a physician and epidemiologist, he could work side by side with vaccination teams in the field. And at WHO headquarters in Geneva, he proved adept at working around bureaucratic roadblocks. These would turn out to be abundant, starting with the $2.4 million budget WHO allocated for the first year of smallpox eradication, to be parceled out among the four regions that still routinely suffered smallpox.[5]

Each region had its own director, and each country within a region had its own national healthcare leaders—many of them capable and committed to eradication, others less so. The entire effort depended on each nation supplying medical expertise and field workers to conduct its own vaccination campaign, with international support as needed. The WHO program focused first on West Africa, where US funding for the combined measles and smallpox program improved the chances of success, and Brazil, which was far enough from other smallpox epicenters to avoid easy reinfection. The strategy was to win over skeptics by scoring key victories early on.[6]

By the 1960s, almost all countries were reporting data on smallpox and other important infectious diseases. But when WHO field teams went out to verify this data, they often found that only one smallpox case in twenty was being reported, and sometimes more like one in one hundred, or even one in one thousand. Much as polio researchers used evidence of lameness to demonstrate incidence of that disease, the WHO field teams used surveys of facial scars to show countries that their smallpox problem was deadlier than they imagined. It was another strategy for enlisting support.[7]

PUTTING OUT FIRES

Until then, mass vaccination was the standard practice for fighting smallpox, followed by "surveillance/containment." The usual goal, vaccinating

80 percent of the population, was an arbitrary number thought to stop or slow the spread of disease by establishing herd immunity. Many countries—notably Peru, Russia, Brazil, and India—had tried to get there unsuccessfully. The American effort in West Africa aimed to do better by introducing the jet injector. Instead of a needle, it used high pressure to shoot a vaccine dose into the skin quickly and painlessly. For work in remote areas, the original electrical version was modified to be operated with a hydraulic pedal.

When a mobile vaccination team visited an area, it was common for families to walk in from miles around to line up for their shots. They knew the horror of smallpox too well. With proper crowd control and a jet injector, an operator could in theory vaccinate one thousand people an hour. But mass vaccination still often failed. At times, too many people showed up for the available vaccine. In Liberia, one mobile team decided to stretch their stock of vaccine by diluting it fifteenfold, and vaccinated the entire population. But smallpox appeared in the immediate aftermath, and people who believed they had protected themselves died instead. Even when it was done right, mass vaccination sometimes failed. In the Nigerian city of Abakaliki in 1967, teams vaccinated 94 percent of the population. But smallpox broke out immediately after—not in one neighborhood that had somehow been overlooked, but scattered all across the city. The victims turned out to be members of a religious congregation opposed to vaccination.

That led CDC-trained physician and epidemiologist William Foege (1936–) to rethink the emphasis on mass vaccination. Was it possible, he wondered, that going straight to surveillance/containment might be more effective? The *surveillance* part meant actively watching to detect any new outbreak as quickly as possible. And *containment* meant rushing a vaccination team there to bottle it up before it could spread. In his youth, Foege (pronounced *FAY-gee*, with a hard *g*) had worked as a smoke jumper fighting forest fires around the American West. That experience would play a key part in what followed.

In Nigeria, Foege noticed that the spread of smallpox was influenced by two cycles, one short term, the other long. The end of the rainy season and the beginning of dry weather determined the short cycle by freeing infected people to travel again and spread the disease. From a smoke jumper's perspective, they were the fire advancing across the landscape. The longer cycle had to do with when the last outbreak had passed through a village, which was plainly visible in the smallpox scars carried by survivors. The absence of scars in young people born since then indicated the growing stock of fresh victims not yet exposed to the disease and thus lacking immunity. They were the fuel. The smoke jumper's perilous job is to cut a firebreak, a line in the forest stripped of all vegetation down to bare earth, to deny a wildfire the fuel it needs to advance. But how to do something like that to stop an advancing epidemic?[8]

Smallpox was easy to detect, like smoke from a distant fire: a new appearance of the disease wrote itself all too plainly in fresh sores on the faces of the infected. Moreover, smallpox only became contagious after those sores appeared. There were no hidden carriers. Fortunately, smallpox was also less contagious than some other infectious diseases. If one member of an unvaccinated household came down with the disease, there was only a 30 percent likelihood that other members of the household would soon follow. Smallpox also had a slow incubation time, typically ten to fourteen days—longer than it took for the vaccine to become effective. So it was possible to vaccinate that person's contacts even several days after exposure and still prevent the disease, or at least make it less virulent. These were vulnerabilities a shrewd adversary could exploit.[9]

One night in December 1966, Foege and a colleague traveled on motorbikes to an outbreak in the village of Ovirpua, in southeastern Nigeria. After examining patients and vaccinating their contacts, Foege sat down that night by the light of a kerosene lantern to talk with missionaries in outlying areas by shortwave radio. With an epidemic raging around them and not enough vaccine to go around, Foege asked the missionaries to send out runners to identify villages with active smallpox outbreaks—that is, places from which the fire now threatened to advance. The vaccination teams focused on those villages first. Then, with the last of their vaccine, they targeted nearby villages considered susceptible based on market and family travel from the infected villages. The outbreak quickly ended. They had broken the chain of transmission, the way a firebreak stops a forest fire, containing the disease before it could reach fresh fuel and become a conflagration. "And we had vaccinated such a small proportion of the population!" said Foege.[10]

After this initial success, the smallpox eradication campaign still had to persuade national governments to accept the shift away from mass vaccination. It was a complicated task because both the WHO and the CDC had previously argued for mass immunization, and they continued to encourage vaccinating as many people as possible. But containing outbreaks became the new priority. Winning over all twenty countries in the West and Central Africa campaign took eighteen months, to mid-1968. But then, Foege recalled, "in country after country, smallpox disappeared," until the region's last recorded case in May 1970. It was one of the poorest areas of the world, with severely limited basic healthcare, and some of the world's worst smallpox incidence. But surveillance/containment had eliminated the disease nineteen months ahead of the ambitious five-year schedule, and under budget. African and expatriate program leaders then moved on to help WHO repeat this success elsewhere, and "countries in other regions were forced to ask why they should lag behind."[11]

LESSONS FROM THE FIELD

Soon after, in April 1971, public health workers eliminated smallpox from Brazil. Next came Indonesia, spread out across seventeen thousand islands, with an estimated twenty thousand cases a year. News that the actual caseload was closer to two hundred thousand cases startled the government into action. With minimal outside financial assistance, Indonesia applied surveillance/containment to reach "target zero" by the end of January 1972. It went on to contribute program leaders to the global effort, along with two key innovations. The first came from a fieldworker responsible for door-to-door searches. He had a puzzling reputation for both laziness, because he was the first one done every day, and effectiveness, because he was a leader at finding villages with outbreaks. On inquiry, he sheepishly admitted skipping door-to-door visits. Instead, he went to grade schools, where he showed children a WHO photo of a smallpox case and asked if they'd seen anything like it. Thereafter, school visits and the "smallpox recognition card" became tools for WHO field teams everywhere. The other innovation came near the end of the Indonesia campaign after a local official tried to suppress word of an outbreak. Authorities responded by offering a transistor radio to members of the public reporting an active smallpox case. Highly publicized rewards became useful in the later stages of smallpox campaigns everywhere, eventually rising to $1,000 as the worldwide eradication campaign approached the finish.[12]

One other tool sped up the eradication effort. Jet injectors had proved temperamental in West Africa and Brazil. They broke down so often that every vaccination team needed a repair person and backup injectors. The bifurcated needle, also an American invention, was infinitely simpler. It consisted of a thin stainless steel rod with a small forked tip. The operator held it between index finger and thumb, dipped it into a vial of vaccine to pick up a droplet between the forks, and rested the heel of the hand on the patient's arm. With the needle at a right angle to the skin, the operator then made a quick motion like tapping a ballpoint pen on a tabletop fifteen times,

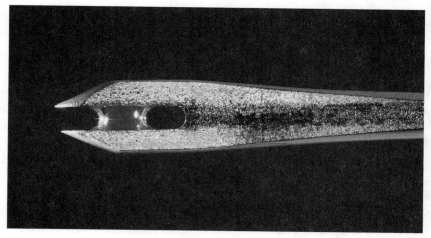

Figure 31.1
The ingeniously simple bifurcated needle became the most efficient tool for eradicating smallpox (CDC/ WHO).

leaving a tight circle of shallow punctures. Then the needle went into a discard bucket to be sterilized and reused the next day. With bifurcated needles, a three-person team averaged 1,500 to 3,000 vaccinations a day—what two people averaged with jet injectors. But bifurcated needles cost much less, never broke down, and could effectively vaccinate one hundred people with the same vial that had previously vaccinated just twenty-five.[13]

DELUSIONAL OPTIMISM

The eradication campaign grew to a multinational army 150,000 strong, moving in small teams across multiple nations by foot, horse, bicycle, car, bus, train, and boat. They traveled by camels across the desert in Sudan, mules in the mountains of northern Ethiopia, and elephants to ford rivers in India. They traveled in floods, droughts, famine, and civil war. At times, they traveled in unmapped regions, where you could be jailed for making a map of your own. They traveled with whatever cash or barter goods they might need because there were no credit cards or cash machines then. Nor were there cellphones or social media to call for help in emergencies, which were a daily routine. In Ethiopia, where a grant enabled the eradication effort to lease three helicopters, rifle fire brought down one. A hand grenade destroyed another on the ground. (The attackers were said to be bandits, or villagers who mistook the helicopters for returning Italian colonizers.) A helicopter pilot who was kidnapped knew the drill and proceeded to vaccinate his captors.[14]

For communicating back and forth with WHO headquarters in Geneva, it was possible to send printed messages by telex. But doing so through a nation's official channels, as protocol demanded, took too long. Henderson's workaround was to honor protocol by sending a telex through the channels while simultaneously telexing or mailing a copy directly to field staff who needed an answer now. One time an urgent telex arrived from Uganda team leaders requesting two million doses of vaccine. The shipment went out by air the next morning. The request arrived through official channels five months later.[15]

Managing this far-flung effort was massively complicated. And yet it did seem somehow to be managed. National programs incorporated experienced leaders from other national programs—a Brazilian in Indonesia, a Sudanese in Afghanistan, an Indian in Ethiopia. "People lost their national identities," said Foege. Best practices accumulated along the way. Standards developed and became more stringent with time. Assessment teams followed behind the vaccinators, sampling representative populations. If the percentage of people vaccinated fell below the standard, the vaccinators had to go back and do it over again.[16]

People of all circumstances and nationalities seemed to subscribe to these standards. They were united by the acute awareness that their common enemy, smallpox, was a monster bent on destroying young lives. This was the moment for ending its ten-thousand-year reign of terror over humanity. Better still, they were part of that moment. Nothing else in their lives would match the sense of accomplishment, assuming they could accomplish it. The moving spirit was "delusional optimism," according to Henderson. A US surgeon general agreed: "The workers in the program were simply too young to know it couldn't be done."[17]

In the first half of 1974, all the obstacles to eradication swirled together ominously in India, where rational minds saw a hopeless cause. The campaign, led by a tight-knit group of epidemiologists from the Indian national government and the WHO, required more than one hundred thousand workers, and the assessment teams alone visited 107,000 villages to check whether vaccination teams had done their work properly. But the ordinary business of life kept tens of millions of Indians on the move by road, rail, and boat. An outbreak in one village could spark another in a village hundreds of miles away.[18]

The worst problems were in the impoverished and densely populated northern states of Uttar Pradesh, West Bengal, and Bihar. In Bihar in May 1974, thirty-six thousand cases turned up. When the eradication team urgently sought the help of several thousand workers hired by the state smallpox program director, it turned out that this workforce existed in name only, with the director pocketing most of the payroll. His political backers prevented his removal for months. To complicate the difficulties, railway workers went on strike. Healthcare workers threatened to follow.[19]

Then monsoon rains caused disastrous flooding. As displaced residents shifted to new locations, they brought smallpox with them. A high-ranking national official ordered abandonment of surveillance/containment and a return to mass immunization. It took a visit by the national minister of health to override him and put surveillance/containment back on track. India's Tata Group, a large industrial presence in Bihar, committed financial and political support. The head of the group, J. R. D. Tata, lobbied his friend, Prime Minister Indira Gandhi, on behalf of the smallpox campaign. She pressured members of her own government and the state to aid the campaign. Extra staff poured into the region from the WHO, the CDC, and elsewhere in India. A major grant also turned up unexpectedly from the Swedish International Authority, and as it had been doing throughout the campaign, the Soviet Union contributed hundreds of millions of doses of vaccine.[20]

Teams searched more than one hundred million households in periodic sweeps. Every new case required a twenty-four-hour guard posted at the house to ensure that the victim remained isolated—together with intensive searches of the surrounding five hundred to one thousand houses. Workers also searched alleyways and railway stations, where the characteristic "dead animal odor" of smallpox, from flesh decaying beneath the pustules, alerted them to homeless victims of the disease. At the end of June 1974, India still had 6,400 villages infected with smallpox. But the intensity of the effort and the effectiveness of multinational collaboration were such that just one year later, on June 30, 1975, the minister of health announced the disease eliminated from India. It was a risky call, just thirty-five days after the last known case. But another two years of constant surveillance, combined with substantial rewards that went unclaimed, demonstrated that India was in fact free of smallpox for the first time in thousands of years.[21]

The smallpox eradication campaign still had hard work to do in Afghanistan, Pakistan, and Bangladesh. Then the focus shifted to the Horn of Africa, where WHO hired local healthcare workers to track down nomadic herders in the Ogaden Desert, an area nearly as big as the state of Kansas on the

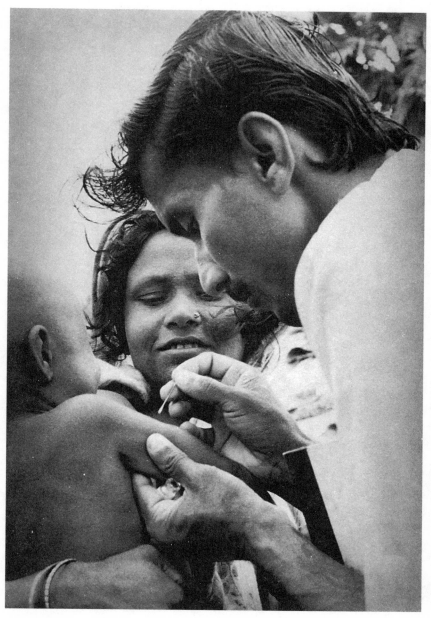

Figure 31.2
During the campaign to eradicate smallpox, the mantra was that only one type of person did not need the vaccination—"a dead person" (Stanley Foster, MD; CDC/WHO).

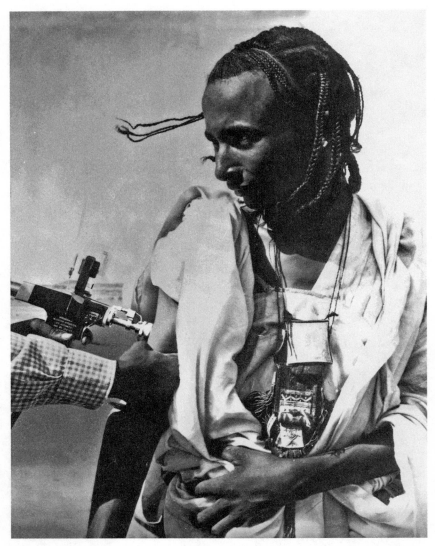

Figure 31.3
Using the jet injector to vaccinate a man in Niger in 1969 (J. D. Millar, MD; CDC/WHO).

border of Somalia and Ethiopia. What appeared to be the world's last small-pox outbreak was soon contained at a nomad encampment in July 1976.

For seven weeks, members of the team held their breath and continued the search. But in September, five more cases occurred in the populous heart of Mogadishu, Somalia's capital city. Smallpox scattered from there across the southern part of the country, as if in a desperate race for survival. The national government declared it a disaster and called for international help. By June 1977, smallpox teams had found 1,400 cases. Heavy summer rains made vehicle travel impossible, but vaccinators continued to crisscross the desert on foot, carrying their supplies on donkeys and camels. Another apparent last outbreak among nomads was rapidly coming under control. In mid-October, a government vehicle brought a badly afflicted six-year-old girl named Habiba Nur Ali and her younger brother into the coastal town of Merca for medical help.[22]

When the driver stopped in town for directions, a twenty-three-year-old hospital cook named Ali Maow Maalin climbed into the vehicle and directed them to the destination, a smallpox isolation camp. Although he had occasionally served as a vaccinator for the WHO campaign, Maalin had somehow avoided being vaccinated himself. When his skin pebbled over several days later with the bead-like pustules of smallpox, he retreated to his room. On October 30, 1977, someone reported the case to collect a reward, and investigators moved Maalin to the same isolation camp where the child Habiba Nur Ali had died, like so many children before her, a few days after arriving. The eradication teams tracked down ninety-one people with whom Maalin had had contact. House-to-house searches led to the vaccination of another fifty-four thousand people. But no further cases occurred. Maalin survived, and entered history as the world's last-known case of naturally acquired smallpox.[23]

THE FINAL INCH

The eradication campaign was not done. Epidemiological practice required two years of continued searching to certify that an area was clear of a disease. Teams of experts traveled everywhere looking for symptoms. "Go anywhere you wish," said Indonesia's health minister, proudly welcoming an early certification team visit in 1974. "Ask anyone any question, examine any document. I am confident that you will find that smallpox has been eliminated from Indonesia." Other nations also opened their doors, proud of having driven an ancient enemy to its death.[24]

But disease bides its time and can sometimes rise from the grave to carry us away. Just one year after Maalin survived the disease, a forty-year-old British medical photographer named Janet Parker was working in her darkroom at the University of Birmingham Medical School. In a laboratory one floor below, a virologist named Henry S. Bedson operated one of a handful of facilities in the world where smallpox virus still survived in captivity. WHO experts had visited a few months earlier and told Bedson to make major biosafety improvements or shut down the laboratory. No improvements occurred, however, and Bedson went on with his research. Early that August of 1978, a few strands of the virus broke loose, became airborne, and found their way up and into Parker's lungs.

A photo survives of her lying on her back in a hospital bed not long afterward, her face turned to the camera. Her dark hair is pulled back, her eyes are serene, though bleary, and she is disturbingly beautiful, except that her face is entirely covered in pustules. A hospital soon sent a sample back for identification at the University of Birmingham, where Bedson himself examined it under an electron microscope. It was of course smallpox. Parker had been vaccinated twelve years earlier, but that was well past the vaccine's expected effectiveness. Further analysis by a researcher in London confirmed that the virus was the specific strain on which Bedson had been working.

The urgent business of tracing contacts turned up 341 people potentially infected by Parker. One of them, a harbinger of a world increasingly connected by jet travel, had gone as far as a farm in North Dakota. The familiar business of vaccinating contacts went forward, with Bedson himself helping for a time. But on September 1, Bedson told his wife he was going out to garden. She followed minutes later and found him lying in a pool of blood on the potting shed floor, with his throat slit and a suicide note at his side. Parker's father became ill a few days later and died of a heart attack. Then her mother came down with smallpox. Finally, Parker herself died on September 11, 1978, the last known smallpox fatality on Earth.

The Birmingham incident led to the destruction of all known smallpox virus stocks, except at two laboratories, one in the United States, and one in Russia. Otherwise, the business of certifying smallpox eradication went forward smoothly. On May 8, 1980, member states of the World Health Organization formally accepted certification and declared "that the world and all its peoples have won freedom from smallpox."[25]

It was three thousand years since the earliest known case of smallpox, based on evidence in Egyptian mummies, and perhaps ten thousand since the disease first afflicted humankind. It was 460 years since the arrival of smallpox in the New World began the annihilation of Native American civilizations. It was 184 years, less six days, since Edward Jenner vaccinated his first patient, eight-year-old James Phipps, against smallpox. The WHO smallpox campaign had missed its wildly ambitious goal of achieving eradication in ten years, but not by much. Privately, Henderson lionized the heroes of the campaign, dubbing hundreds of his fellow pox hunters as members of the "Order of the Bifurcated Needle." For many, it would be the great honor of their lives.[26]

In the United States, which had not seen a case of smallpox since 1949, the *New York Times* reported the official announcement of eradication on page A21, at the bottom of a column, beside a department store ad for a Mother's Day nightgown. Smallpox was already being forgotten, and fading into history. It was the blessing and the curse of all great cures: to defeat a disease so thoroughly it could seem as if it had never existed in the first place. Eradication freed us to drift for a time in a comfortable sense of freedom from our most ancient mortal enemies. But new destroying angels—HIV/AIDS, Ebola, and others still unnamed—were already taking wing in the far corners of the earth.[27]

EPILOGUE: THE PLAGUE NEXT TIME

Over the past three years, 6.6 million people have died from COVID-19. With vaccination rates lagging in many areas, we may continue to die for some time to come. But COVID-19 has also reminded me just how lucky we are, how much better off even now than humans who have lived at any other moment in history. Working on this book has helped me to see both where that good fortune has come from and how fragile it may yet prove to be.

Let's start with our good fortune. Go back to 1800, when England was one of the world's most prosperous nations, and life expectancy at birth was just forty years. Worldwide, it was more like thirty. Today, it's seventy-three years worldwide, and well into the mid-eighties in a few countries. This doubling of the average lifespan within a few generations is "arguably the most important single historical change of the last two hundred years," according to Cambridge University historian Leigh Shaw-Taylor.[1]

It's not that anyone has made great progress at the dreamy business of life extension. We just don't die prematurely as much. Go back to 1900, and one child in three died before age five. By the start of the twenty-first century, that was down to one child in twenty-seven, and in developed countries one in one hundred. This dramatic transformation in the character of childhood, family life, and human society—dubbed the *mortality revolution*—has attracted surprisingly little public attention. Viewed in historical terms, it was a lightning stroke, it was the eruption of Krakatoa, it was the Chicxulub asteroid. But to our eyes, it hardly seemed to happen at all.

And yet we know what it means in our personal lives: When parents feel confident that each child will survive to maturity, they also feel confident in having fewer children. Declining child mortality has led to declining birth rates almost everywhere. (Sub-Saharan Africa is no exception, but a third of young mothers in some countries still suffer the devastating loss of a child. That contributes to persistently high birth rates there.) Confidence about survival also frees prospective parents to delay child-rearing and devote more effort to schooling and careers. Studies suggest that children benefit, too, from increased parental attention and resources. That translates in turn to national economies: countries with a falling birth rate tend to prosper over the following decades, a global phenomenon known as the *demographic dividend*. Freed of the heartbreaking burden of raising children only to see them die, parents and nations alike steer their energies in new directions.[2]

We owe this good fortune to many of the successes already detailed in this book. One of the lasting benefits of the smallpox eradication campaign, for instance, was the recognition by nations everywhere that vaccines save lives. A direct result, the WHO's Expanded Program on Immunization, begun in 1974, has helped to boost uptake of six basic childhood vaccines from less than 5 percent of children in many countries to 86 percent or better in almost all countries, with a corresponding reduction in disease. New vaccines have also become widely available against pathogens that once routinely killed children, though most parents have never heard of them: *Haemophilus influenzae* type B (Hib) was a major cause of childhood meningitis, pneumonia, and sepsis. Rotavirus was the leading cause of severe infant diarrhea. Both are now rapidly vanishing.[3]

So where's the fragility? Progress has come more slowly on other factors directly affecting death from infectious diseases. Worldwide, 2.1 billion people still lack access to safe drinking water at home, and 4.5 billion lack adequate sanitation. Better preventive measures, including more precise mosquito control, have cut malaria mortality in half over the past two decades. But more than 627,000 people, mostly children in Africa and India, still died of the disease in 2020. Antibiotics and other pharmaceutical interventions have improved treatment of diseases. But cost and the emergence of multi-drug-resistant pathogens have hampered their effectiveness. It's a major reason tuberculosis, that disease of nineteenth-century poets, still kills 1.4 million people a year in the twenty-first century.[4]

Our biggest vulnerability, however, is almost certainly our stubborn, stupid sense that we have somehow become invulnerable. It's why we resist vaccines in the face of overwhelming scientific evidence of their safety and life-saving effectiveness. It's why, as a result, we have allowed measles to return to the United States and Europe not long after vaccines eliminated the disease there. It's why healthcare workers have endured angry COVID-19 denial even from patients dying of the disease. It's why people have experienced assault for wearing face masks. We have become so accustomed to the absence of contagion that even *other people inconveniencing themselves* to protect us somehow seems like an attempt to impose political control.

The reality is that victory over infectious diseases was never a done deal, and society will inevitably require new and inconvenient forms of protection to prevent future pandemics. We remain vulnerable partly because old diseases can learn new tricks. A more virulent form of scarlet fever, for instance, has recently evolved in northern China and spread to other countries, causing a fivefold increase in the disease after a long period of decline. Entirely new "indefinable Somethings" have also continued to appear throughout what seemed like the golden age of infectious disease control. According to one study, 183 new pathogens emerged between 1940 and 2004, notably including HIV/AIDS and Ebola. More of them are infecting humans with each passing decade, leading Michael Ryan, executive director of the WHO's Health Emergencies Program, to suggest that we have entered "a very new phase of high impact epidemics." Specialists worry that epidemics have begun to "overlap and run into each other."[5]

It's a familiar story of converging risks: Populations increase. People push deeper into remote habitats. They encounter wildlife pathogens formerly beyond human reach. Those pathogens find their way to urban boomtowns, where people living in squalid conditions become unwilling incubators. Or the wildlife itself spends time in urban markets, side by side with other species never encountered in the wild. Alien viruses comingle and exchange genetic segments within the bodies of living animals, which also become incubators. Novel pathogens spread to larger cities because everything is so mobile now. Then they find their way onto international flights and become pandemic.

That scenario has already happened in the modern era with HIV/AIDS, SARS, and COVID-19. Ebola came close in 2014, with local transmissions in the United States and Spain. Only rapid isolation of the victims and intensive contact tracing prevented a larger outbreak. By enabling mosquito vectors to expand their range, climate change has contributed to temperate zone outbreaks of otherwise tropical diseases, including Zika, chikungunya, and dengue viruses. Fatal cases of West Nile virus have become routine worldwide.

Countering these forces will require a unified global disease-fighting effort on a scale and intensity well beyond the pox-hunting labors of the Order of the Bifurcated Needle—perhaps even beyond the abilities of the WHO. Nothing about it will be simple. Shutting down live wildlife markets sounds easy, for instance. But it requires enforcement to keep the trade from moving online or underground, and it will necessitate finding alternative protein sources for people who now depend on bushmeat to feed their families. Detecting pathogens before they spread may sound practical because we can deploy portable PCR screening equipment. But it requires training and supporting multinational teams of virus hunters to put that equipment to good use. It means enlisting community workers to detect incidents—three monkeys found dead in a forest, a sudden die-off at a small pig farm—warning of pathogens that might spill over to humans. A pilot project in the Republic of the Congo has already put such teams to work detecting Ebola and primate anthrax. It will take a major investment to expand that effort to hot zones for pathogen emergence elsewhere.

Surveillance and containment can work on the global scale. But smallpox was a single well-known pathogen. It's much harder to identify the threat that matters in an entire, rapidly evolving planet of viral and bacterial strains. Government programs to identify and control emerging biological threats have existed for years. But they did little to stop the COVID-19 pandemic, despite early warning from recent outbreaks of other coronaviruses.[6]

There's plenty of reason to fear governments will do no better next time. Economic austerity may discourage large-scale international investment in disease prevention. National leaders may treat efforts to improve basic healthcare and vaccination coverage in the developing world as merely altruistic, rather than as a self-interested way to prevent the emergence and spread of disease variants. Political disdain for scientists may result in failure to train or support future Jenners, future Pearl Kendricks and Isabel Morgans. Governments may fail at the intellectual and emotional challenge of prevention as a full-time, never-ending endeavor. Spending $13 billion to buy an aircraft carrier, largely in the service of preventing armed conflict, can seem "realistic" because there are jobs to be had at shipyards, as well as at sea. Spending to prevent disease, on the other hand, provides no heroic physical object, just the unsatisfying knowledge that the catastrophe we feared did not happen.

Disease prevention efforts will also run up against highly profitable and powerful business interests. A major pathway to preventing the emergence of new pathogens, for instance, is to keep remaining large forest blocks intact. But logging, mining, fossil fuel, and agribusiness industries have been highly successful up to now in bypassing such initiatives, even in national parks and UNESCO Natural World Heritage sites.[7]

How do we shift the focus from short-term profits to long-term survival? One answer is to require that the price of products include costs currently imposed on society at large and on future generations. If a logging project will cause local malaria incidence to rise by 48 percent, as one study found, the logger should pay nearby health districts to eliminate that risk. Or go somewhere else. Climate and biodiversity damage should also be part of the accounting because both contribute to the risk of disease. Accounting for this true cost will put some forms of business off-limits in certain areas or make them untenable anywhere. It will make many products more expensive for all of us. Accounting for the climate cost of livestock production, for instance, would more than double the price of every pound of meat or dairy product.[8]

These added costs won't come close, however, to the appalling scale of the loss when we fail to prevent disease. Think first of the people singled out by COVID-19 for such terrible, lonely deaths. We also need to remind political leaders, loudly and often, of the financial cost—the *business cost*—of failing to prevent disease. The losses from the COVID-19 pandemic will run to the *tens of trillions* of dollars. Those losses have hit every business, every job holder, every family on earth. But the next pandemic could easily prove costlier and more destructive.

One person with the COVID-19 omicron variant typically infected 3.2 other people, still a relatively low infection rate. By comparison, a person with measles infects twelve to eighteen others. Moreover, fewer than 3 percent of all COVID-19 cases have ended in death in most countries, though with some stark differences by age, race, or economic status. That's a polite little *memento mori* compared with the 60 to 90 percent fatality rate of the Black Death. And this is the real worry: the pathogen next time could easily combine high infectiousness like measles with high mortality like plague.

Humankind could revert to our long history of endless epidemics. Life, which now seems to begin at thirty, could once again end there instead. The freedom from disease we have taken for granted our entire lives could vanish and seem in retrospect like a wondrous dream, a *pax medica*, with a raging storm of disease on either side. We could yet face mass die-offs or even extinction. The combination of the pandemic with increasingly fierce manifestations of climate change has moved this fear from the fringes to the mainstream.

This is a massively larger challenge than what past medical researchers faced. They set out to accomplish the impossible by understanding individual diseases and preventing them. And what they achieved changed our world. But the job now is to protect not just the human species but the world itself. It will take "delusional optimism" on a global scale.

It will take an army of young people who do not know it cannot be done.

Acknowledgments

A generous fellowship from the Alfred P. Sloan Foundation made the research and writing of this book possible. In addition, I owe special thanks to David Skelly, an ecology professor at Yale and director of the Peabody Museum of Natural History; Fred Strebeigh, a teacher of generations of writers at Yale; and prize-winning historian Geoffrey C. Ward.

Among the many others who helped in the production of this book, I am grateful to librarians and archivists everywhere, for preserving research material and often making it easily available (even in the middle of a pandemic!) via the Wellcome Collection, the Royal Society, the Pasteur Institute, the Bibliothèque Nationale de France, and other institutions. In particular, Christopher Zollo, Melissa Grafe, and other staff at the Yale Medical Historical Library helped keep my work going throughout.

Researchers and medical practitioners who generously answered my questions include medical historian Sanjoy Bhattacharya at York University; William E. Browne at the University of Miami; James F. Conniff at the University of Minnesota; Stephen Calderwood at Massachusetts General Hospital/Harvard Medical School; Joseph Gal at the University of Colorado-Denver; Joseph Hinnebusch at the National Institute of Allergy and Infectious Diseases; Axel C. Hüntelmann at the University of Berlin; Walter A. Orenstein at Emory University; author Robert Poole; Adrian Raftery at the University of Washington; Lesley A. Robertson at Delft University of Technology; Nils Roll-Hansen at the University of Oslo; Lukas Rieppel at Brown University; Gilbert Shama at Loughborough University; Emily

Smith-Greenaway at the University of Southern California; Andreas Fast at the Friedrich Loeffler Institut; Peter Vinten-Johansen at Michigan State University; and Liz McGow at the Linnean Society of London. Thanks also to Gregory F. X. Conniff for editorial suggestions; and to intern Akash Naga-purkar at New York University for help with footnoting and fact-checking.

For their support on excerpts from this book, thanks to editor Jennie Rothenberg Gritz at *Smithsonian* magazine; and to editors Glenn Oeland, Peter Gwin, and John Hoeffel and researcher Heidi Schultz at *National Geographic* magazine.

Thanks finally to editors Robert Prior, Anne-Marie Bono, Kathleen A. Caruso, and Melinda Rankin at the MIT Press, to John Thornton at the Spieler Agency, and to the many friends and family who supported me through Patreon and in person. Good health and blessings upon you all.

Notes

More complete references, with online links, are available at https://mitpress.mit.edu/ending-epidemics, and at the Ending Epidemics website, www.endingepidemics.com.

PREFACE

1. A. Feuer and W. K. Rashbaum, "'We Ran Out of Space': Bodies Pile Up as N.Y. Struggles to Bury Its Dead," *New York Times*, April 2, 2020.

2. S. W. Roush and T. V. Murphy, "Historical Comparisons of Morbidity and Mortality for Vaccine-Preventable Diseases in the United States," *JAMA* 298, no. 18 (2007): 2155–2163.

3. W. Churchill, *Europe Unite: Speeches, 1947 and 1948* (Boston: Cassell, 1950), 138.

4. J. Paget, *Memoirs and Letters of James Paget*, ed. S. Paget (London: Longmans, Green, 1901), 55.

CHAPTER 1

1. C. Dobell, *Antoni van Leeuwenhoek and His "Little Animals"* (New York: Harcourt, Brace, 1932), 28–37.

2. R. Hooke, preface to *Micrographia* (London: James Allestry, 1665).

3. S. Pepys, *The Diary of Samuel Pepys*, ed. H. B. Wheatley (London: George Bell, 1893), v, iv, 338; H. Gest, "The Discovery of Microorganisms by Robert Hooke and Antoni Van Leeuwenhoek, Fellows of the Royal Society," *Notes and Records of the Royal Society of London* 58, no. 2 (2004): 187–201.

4. H. Gest, "Homage to Robert Hooke (1635–1703): New Insights from the Recently Discovered Hooke Folio," *Perspectives in Biology and Medicine* 52, no. 3 (2009): 392–399; L. Robertson, J. Backer, C. Biemans, J. v. Doorn, K. Krab, W. Reijnders, H. Smit, and P. Willemsen, *Antoni Van Leeuwenhoek: Master of the Minuscule* (Leiden: Brill, 2016), 7–9, 21–30, 54.

5. L. J. Snyder, *Eye of the Beholder: Johannes Vermeer, Antoni Van Leeuwenhoek, and the Reinvention of Seeing* (New York: W. W. Norton: 2015).

6. A. v. Leeuwenhoek, *Alle de Brieven van Antoni van Leeuwenhoek/The Collected Letters of Antoni van Leeuwenhoek*, vol. 2: 1676–1679 (Amsterdam: Swets and Zeitlinger, 1939), 79; Robertson et al., *Antoni Van Leeuwenhoek*, 60.

7. A. v. Leeuwenhoek, *Alle de Brieven van Antoni van Leeuwenhoek/The Collected Letters of Antoni van Leeuwenhoek*, vol. 1: 1673–1676 (Amsterdam: Swets and Zeitlinger, 1939), 165; Dobell, *Antoni van Leeuwenhoek*, 109.

8. Leeuwenhoek, *Collected Letters*, 2:71, 2:73, 2:75.

9. Dobell, *Antoni van Leeuwenhoek*, 71.

10. Robertson et al., *Antoni Van Leeuwenhoek*, 95–96; Leeuwenhoek, *Collected Letters*, 2:285.

11. Dobell, *Antoni van Leeuwenhoek*, 58, 64, 71.

12. Leeuwenhoek, *Collected Letters*, 1:279.

13. Dobell, *Antoni van Leeuwenhoek*, 112.

14. Leeuwenhoek, *Collected Letters*, 2:81, 2:171; emphasis in original. [Note from author: Here and throughout, I have aimed as much as practical to follow the spelling and italicized emphasis from the original document.]

15. Leeuwenhoek, 2:95, 2:99, 2:115.

16. Leeuwenhoek, 2:199, 2:207; Dobell, *Antoni van Leeuwenhoek*, 177.

17. R. Hooke, *Lectiones Cutlerianæ* (London: John Martyn, 1679), 82, 83.

18. Dobell, *Antoni van Leeuwenhoek*, 184.

19. Dobell, 50.

CHAPTER 2

1. "Some Considerations of an Observing Person in the Country," *Philosophical Transactions of the Royal Society* 12, no. 136 (1677): 890–892.

2. A. v. Leeuwenhoek, *Alle de Brieven van Antoni van Leeuwenhoek/The Collected Letters of Antoni van Leeuwenhoek*, vol. 3: 1679–1682 (Amsterdam: Swets and Zeitlinger, 1939), 365–367; Dobell, *Antoni van Leeuwenhoek*, 224n.

3. Dobell, *Antoni van Leeuwenhoek*, 245; A. v. Leeuwenhoek, *Alle de Brieven van Antoni van Leeuwenhoek/The Collected Letters of Antoni van Leeuwenhoek*, vol. 4: 1683–1684 (Amsterdam: Swets and Zeitlinger, 1939), 131–135.

4. H. Newton, "'Nature Concocts & Expels': The Agents and Processes of Recovery from Disease in Early Modern England," *Social History of Medicine* 28, no. 3 (2015): 465–486.

5. C. E. A. Winslow, *The Conquest of Epidemic Disease: A Chapter in the History of Ideas* (Madison: University of Wisconsin Press, 1980), 56.

6. C. Richet, "An Address on Ancient Humorism and Modern Humorism," *British Medical Journal* 2 (1910): 921–926.

7. E. Jorpes, "Robin Fåhraeus and the Discovery of the Erythrocyte Sedimentation Test," *Acta Medica Scandinavica* 185 (1969): 23–26; R. Fåhraeus, "The Suspension Stability of the Blood," *Physiological Reviews* 9, no. 2 (1929): 241–274; M. Lister, "A Remarkable Relation of a Man Bitten with a Mad Dog, and Dying of the Disease Called Hydrophobia," *Philosophical Transactions of the Royal Society* 13 (1683):162–170.

8. Winslow, *Conquest of Epidemic Disease*, 182.

CHAPTER 3

1. A. Koch, C. Brierley, M. Maslin, and S. Lewis, "Earth System Impacts of the European Arrival and Great Dying in the Americas after 1492," *Quaternary Science Reviews* 207 (2019): 13–36.

2. E. W. Stearn and A. E. Stearn, *The Effect of Smallpox on the Destiny of the Amerindian* (Boston: B. Humphries, 1945), 14–15; N. D. Cook, *Born to Die: Disease and New World Conquest, 1492–1650* (Cambridge: Cambridge University Press, 2004), 23–24.

3. F. N. Thorpe, *The Federal and State Constitutions, Colonial Charters, and Other Organic Laws of the State, Territories, and Colonies Now or Heretofore Forming the United States of America* (Washington, DC: US Government Printing Office, 1909), 3:1828–1829; C. Mather, *Magnalia Christi Americana: Or, the Ecclesiastical History of New-England* (London: Thomas Parkhurst, 1702), 1:7.

4. R. G. Thwaites, *Jesuit Relations and Allied Documents: Travels and Explorations of the Jesuit . . . Missionaries in New France, 1610–1791* (Cleveland, OH: Burrows Brothers, 1899), 47:193; G. L. Leclerc, *Natural History, General and Particular*, trans. W. Smellie (London: W. Strahan & T. Cadell, 1785), 5:135–136.

5. U. V. Hutten, *De Morbo Gallico: A Treatise of the French Disease* (London: John Clarke, 1730), 3.

6. E. Tognotti, "The Rise and Fall of Syphilis in Renaissance Europe," *Journal of Medical Humanities* 30, no. 2 (2009): 99–113.

7. E. L. Abel, "Syphilis: The History of an Eponym," *Names* 66, no. 2 (2018): 96–102; G. Fracastoro, *Syphilis, from the Original Latin. A Translation in Prose of Fracastor's Immortal Poem*, trans. S. C. Martin (St. Louis: Philmar Company, 1911); V. Iommi Echeverría, "Girolamo Fracastoro and the Invention of Syphilis," *História, Ciências, Saúde*, 17, no. 4 (2010), https://www.scielo.br/j/hcsm/a/Lz54jdJJTnKxNb8N5WwtR8M/?format=pdf&lang=en.

8. S. E. Morison, *Admiral of the Ocean Sea* (Boston: Little, Brown, 1942), 2:202–204; C. Quétel, *History of Syphilis*, trans. J. Braddock and B. Pike (Cambridge: Polity Press, 1990), 9–16.

9. B. Boehrer, "Early Modern Syphilis," *Journal of the History of Sexuality* 1, no. 2 (1990): 197–214; K. Sudhoff, *The Earliest Printed Literature on Syphilis*, ed. C. Singer (Florence: Lier, 1925), xi, xvi; Tognotti, *Rise and Fall of Syphilis*.

10. Hutten, *De Morbo Gallico*, 8–11.

11. Hutten, 10–11, 30, 86.

12. A. Boorde, *The Breviary of Helthe* (London: W. Middleton, 1547), 195; Hutten, 4; Tognotti, *Rise and Fall of Syphilis*.

13. W. Schleiner, "Moral Attitudes toward Syphilis and Its Prevention in the Renaissance," *Bulletin of the History of Medicine* 68, no. 3 (1994): 389–410.

14. Hutten, *De Morbo Gallico*, 90; Schleiner, "Moral Attitudes"; M. K. DeLacy, *The Germ of an Idea* (London: Palgrave Macmillan, 2016), 43.

15. Hutten, *De Morbo Gallico*, 14–22, 81–82.

16. R. Munger, "Guaiacum, the Holy Wood from the New World," *Journal of the History of Medicine and Allied Sciences* 4, no. 2 (1949): 196–229.

17. D. F. Strauss and J. Sturge, *Ulrich von Hutten, His Life and Times* (London: Daldy Isbister, 1874), 352.

CHAPTER 4

1. G. Fracastoro, "Contagion, Contagious Diseases and Their Treatment," in *Milestones in Microbiology*, ed. T. D. Brock (Englewood Cliffs, NJ: Prentice-Hall, 1961), 69–75. First published 1546.

2. V. Nutton, "The Reception of Fracastoro's Theory of Contagion: The Seed That Fell among Thorns?," *Osiris* 6 (1990): 196–234; DeLacy, *Germ of an Idea*, 9.

3. F. Garrison, "Fracastorius, Athanasius Kircher and the Germ Theory of Disease," *Science* 31, no. 796 (1910): 500–502; T. D. Brock, ed., *Milestones in Microbiology* (Englewood Cliffs, NJ: Prentice-Hall, 1961), 75.

4. H. Torrey, "Athanasius Kircher and the Progress of Medicine," *Osiris* 4 (1938): 246–275.

5. C. Singer, *The Development of the Doctrine of Contagium Vivum 1500–1750* (London: Royal College of Surgeons of England, 1913), 10.

6. Torrey, "Athanasius Kircher"; E. Fletcher and A. Kircher, *A Study of The Life and Works of Athanasius Kircher, "Germanus Incredibilis"* (Leiden: Brill, 2011), 118.

7. P. Gottdenker, "Francesco Redi and the Fly Experiments," *Bulletin of the History of Medicine* 53, no. 4 (1979): 575–592.

8. F. Redi, *Experiments on the Generation of Insects*, trans. M. K. Bigelow (New York: Kraus Reprint, 1969).

9. E. G. Ruestow, "Leeuwenhoek and the Campaign against Spontaneous Generation," *Journal of the History of Biology* 17, no. 2 (1984): 225–248.

CHAPTER 5

1. J. R. Busvine, *Insects, Hygiene and History* (London: Athlone Press, 1976), 204–206, 215–217; J. Romaní and M. Romaní, "Causes and Cures of Skin Diseases in the Work of Hildegard of Bingen," *Actas Dermosifiliogr.* 108, no. 6 (2017): 538–543.

2.   G. C. Bonomo, "An Abstract of Part of a Letter from Dr Bonomo to Signor Redi, Containing Some Observations Concerning the Worms of Humane Bodies," trans. R. Mead, *Philosophical Transactions (1683–1775)* 23 (1702): 1296–1299.

3.   M. A. Montesu and F. Cottoni, "G. C. Bonomo and D. Cestoni: Discoverers of the Parasitic Origin of Scabies," *American Journal of Dermatopathology* 13, no. 4 (1991): 425–427.

4.   L. Wilkinson, "Rinderpest and Mainstream Infectious Disease Concepts in the Eighteenth Century," *Medical History* 28, no. 2 (1984): 129–150.

5.   DeLacy, *Germ of an Idea*, 76–77.

6.   Wilkinson, "Mainstream Infectious Disease."

7.   G. M. Lancisi, "The Draining of Swamps as a Key to the Elimination of Disease," in *Tropical Medicine and Parasitology: Classic Investigations*, ed. B. H. Kean, K. E. Mott, and A. J. Russell (Ithaca, NY: Cornell University Press, 1978), 22. First published 1717.

8.   DeLacy, *Germ of an Idea*, 82.

9.   C. F. Cogrossi, *New Theory of the Contagious Disease among Oxen*, trans. D. M. Schullian (Rome: Sixth International Congress of Microbiology, 1953), 1.

10. Cogrossi, *New Theory*, 9, 4–5, 6–7.

11. Cogrossi, 7, 15, 32, 17.

12. Congrossi, 18, 13, 28; C. A. Spinage, *Cattle Plague: A History* (New York: Kluwer Academic/Plenum, 2003), 61.

13. Wilkinson, "Mainstream Infectious Disease."

CHAPTER 6

1.   C. Mather, *Diary of Cotton Mather* (Boston: Massachusetts Historical Society, 1911), 8:657–658.

2.   S. Coss, *The Fever of 1721* (New York: Simon & Schuster, 2016), 183; K. Silverman, *The Life and Times of Cotton Mather* (New York: Harper & Row, 1984), 221; Mather, *Diary of Cotton Mather*, 2:216–217.

3.   Z. Boylston, *An Historical Account of the Small-Pox Inoculated in New-England* (London: S. Chandler, 1726), 44.

4.   Boswell Collection, box 58, folder 1220, General Collection, Beinecke Rare Book and Manuscript Library. Boswell's Memorial for Sir John Pringle, n.d.

5.   O. T. Beall and R. H. Shryock, *Cotton Mather: First Significant Figure in American Medicine* (Baltimore: Johns Hopkins University Press, 1954), 52ff.

6.   C. Mather, E. Timonius, and J. Pylarinus, *Some Account of What Is Said of Inoculating or Transplanting the Small Pox* (Boston: Z. Boylston, 1721), 8.

7.   G. L. Kittredge, *Some Lost Works of Cotton Mather* (Cambridge, MA: John Wilson & Son, 1912), 422, 431–432.

8. B. Colman, *Some Observations on the New Method of Receiving the Small-Pox by Ingrafting or Inoculating* (Boston: Gerrish, 1721), 15–16.

9. Boylston, *An Historical Account*; Mather, *Diary of Cotton Mather*, 2:632.

10. M. W. Montagu, *Essays and Poems, and Simplicity: A Comedy*, ed. R. Halsband and I. Grundy (Oxford: Clarendon Press, 1977), 204; C. Maitland, *Mr. Maitland's Account of Inoculating the Small Pox Vindicated* (London: J. Peele, 1722), 7.

11. I. Grundy, *Lady Mary Wortley Montagu* (Oxford: Oxford University Press, 2004), 209–210.

12. Montagu, *Essays and Poems*, 35–36; W. Wagstaffe, *A Letter to Dr. Freind: Shewing the Danger and Uncertainty of Inoculating the Small Pox* (London: Samuel Butler, 1722), 5–6, 36; W. Douglass, *Inoculation of the Small Pox as Practised in Boston: Consider'd in a Letter to A—S—M.D. & F.R.S. in London* (Boston: J Franklin, 1722).

13. Douglass, *Inoculation of the Small Pox*, 7.

14. J. B. Blake, *Public Health in the Town of Boston, 1630–1822* (Cambridge MA: Harvard University Press, 1959), 57–58.

15. DeLacy, *Germ of an Idea*, 4–5.

16. J. Jurin, "A Letter to the Learned Dr. Caleb Cotesworth," *Philosophical Transactions of the Royal Society* 32, no. 374 (1723): 213–227; R. A. Weiss and J. Esparza, "The Prevention and Eradication of Smallpox," *Philosophical Transactions of the Royal Society B* 370 (2015): 20140378; P. E. Razzell, *The Conquest of Smallpox: The Impact of Inoculation on Smallpox Mortality In Eighteenth Century Britain* (Firle, UK: Caliban Books, 2003), 94.

17. L. Stewart, "The Edge of Utility: Slaves and Smallpox in the Early Eighteenth Century," *Medical History* 29, no. 1 (1985): 54–70; Douglass, *Inoculation of the Small Pox*, 20.

18. C. Mather, *The Angel of Bethesda* (Worcester, MA: American Antiquarian Society, 1972), 43–44.

19. B. Marten, *A New Theory of Consumptions: More Especially of a Phthisis, or Consumption of the Lungs* (London: R. Knaplock, 1720), 45, 56.

20. J. Jurin, *The Correspondence of James Jurin (1684–1750): Physician and Secretary to the Royal Society* (Amsterdam: Rodopi, 1996), 100–106.

CHAPTER 7

1. J. C. Moore, *The History and Practice of Vaccination* (London: J. Callow, 1817), 4; J. Baron, *The Life of Edward Jenner: With Illustrations of His Doctrines, and Selections from His Correspondence* (London: Colburn, 1838), 1:1–6, 1:88.

2. W. Moore, *The Knife Man: The Extraordinary Life and Times of John Hunter, Father of Modern Surgery* (New York: Broadway Books, 2005), 4, 239.

3. "Letter: From John Hunter to Edward Jenner, 2nd August 1775," *Annals of the Royal College of Surgeons of England* 54, no. 3 (1974):149.

4. J. Oppenheimer, "Anne Home Hunter and Her Friends," *Journal of the History of Medicine and Allied Sciences* 1, no. 3 (1946): 434–445.

5. T. D. Fosbroke and J. Smyth, *Berkeley Manuscripts: Abstracts and Extracts of Smyth's Lives of the Berkeleys . . . and Biographical Anecdotes of Dr. Jenner, Etc.* (London: John Nichols, 1821), 230; R. B. Fisher, *Edward Jenner 1749–1823* (London: André Deutsch, 1991), 31; Baron, *Life of Edward Jenner*, 1:20, 1:26, 1:71.

6. Baron, *Life of Edward Jenner*, 1:15–16; T. D. Fosbroke, *A Picturesque and Topographical Account of Cheltenham and Its Vicinity: To which Are Added Contributions towards the Medical Topography, Including the Medical History of the Waters* (Cheltenham, UK: S. C. Harper, 1826), 276–277.

7. Baron, *Life of Edward Jenner*, 1:16; Fisher, *Edward Jenner 1749–1823*, 45–46, 52–53.

8. E. Scott, "Edward Jenner, F.R.S. and the Cuckoo," *Notes and Records of the Royal Society of London* 28, no. 2 (1974): 235–240.

9. C. Creighton, *Jenner and Vaccination: A Strange Chapter of Medical History* (London: Swan Sonnenschein, 1889), 14, 17; Scott, "Edward Jenner."

10. Fosbroke and Smyth, *Berkeley Manuscripts*, 221–222; Baron, *Life of Edward Jenner*, 2:427–428.

11. A. W. Boylston, "The Myth of the Milkmaid," *New England Journal of Medicine* 378, no. 5 (2018): 414–415; R. Jesty and G. Williams, "Who Invented Vaccination?," *Malta Medical Journal* 23, no. 2 (2011): 29–32.

12. Baron, *Life of Edward Jenner*, 1:122, 1:125, 1:493; Moore, *History and Practice of Vaccination*, 19.

13. Fisher, *Edward Jenner 1749–1823*, 61, 55–56.

14. E. Jenner, *An Inquiry into the Causes and Effects of the Variolæ Vaccinæ* (London: Sampson Low, 1798), 32, 34; Baron, *Life of Edward Jenner*, 2:303–304.

CHAPTER 8

1. J. Banks, *Scientific Correspondence of Sir Joseph Banks, 1765–1820*, ed. N. Chambers (London: Pickering & Chatto, 2007), 4:474–475.

2. Baron, *Life of Edward Jenner*, 2:167–169; E. Jenner, *On the Origin of Vaccine Inoculation* (London: D. N. Shury, 1801), 10.

3. Jenner, *Inquiry into Causes and Effects*, 44; Baron, *Life of Edward Jenner*, 1:141.

4. Jenner, *Inquiry into Causes and Effects*, 66–68.

5. Jenner, *Inquiry into Causes and Effects*, 37; E. Jenner, *Further Observations on the Variolæ Vaccinæ, or Cow Pox* (London: Sampson Low, 1799), 4; J. Austen, *My Dear Cassandra: The Letters of Jane Austen*, ed. P. Hughes-Hallett (New York: Potter, 1991), 36.

6. Baron, *Life of Edward Jenner*, 1:307–314.

7. Moore, *History and Practice of Vaccination*, 22–25, 25n; G. Pearson, *An Inquiry Concerning the History of the Cowpox: Principally with a View to Supersede and Extinguish the Smallpox* (London: J. Johnson, 1798), 3; Fisher, *Edward Jenner 1749–1823*, 96.

8. Fisher, *Edward Jenner 1749–1823*, 127–131; Banks, *Scientific Correspondence*, 5:217.

9. Baron, *Life of Edward Jenner*, 1:155–156.

10. G. Miller, *Letters of Edward Jenner and Other Documents Concerning the Early History of Vaccination* (Baltimore: Johns Hopkins University Press, 1983), 11–12; E. J. Edwardes, *A Concise History of Small-Pox and Vaccination in Europe* (London: H. K. Lewis, 1902), 42; Baron, *Life of Edward Jenner*, 2:53.

11. Baron, *Life of Edward Jenner*, 1:453, 1:403; M. Few, "Circulating Smallpox Knowledge: Guatemalan Doctors, Maya Indians and Designing Spain's Smallpox Vaccination Expedition, 1780–1803," *British Journal for the History of Science* 43, no. 4 (2010): 519–537.

12. A. Rusnock, "Catching Cowpox: The Early Spread of Smallpox Vaccination, 1798–1810," *Bulletin of the History of Medicine* 83, no. 1 (2009): 17–36.

13. Baron, *Life of Edward Jenner*, 1:410–411, 1:413.

14. Fisher, *Edward Jenner 1749–1823*, 110–111; T. Jefferson, *The Papers of Thomas Jefferson*, ed. B Oberg (Princeton, NJ: Princeton University Press, 2008), 40:179.

15. C. Mark and J. G. Rigau-Pérez, "The World's First Immunization Campaign: The Spanish Smallpox Vaccine Expedition, 1803–1813," *Bulletin of the History of Medicine* 83, no. 1 (2009): 63–94.

16. Jenner, *Origin of Vaccine Inoculation*.

17. *Thomas Jefferson to G. C. Edward Jenner*, May 14, 1806, manuscript/mixed material, https://www.loc.gov/item/mtjbib016128/.

CHAPTER 9

1. B. Lewis, "The Sewer and the Prostitute in Les Misérables: From Regulation to Redemption," *Nineteenth-Century French Studies* 44, no. 3–4 (2016): 266–278.

2. A. S. Wohl, *Endangered Lives: Public Health in Victorian Britain* (Cambridge, MA: Harvard University Press, 1983), 88.

3. R. A. Lewis, *Edwin Chadwick and the Public Health Movement, 1832–1854* (New York: Kelley, 1970), 3.

4. B. W. Richardson, *The Health of Nations: A Review of the Works of Edwin Chadwick* (London: Longmans, Green, 1887), xxi.

5. Lewis, *Public Health Movement*, 3.

6. S. Litsios, "Charles Dickens and the Movement for Sanitary Reform," *Perspectives in Biology and Medicine* 46, no. 2 (2003): 183–199.

7. Lewis, *Public Health Movement*, 12, 22, 34–39; S. E. Finer, *The Life and Times of Sir Edwin Chadwick* (London: Methuen, 1952), 163, 209–210.

8. Wohl, *Endangered Lives*, 147–148.

9. E. Chadwick, *Report to Her Majesty's Principal Secretary of State for the Home Department, from the Poor Law Commissioners, on an Inquiry into the Sanitary Condition of the Labouring Population of Great Britain* (London: HMSO, 1842), 24, 47, 34, 3, 158, 176–177, 369. Lewis, *Public Health Movement*, 63

10. Litsios, "Sanitary Reform"; C. Dickens, *Dombey and Son* (London: Bradbury & Evans, 1848), 359.

11. C. Dickens, "To Working Men," *Household Words: A Weekly Journal* 10 (1850): 170.

12. E. Chadwick, *A Supplementary Report on the Results of a Spiecal [sic] Inquiry into the Practice of Interment in Towns* (London: HMSO, 1843), 25, 35.

13. *First Report of the Commissioners for Inquiring into the State of Large Towns and Populous Districts* (London: HMSO, 1844); *Second Report of the Commissioners for Inquiring into the State of Large Towns and Populous Districts* (London: HMSO, 1845), 11–12, 25, 122.

14. S. Halliday, *The Great Filth: Disease, Death and the Victorian City* (Gloucestershire, UK: History Press, 2011), 25.

15. Lewis, *Public Health Movement*, 181.

16. Wohl, *Endangered Lives*, 151; *Report of the Health of London Association on the Sanitary Condition of the Metropolis* (London: Health of Towns Association, 1847), vii.

17. Lewis, *Public Health Movement*, 315–316, 339-340; *Report of the General Board of Health on the Administration of the Public Health Act . . . from 1846 to 1854* (London: HMSO, 1854), 14, 28–30.

18. A. Brundage, *England's "Prussian Minister": Edwin Chadwick and the Politics of Government Growth, 1832–1854* (University Park: Pennsylvania State University Press, 1988), 140, 153.

19. "If There Is Such a Thing as a Political Certainty," *Times* (London), August 1, 1854, 8 (col. 6), http://tinyurl.galegroup.com/tinyurl/BSPBP0 (accessed July 30, 2019).

CHAPTER 10

1. Wohl, *Endangered Lives*, 118–119.

2. W. T. Gairdner, *Public Health in Relation to Air and Water* (Edinburgh: Edmonston and Douglas, 1862), 15-16.

3. R. Pollitzer, "Cholera Studies: 1: History of the Disease," *Bulletin of the World Health Organization* 10, no. 3 (1954): 421–461.

4. W. Macmichael, "A Brief Sketch of the Progress of Opinion on the Subject of Contagion," *The Pamphleteer* 15, no. 1 (1825): 519–531.

5. R. H. Major, "Agostino Bassi and the Parasitic Theory of Disease," *Bulletin of the History of Medicine* 16, no. 2 (1944): 97–107.

6. J. R. Porter, "Agostino Bassi Bicentennial (1773–1973)," *Bacteriological Reviews* 37, no. 3 (1973): 284–288.

7. Major, "Agostino Bassi and the Parasitic Theory of Disease."

8. W. C. Campbell, "History of Trichinosis: Paget, Owen and the Discovery of *Trichinella spiralis*," *Bulletin of the History of Medicine* 53, no. 4 (1979): 520–552.

9. J. Paget, *Memoirs and letters of Sir James Paget* (London: Longmans, 1901), 55.

10. Campbell, "History of Trichinosis."

11. W. C. Campbell, "A Historic Photomicrograph of a Parasite (*Trichomonas vaginalis*)," *Trends in Parasitology* 17, no. 10 (2001): 499–500; A. L. Thorburn, "Alfred François Donné, 1801–1878, Discoverer of *Trichomonas vaginalis* and of Leukaemia," *British Journal of Venereal Diseases* 50, no. 5 (1974): 377–380.

CHAPTER 11

1. K. C. Carter and B. R. Carter, *Childbed Fever: A Scientific Biography of Ignaz Semmelweis* (Westport, CT: Greenwood Press, 1994), 21–24, 44–45.

2. I. Semmelweis, *Etiology, Concept and Prophylaxis of Childbed Fever*, trans. K. C. Carter (Madison: University of Wisconsin Press, 1983), 87–89, 122, 98.

3. Semmelweis, *Childbed Fever*, 89–92.

4. O. W. Holmes, "The Contagiousness of Puerperal Fever," *New England Quarterly Journal of Medical Surgery* (1843): 1:503–530; C. D. Meigs, *On the Nature, Signs, and Treatment of Childbed Fevers* (Philadelphia: Blanchard and Lea, 1854), 104; W. J. Sinclair, *Semmelweis: His Life and Doctrine: A Chapter in the History of Medicine* (Manchester: University Press, 1909), 1.

5. K. C. Carter, "Ignaz Semmelweis, Carl Mayrhofer, and the Rise of Germ Theory," *Medical History* 29, no. 1 (1985): 33–53; Semmelweis, *Childbed Fever*, 37.

6. Carter and Carter, *Childbed Fever*, 72–73.

7. Sinclair, *Semmelweis*, 81, 93; Carter and Carter, *Childbed Fever*, 69, 64.

8. Sinclair, *Semmelweis*, 250–251, 247; O. W. Holmes, *Medical Essays, 1842–1882* (Boston: Houghton, Mifflin, 1883), 128.

9. Carter, "Rise of Germ Theory"; Sinclair, *Semmelweis*, 55, 290–291.

10. K. Carter, S. Abbott, and J. Siebach, "Five Documents Relating to the Final Illness and Death of Ignaz Semmelweis," *Bulletin of the History of Medicine* 69, no. 2 (1995): 255–270.

11. Sinclair, *Semmelweis*, 367.

CHAPTER 12

1. M. Bentivoglio and P. Pacini, "Filippo Pacini: A Determined Observer," *Brain Research Bulletin* 38, no. 2 (1995): 161–165.

2. C. Pogliano, "Eye, Mind, Hand: Filippo Pacini's Microscopy," *Nuncius* 28, no. 2 (2013): 313–344.

3. D. Lippi and E. Gotuzzo, "The Greatest Steps towards the Discovery of *Vibrio cholerae*," *Clinical Microbiology and Infection* 20, no. 3 (2014): 191–195.

4. N. Howard-Jones, *The Scientific Background of the International Sanitary Conferences: 1851–1938* (Geneva: World Health Organization, 1975).

5. "Microscopic Observations and Pathological Deductions on Asiatic Cholera," *British and Foreign Medico-Chirurgical Review* 16, no. 31 (July 1855): 144–145.

6. "A Treatise on the Specific Cause of Cholera, Its Pathology and Cure," *British and Foreign Medico-Chirurgical Review* 38 (July 1866): 167–168.

7. Pogliano, "Eye, Mind, Hand"; Howard-Jones, *Scientific Background*.

8. J. Snow, *On the Mode of Communication of Cholera* (London: John Churchill, 1855), 20.

9. P. Vinten-Johansen, H. Brody, N. Paneth, S. Rachman, and M. Rip, *Cholera, Chloroform, and the Science of Medicine: A Life of John Snow* (Oxford: Oxford University Press, 2003), 165–166.

10. J. F. Newton, *The Return to Nature: or, A Defence of the Vegetable Regimen* (London: Cadell & Davies, 1811), 37–43, 137.

11. "The Splendid Report on Cholera," *Lancet* 62, no. 1573 (1853): 393–394.

12. Snow, *On the Mode of Communication of Cholera* (London: John Churchill, 1849), 8–18; Vinten-Johansen et al., *Science of Medicine*, 202–210.

13. General Board of Health, *Report of the General Board of Health on the Epidemic Cholera of 1848 & 1849* (London: HMSO, 1850), 56–57.

14. Snow, *Communication of Cholera* (1849), 30.

15. M. Worboys, *Spreading Germs: Disease Theories and Medical Practice in Britain, 1865–1900* (Cambridge: Cambridge University Press, 2006), 41.

16. W. Heath, *Monster Soup Commonly Called Thames Water* (London: Thomas McLean, 1828); "Dirty Father Thames," *Punch* 15, October 7, 1848, 152; A. H. Hassall, "The Filtration of Water," *Morning Post*, April 11, 1850.

17. Vinten-Johansen et al., *Science of Medicine*, 261; J. Farr, "Cholera and the London Water Supply," *Registrar General's Weekly Return of Births and Deaths, 1850–1886*, November 19, 1854, 401, 409; Snow, *Communication of Cholera* (1855), 75.

18. Vinten-Johansen et al., *Science of Medicine*, 267–270.

CHAPTER 13

1. Snow, *Communication of Cholera* (1855), 15, 38–39, 52.

2. H. Brody, M. Rip, P. Vinten-Johansen, N. Paneth, and S. Rachman, "Map-Making and Myth-Making in Broad Street: The London Cholera Epidemic, 1854," *Lancet* 356, no. 9223 (2000): 64–68; J. Snow, *Snow on Cholera, Being a Reprint of Two Papers*, ed. W. H. Frost (New York: Commonwealth Fund, 1936), ix.

3. Brody et al., "Map-Making"; Vinten-Johansen et al., *Science of Medicine*, 328–337.

4. Snow, *Communication of Cholera* (1855), 40–44, 67; Vinten-Johansen et al., *Science of Medicine*, 245, 316–317.

5. H. Whitehead, "The Broad Street Pump," *Macmillan's Magazine* (December 1865): 113–122; "The Broad-Street Pump," *The Examiner* (London), November 24, 1855, 738–739.

6. A. B. Hill, "Snow—An Appreciation," *Proceedings of the Royal Society of Medicine* 48, no. 12 (1955): 1008–1012; Whitehead, "Broad Street Pump."

7. Whitehead, "Broad Street Pump."

8. Snow, *Communication of Cholera* (1855), 83; T. Koch, "Commentary: Nobody Loves a Critic: Edmund A. Parkes and John Snow's Cholera," *International Journal of Epidemiology* 42, no. 6 (2013): 1553–1559.

9. E. A. Parkes, "Mode of Communication of Cholera," *British and Foreign Medico-Chirurgical Review* 15, no. 30 (April 1855): 449–463.

10. D. E. Lilienfeld, "John Snow: The First Hired Gun?," *American Journal of Epidemiology* 152, no. 1 (2000): 4–9.

11. "It Is the Misfortune of Medicine," *Lancet* 65, no. 1660 (1855): 634–635.

12. E. H. Greenhow, *Papers Relating to the Sanitary State of the People of England* (London: Eyre & Spottiswoode, 1858), xiv–xv.

13. Howard-Jones, *Scientific Background*.

14. General Register Office, *Report on the Cholera Epidemic of 1866 in England: Supplement to the Twenty-Ninth Annual Report of the Registrar-General of Births, Deaths, and Marriages in England* (London: Eyre & Spottiswoode, 1868), 85–95, 100–101, 147.

15. General Register Office, *Cholera Epidemic*, 302; S. Halliday, "William Farr: Campaigning Statistician," *Journal of Medical Biography* 8, no. 4 (2000): 220–227; "Medical Annotations," *Lancet* 88, no. 2248 (1866): 363–364; Vinten-Johansen et al., *Science of Medicine*, 394.

16. Howard-Jones, *Scientific Background*; J. P. Vandenbroucke, H. M. E. Rooda, and H. Beukers, "Who Made John Snow a Hero?," *American Journal of Epidemiology* 133, no. 10 (1991): 967–973.

CHAPTER 14

1. P. Debré, *Louis Pasteur* (Baltimore: Johns Hopkins University Press, 2000), 6, 54, 183–184.

2. L. Geison, *Private Science of Louis Pasteur* (Princeton, NJ: Princeton University Press, 1995), 25; Debré, *Louis Pasteur*, xxiv, 86, 140–141, 208.

3. Debré, *Louis Pasteur*, 12, 4, 74, 38–39.

4. J. Gal, "In Defense of Louis Pasteur: Critique of Gerald Geison's Deconstruction of Pasteur's Discovery of Molecular Chirality," *Chirality* 31, no. 4 (2019): 261–282; Debré, 46–51.

5. Geison, *Private Science*, 96; Debré, *Louis Pasteur*, 76.

6. Debré, *Louis Pasteur*, 103, 87; Geison, *Private Science*, 94.

7. Debré, *Louis Pasteur*, 90–93.

8. Geison, *Private Science*, 96.

9. Debré, *Louis Pasteur*, 106–108.

10. Geison, *Private Science*, 90–91.

11. R. J. Dubos, *Pasteur and Modern Science*, ed. T. D. Brock (Madison, WI: Science Tech, 1988); Debré, *Louis Pasteur*, 101.

12. Debré, *Louis Pasteur*, 148; L. Pasteur, "On the Organized Bodies Which Exist in the Atmosphere; Examination of the Doctrine of Spontaneous Generation," in Brock, *Milestones in Microbiology*, 44. First published 1861.

13. Debré, *Louis Pasteur*, 158.

14. N. Roll-Hansen, "Revisiting the Pouchet–Pasteur Controversy over Spontaneous Generation: Understanding Experimental Method," *History and Philosophy of the Life Sciences* 40, no. 4 (2018), https://doi.org/10.1007/s40656-018-0229-7.

15. L. Pasteur and L. P. Vallery-Radot, *Oeuvres de Pasteur* (Paris: Masson et cie, 1922), 2:237, 2:315, 2:343.

16. Debré, *Louis Pasteur*, 166.

17. Pasteur and Vallery-Radot, *Oeuvres de Pasteur*, 2:190.

18. Geison, *Private Science*, 124, 130; Roll-Hansen, "Spontaneous Generation."

19. Pasteur and Vallery-Radot, *Oeuvres de Pasteur*, 2:328–338; Debré, *Louis Pasteur*, 159; Geison, *Private Science*, 130.

20. R. Vallery-Radot, *La Vie de Pasteur* (Paris: Hachette, 1900); Debré, *Louis Pasteur*, 128.

CHAPTER 15

1. M. Davidson, "Pioneers in Optics: Joseph Jackson Lister and Maksymilian Pluta," *Microscopy Today* 19, no. 3 (2011): 54–56; R. B. Fisher, *Joseph Lister* (London: MacDonald and Jane's, 1977), 21.

2.   F. Treves, *The Elephant Man and Other Reminiscences* (London: Cassell, 1923), 56; Fisher, *Joseph Lister*, 124.

3.   J. Lister, "On a New Method of Treating Compound Fracture, Abscess, Etc.," *Lancet* 89, no. 2272 (1867): 326–329; J. Lister, "Illustrations of the Antiseptic System of Treatment in Surgery," *Lancet* 90, no. 2309 (1867): 668–669.

4.   Lister, "New Method."

5.   Lister, "New Method"; Fisher, *Joseph Lister*, 136.

6.   Fisher, *Joseph Lister*, 145; Lister, "Antiseptic System."

7.   T. Nunneley, "Address in Surgery," *British Medical Journal* 2, no. 449 (1869): 143–156; L. Tait, "Effects of Carbolic Acid," *Medical Times and Gazette* 2 (1868): 465.

8.   Treves, *Elephant Man*, 56; J. Waller, *Fabulous Science: Fact and Fiction in the History of Scientific Discovery* (New York: Oxford University Press, 2002), 166.

9.   P. Banks, "The Lost World of Lord Lister," *Canadian Medical Association Journal* 135, no. 9 (1986): 1027–1030.

10. R. Richardson, "Joseph Lister's Domestic Science," *Lancet* 382, no. 9898 (2013): 8–9.

11. M. Santer, "Joseph Lister: First Use of a Bacterium as a 'Model Organism' to Illustrate the Cause of Infectious Disease of Humans," *Notes and Records of the Royal Society Journal of the History of Science* 64, no. 1 (2009): 59–65; J. Lister, "On the Lactic Fermentation and Its Bearings on Pathology," *Transactions of the Pathological Society of London* 29 (1878): 425–467; Richardson, "Lister's Domestic Science."

12. Fisher, *Joseph Lister*, 176.

13. U. Tröhler, "Statistics and the British Controversy about the Effects of Joseph Lister's System of Antisepsis for Surgery, 1867–1890," *Journal of the Royal Society of Medicine* 108, no. 7 (2015): 280–287.

14. L. Tait, "Clinical Lecture on the Details Necessary in the Performance of Abdominal Section," *Lancet* 138, no. 3550 (1891): 597–599.

CHAPTER 16

1.   Debré, *Louis Pasteur*, 303.

2.   G. B. Webb, "Robert Koch 1843–1910," *Annals of Medical History* 4 (1932): 509–523; T. D. Brock, *Robert Koch, a Life in Medicine and Bacteriology* (Madison, WI: Science Tech Publishers and Berlin: Springer, 1988), 23, 31.

3.   Brock, *A Life*, 11–12; K. C. Carter, "Koch's Postulates in Relation to the Work of Jacob Henle and Edwin Klebs," *Medical History* 29, no. 4 (1985): 353–374.

4.   Brock, *A Life*, 31.

5.   Brock, 33–34, 46–47, 94.

CHAPTER 17

1. Geison, *Private Science*, 159.

2. A. Cadeddu, "Pasteur et le Choléra des Poules: Révision Critique d'un Récit Historique," *History and Philosophy of the Life Sciences* 7, no. 1 (1985): 87–104.

3. Cadeddu, "Pasteur et le Choléra des Poules"; Debré, *Louis Pasteur*, 379

4. Cadeddu, "Pasteur et le Choléra des Poules"; Geison, *Private Science*, 40, 167.

5. Cadeddu, "Pasteur et le Choléra des Poules"; Debré, *Louis Pasteur*, 379; L. Pasteur, "The Attenuation of the Causal Agent of Fowl Cholera," in Brock, *Milestones in Microbiology*, 126–130. First published 1880.

6. Cadeddu, "Pasteur et le Choléra des Poules"; Brock, *Milestones in Microbiology*, 130.

7. Debré, *Louis Pasteur*, 389.

8. Geison, *Private Science*, 163–171, 287–291, appendix E, 294–295, appendix I.

9. L. Pasteur, Chamberland, and Roux, "Summary Report of the Experiments Conducted at Pouilly-le-Fort, 1881," *Yale Journal of Biology and Medicine* 75, no. 1 (2002): 59–62.

10. Debré, *Louis Pasteur*, 396.

11. A. Cadeddu, "Pasteur et la Vaccination Contre le Charbon: Une Analyse Historique et Critique," *History and Philosophy of the Life Sciences* 9, no. 2 (1987): 255–276.

12. Debré, *Louis Pasteur*, 397–399.

13. C. Nicolle, *Biologie de l'Invention* (Paris: Librairie Félix Alcan, 1932), 64.

14. Debré, *Louis Pasteur*, 400–401; "From Our Correspondents: France," *Times* (London), June 3, 1881, 5.

15. Pasteur, Chamberland, and Roux, "Summary Report"; Geison, *Private Science*, 173.

16. J. Cavaillon and S. Legout, "Duclaux, Chamberland, Roux, Grancher, and Metchnikoff: The Five Musketeers of Louis Pasteur," *Genes & Immunity* 20, no. 5 (2019): 344–356.

17. Geison, *Private Science*, 175.

CHAPTER 18

1. Brock, *A Life*, 56, 65, 72.

2. V. Jay, "The Legacy of Robert Koch," *Archives of Pathology & Laboratory Medicine* 125, no. 9 (2001): 1148–1149; Brock, *A Life*, 22–23, 54–69.

3. "The Mauve Measles," *Punch* 37, August 20, 1859, 81–81.

4. Brock, *A Life*, 76.

5. S. Bradbury, *The Evolution of the Microscope* (Oxford: Pergamon, 1968), 245–250; Brock, *A Life*, 66–69, 76.

6. R. Koch, "Methods for the Study of Pathogenic Organisms," in Brock, *Milestones in Microbiology*, 101–108. First published 1881.

7. Brock, *A Life*, 100; Brock, *Milestones in Microbiology*, 108; A. Ullman, "Pasteur-Koch: Distinctive Ways of Thinking about Infectious Diseases," *mBio*, 2, no. 8 (2007): 383–387.

8. Debré, *Louis Pasteur*, 361–363; Brock, *A Life*, 73.

9. Koch, "Methods," in Brock, *Milestones in Microbiology*, 107–108.

CHAPTER 19

1. Brock, *A Life*, 72, 117; J. B. Huber, *Consumption, Its Relation to Man and His Civilization, Its Prevention and Cure* (Philadelphia: J. B. Lippincott, 1906), 18, 41.

2. T. Moore, *Memoirs, Journal and Correspondence of Thomas Moore* (London: Longman, Brown, Green, and Longmans, 1853), 461.

3. D. Thomas and D. K. Jackson, *The Poe Log: A Documentary Life of Edgar Allan Poe, 1809–1849* (New York: G. K. Hall, 1987), 519; H. Allen, *Israfel: The Life and Times of Edgar Allan Poe* (New York: George H. Doran, 1926), 2:519–521.

4. R. W. Emerson, *The Letters of Ralph Waldo Emerson*, ed. R. L. Rusk (New York: Columbia University Press, 1939), 1:233.

5. Brock, *A Life*, 118–119, 126.

6. Brock, 119–120.

7. R. Koch, "The Etiology of Tuberculosis [Koch's Postulates]," in Brock, *Milestones in Microbiology*, 109–115. First published 1882.

8. J. M. Grange and P. J. Bishop, "'Über Tuberkulose': A Tribute to Robert Koch's Discovery of the Tubercle Bacillus, 1882," *Tubercle* 63, no. 1 (1982): 3–17.

9. Koch, "Etiology," 110–115.

10. R. Koch, "Die Ätiologie der Tuberkulose," *Berliner Klinische Wochenschrift*, no. 15 (April 10, 1882): 221–230.

11. Brock, *A Life*, 129.

12. "Supplying a Last Link," *New York Times*, May 3, 1882; "New Parasites," *New York Times*, May 5, 1882; "Dr. Koch's Discovery," *New York Times*, May 7, 1882.

13. T. M. Prudden, *Dust and Its Dangers* (New York: G. P. Putnam's Sons, 1890), 60–61, 70, 77–78.

14. F. M. Snowden, *Epidemics and Society: From the Black Death to the Present* (New Haven, CT: Yale University Press, 2019), 299.

15. L. E. Holt, *The Care and Feeding of Children* (New York: D. Appleton, 1914), 176.

16. L. G. Wilson, "The Historical Decline of Tuberculosis in Europe and America: Its Causes and Significance," *Journal of the History of Medicine and Allied Sciences* 45, no. 3 (1990): 366–396.

17. Koch, "Etiology," 116–118.

CHAPTER 20

1. "Cholera in Egypt," *British Medical Journal* 2, no. 1185 (September 15, 1883): 541–542.

2. Debré, *Louis Pasteur*, 342.

3. Debré, 406; Brock, *A Life*, 171–175.

4. Howard-Jones, *Scientific Background*; Brock, *A Life*, 142–146.

5. "Report of the German Cholera Commission," *Science* 2, no. 42 (November 23, 1883), 675–678; Howard-Jones, *Scientific Background*.

6. Brock, *A Life*, 151–158; Debré, *Louis Pasteur*, 342.

7. R. Koch, "Dr. Koch on the Cholera," *Lancet* 124, no. 3180 (1884): 292–295.

8. Brock, *A Life*, 160.

9. Howard-Jones, *Scientific Background*.

10. R. Koch and J. Schwalbe, *Gesammelte Werke von Robert Koch* (Leipzig: Georg Thieme, 1912), 13–17.

11. Brock, *A Life*, 176–177.

CHAPTER 21

1. Debré, *Louis Pasteur*, 417, 420–430; Geison, *Private Science*, 187–192.

2. L. Pasteur and J. J. Pasteur, *Correspondance de Pasteur 1840–1895*, ed. P. Vallery-Radot (Paris: Flammarion, 1940), 3:438; Debré, *Louis Pasteur*, 434–435.

3. Geison, *Private Science*, 236.

4. Debré, *Louis Pasteur*, 426–427.

5. Debré, 435; Geison, *Private Science*, 254–255.

6. Debré, *Louis Pasteur*, 426–440; Geison, *Private Science*, 193–205, 236–243, 254–255.

7. L. Pasteur, *Œuvres de Pasteur* (Paris: Masson et cie, 1922), 6:609–611.

8. "One of Pasteur's Patients Dies," *New York Times*, December 8, 1885, 1; Debré, *Louis Pasteur*, 445.

CHAPTER 22

1. E. Caufield, "A True History of the Terrible Epidemic Vulgarly Called the Throat Distemper which Occurred in His Majesty's New England Colonies between the Years 1735 and 1740," *Yale Journal of Biology and Medicine* 11, no. 3 (1939): 219; W. Brown, *History of Hampton Falls* (Concord, NH: Rumford Press, 1900), 1:301.

2. J. Duffy, *A History of Public Health in New York City, 1866–1966* (New York: Russell Sage Foundation, 1974), 154–155; A. C. Hüntelmann, *Diphtheria Serum and Serotherapy: Development, Production and Regulation in Fin de Siècle Germany* (Dynamis: Acta Hispanica ad Medicinae Scientiarumque Historiam Illustrandam, 2007), 27:107–131.

3. F. Winau and R. Winau, "Emil von Behring and Serum Therapy," *Microbes and Infection* 4, no. 2 (2002): 185–188.

4. É. Roux and A. Yersin, "Contribution à l'Étude de la Diphthérie," *Annales de l'Institut Pasteur* (1888) 2, 629–661; and "Contribution à l'Étude de la Diphthérie" (2e memoire), *Annales de l'Institut Pasteur* (1889) 3: 273–288.

5. Winau and Winau, "Serum Therapy."

6. Brock, *A Life*, 226; E. v. Behring and S. Kitasato, "The Mechanism of Immunity in Animals to Diphtheria and Tetanus," in Brock, *Milestones in Microbiology*, 138–144 (first published 1890); S. H. Kaufmann, "Remembering Emil von Behring: From Tetanus Treatment to Antibody Cooperation with Phagocytes," *mBio* 8, no. 1 (2017): e00117-17.

7. Brock, *A Life*, 196, 205; A. C. Doyle, "Character Sketch," *Review of Reviews*, December 1890, 551.

8. E. M. Hammonds, *Childhood's Deadly Scourge: The Campaign to Control Diphtheria in New York City, 1880–1930* (Baltimore: Johns Hopkins University Press, 1999), 92.

9. H. F. Dowling, *Fighting Infection: Conquests of the Twentieth Century* (Cambridge, MA: Harvard University Press, 1977), 37; "La Guérison Du Croup," *Le Figaro*, September 6, 1894, 1.

10. D. S. Linton, *Emil von Behring: Infectious Disease, Immunology, Serum Therapy* (Philadelphia: American Philosophical Society, 2005), 171–172.

11. Linton, *Emil von Behring*, 397–403.

12. J. Cavaillon and S. Legout, "Centenary of the Death of Elie Metchnikoff: A Visionary and an Outstanding Team Leader," *Microbes and Infection* 18, no. 10 (2016): 577–594.

13. A. I. Tauber, "The Birth of Immunology," *Cellular Immunology* 139, no. 2 (1992): 505–530.

14. Cavaillon and Legout, "Death of Elie Metchnikoff."

15. S. H. Kaufmann, "Immunology's Foundation: The 100-Year Anniversary of the Nobel Prize to Paul Ehrlich and Elie Metchnikoff," *Nature Immunology* 9, no. 7 (2008): 705–712.

16. A. E. Wright and S. R. Douglas, "An Experimental Investigation of the Role of the Blood Fluids in Connection with Phagocytosis," *Proceedings of the Royal Society of London* 72 (1904): 357–370; B. Shaw, *The Doctor's Dilemma, Getting Married, and the Shewing-Up of Blanco Posnet* (London: Constable, 1911), 10.

CHAPTER 23

1. P. H. Manson-Bahr, *Patrick Manson, the Father of Tropical Medicine* (London: Thomas Nelson, 1962), 10; D. M. Haynes, *Imperial Medicine: Patrick Manson and the Conquest of Tropical Disease* (Philadelphia: University of Pennsylvania Press, 2013), 39–41.

2. P. Manson, "On the Development of *Filaria sanguinis hominis*, and on the Mosquito Considered as a Nurse," *Zoological Journal of the Linnean Society* 14, no. 75 (1878): 304–311.

3. C. A. Gordon, *An Epitome of the Reports of the Medical Officers to the Chinese Imperial Maritime Customs Service, From 1871 to 1882* (London: Baillière, Tindall, 1884), 204.

4. C. L. Laveran, "A Newly Discovered Parasite in the Blood of Patients Suffering from Malaria," in *Tropical Medicine and Parasitology: Classic Investigations*, ed. B. H. Kean, K. E. Mott, and A. J. Russell (Ithaca, NY: Cornell University Press, 1978), 23–26. First published in 1880.

5. A. F. King, "The Prevention of Malarial Disease," *Popular Science* 23 (1883): 644–658.

6. C. J. Finlay, "The Mosquito Hypothetically Considered as the Agent of Transmission of Yellow Fever," *New Orleans Medical and Surgical Journal* 34 (1882): 600–616; C. J. Finlay, "Inoculations for Yellow Fever by Means of Contaminated Mosquitoes," *American Journal of the Medical Sciences* 102, no. 3 (1891): 264–268.

7. US Department of Agriculture, *Report of the Commissioner of Agriculture on the Diseases of Cattle in the United States* (Washington, DC: US Government Printing Office, 1871), 88, 118, 132.

8. T. Smith and F. L. Kilborne, *Investigations into the Nature, Causation, and Prevention of Texas or Southern Cattle Fever* (Washington, DC: US Government Printing Office, 1893), 94.

9. D. P. Anderson, A. D. Hagerman, P. D. Teel, G. G. Wagner, J. L. Outlaw, and B. K. Herbst, *Economic Impact of Expanded Fever Tick Range* (College Station: Agricultural and Food Policy Center, Texas A&M University, 2010).

10. P. Manson, "On the Nature and Significance of the Crescentic and Flagellated Bodies in Malarial Blood," *British Medical Journal* 2, no. 1771 (1894): 1306–1308.

CHAPTER 24

1. W. F. Bynum and C. Overy, *The Beast in the Mosquito: The Correspondence of Ronald Ross and Patrick Manson* (Netherlands: Rodopi, 1988), x–xi; Haynes, *Imperial Medicine*, 101.

2. Laveran, "Newly Discovered Parasite."

3. A. Bignami, J. Mannaberg, and E. Marchiafava, *Two Monographs on Malaria and the Parasites of Malarial Fevers*, trans. H. J. Thompson (London: New Sydenham Society, 1894), 272.

4. Bynum and Overy, *Beast in the Mosquito*, xii, 2–3; W. Bynum, "Experimenting with Fire: Giving Malaria," *Lancet* 376, no. 9752 (2010): 1534–1535.

5. Bynum and Overy, *Beast in the Mosquito*, 5–8, 31.

6. R. Ross, "On Some Peculiar Pigmented Cells Found in Two Mosquitos Fed on Malarial Blood," *British Medical Journal* 2, no. 1929 (1897): 1786–1788.

7. W. G. McCallum, "On the Flagellated Form of the Malarial Parasite," *Lancet* 2 (1897): 1240–1241; W. T. Longcope, *Biographical Memoir of William George MacCaullum, 1874–1944* (Washington, DC: National Academy of Sciences of the United States of America, 1945); R. Ross, *Memoirs: With a Full Account of the Great Malaria Problem and Its Solution* (London: J. Murray, 1923), 353.

8. Haynes, *Imperial Medicine*, 114–117.

9. Bynum and Overy, *Beast in the Mosquito*, 331–344.

10. P. Manson, "Surgeon-Major Ronald Ross's Recent Investigations on the Mosquito-Malaria Theory," *British Medical Journal* 1, no. 1955 (1898): 1575–1577.

11. Ross, *Memoirs*, 306; Bynum and Overy, *Beast in the Mosquito*, 401.

12. G. Bastianelli, A. Bignami, and B. Grassi, *Coltivazione delle Semilune Malariche dell' uomo nell' Anopheles claviger Fabr. (sinonimo: Anopheles masculipennis Meig.)* (Rome: Rendiconti, Accademia Nazionale dei Lincei, 1898).

13. Bynum and Overy, *Beast in the Mosquito*, 389.

14. J. Guillemin, "Choosing Scientific Patrimony: Sir Ronald Ross, Alphonse Laveran, and the Mosquito-Vector Hypothesis for Malaria," *Journal of the History of Medicine and Allied Sciences* 57, no. 4 (2002): 385–409.

15. P. Manson, "Experimental Proof of the Mosquito-Malaria Theory," *Lancet* 156, no. 4022 (1900): 923–925.

16. Guillemin, "Choosing Scientific Patrimony."

17. R. Ross, "Malaria and Mosquitoes 1," *Nature* 61, no. 1587 (1900): 522–527.

18. R. Ross, *Researches on Malaria, Being the Nobel Medical Prize Lecture for 1902* (Stockholm: Kungl, Boktryckeriet, 1904), 2.

19. Ross, *Memoirs*, 351–352, 354, 398, 402, 407, 413; Guillemin, "Choosing Scientific Patrimony."

CHAPTER 25

1. M. C. Walther, "Note sur l'Épidémiologie et la Prophylaxie du Tétanos," *Bulletin de l'Académie Nationale de Médecine* 72 (1914): 109–113; L. Bazy, "What the War Has Taught Us about Tetanus," *Lancet* 192, no. 4964 (1918): 523–526.

2. B. Moynihan, "An Address on the Treatment of Gunshot Wounds," *British Medical Journal* 1, no. 2879 (1916): 333–337.

3. P. C. Wever, and L. v. Bergen, "Prevention of Tetanus during the First World War," *Medical Humanities* 38, no. 2 (2012): 78–82.

4. J. Winter, "Demography," in *A Companion to World War I*, ed. J. Horne (Chichester, UK: Wiley-Blackwell, 2012), 249–250; Bergen and Wever, "Prevention of Tetanus."

5. W. Eckart, "The Colony as Laboratory: German Sleeping Sickness Campaigns in German East Africa and in Togo, 1900–1914," *History & Philosophy of the Life Sciences* 24, no. 1 (2002): 69–89.

6. W. Bäumler, *Paul Ehrlich: Scientist for Life*, trans. G. Edwards (New York: Holmes & Meier, 1984), 150, 167, 181; M. Marquardt, *Paul Ehrlich* (New York: Henry Schuman, 1951), 151, 173–174.

7. T. W. Gibbard and L. W. Harrison, "Further Investigations on the Use of Salvarsan in Syphilis," in *Collected Papers Reprinted from the Journal of the Royal Army Medical Corps* (London:

John Bale, 1912), 1:128; L. W. Harrison, "Ehrlich versus Syphilis," *British Journal of Venereal Diseases* 30, no. 1 (1954): 2–6.

8. H. Zinsser, *Rats, Lice, and History* (London: George Routledge, 1935), 221.

9. K. Pelis, *Charles Nicolle, Pasteur's Imperial Missionary: Typhus and Tunisia* (Rochester, NY: University of Rochester Press, 2013), 57–64.

10. W. Hutchinson, *The Doctor in War* (Boston: Houghton Mifflin, 1918), 4–5.

11. C. Nicolle, "Nobel Lecture: Investigations on Typhus," The Nobel Foundation, 1928, https://www.nobelprize.org/prizes/medicine/1928/nicolle/lecture/.

12. US Army Medical Research & Materiel Command, *Typhoid Vaccine Information Paper* (Washington, DC: 2006); W. S. Churchill, *London to Ladysmith via Pretoria* (London: Longmans, Green, 1900), 10–11.

13. V. D. Allison, "Personal Recollections of Sir Almroth Wright and Sir Alexander Fleming," *Ulster Medical Journal* 43, no. 2 (1974): 89–98; A. Hardy, "'Straight Back to Barbarism': Antityphoid Inoculation and the Great War, 1914," *Bulletin of the History of Medicine* 74, no. 2 (2000): 265–290.

14. W. Osler, "Compulsory Anti-Typhoid Vaccination," *Times* (London), August 29, 1914, 6; Hardy, "Back to Barbarism"; W. G. Macpherson, W. B. Leishman, and S. L. Cummins, *Medical Services: Pathology* (London: HMSO, 1923), 211.

15. J. Winter, "Demography," 250.

CHAPTER 26

1. E. Tognotti, "Scientific Triumphalism and Learning from Facts: Bacteriology and the 'Spanish Flu' Challenge of 1918," *Social History of Medicine* 16, no. 1 (2003): 97–110.

2. L. Wilkinson, "The Development of the Virus Concept as Reflected in Corpora of Studies on Individual Pathogens," *Medical History* 18, no. 3 (1974): 211–221.

3. J. K. Taubenberger, J. V. Hultin, and D. M. Morens, "Discovery and Characterization of the 1918 Pandemic Influenza Virus in Historical Context," *Antiviral Therapy* 12, no. 4B (2007): 581–591.

4. T. Yamanouchi, "The Infecting Agent in Influenza: An Experimental Research," *Lancet* 193, no. 4997 (1919): 971.

5. M. Bresalier, "Uses of a Pandemic: Forging the Identities of Influenza and Virus Research in Interwar Britain," *Social History of Medicine* 25, no. 2 (2011): 400–424.

6. MRC, *Report of the Medical Research Council for the Year 1921–1922* (London: HMSO, 1923), 12.

7. T. M. Rivers, "Filterable Viruses: A Critical Review," *Journal of Bacteriology* 14 (1927): 217–258.

8. "Influenza Again," *Times* (London), December 29, 1932, 9.

CHAPTER 27

1. G. Eldering, "Symposium on Pertussis Immunization, in Honor of Dr. Pearl Kendrick," *Health Laboratory Science* 8 (1971): 200–205.

2. C. Locht, pers. comm.

3. Roush and Murphy, "Historical Comparisons."

4. W. H. Welch, "Contribution of Bryn Mawr College to the Higher Education of Women," *Science* 56, no. 1436 (July 7, 1922): 1–8.

5. C. G. Shapiro-Shapin, "'A Whole Community Working Together': Pearl Kendrick, Grace Eldering, and the Grand Rapids Pertussis Trials, 1932–1939," *Michigan Historical Review* 33, no. 1 (2007): 59–85.

6. H. M. Marks, "The Kendrick-Eldering-(Frost) Pertussis Vaccine Field Trial," *Journal of the Royal Society of Medicine* 100, no. 5 (2007): 242–247.

7. C. G. Shapiro-Shapin, "Pearl Kendrick, Grace Eldering, and the Pertussis Vaccine," *Emerging Infectious Diseases* 16, no. 8 (2010): 1273–1278.

8. C. G. Shapiro-Shapin, "Interview with Loney Clinton Gordon, Pearl Kendrick & Grace Eldering," Michigan Women and the Whooping Cough Vaccine Collection 328, Grand Rapids Public Library, 1998.

9. M. Lohr, "Local Vaccine Developer Welcomes New Version," *Grand Rapids Press*, March 10, 1985, A16.

10. T. Labelle, "Pearl Kendrick and the Feminine Mystique," *Grand Rapids Press*, December 12, 1975, A7; S. Redland, pers. comm.

11. C. G. Shapiro-Shapin, pers. comm.

CHAPTER 28

1. M. Gilbert, *Winston S. Churchill: Road to Victory: 1941–1945* (Boston: Houghton Mifflin, 1986), 7:603–612.

2. R. M. Langworth, *Winston Churchill, Myth and Reality: What He Actually Did and Said* (Jefferson, NC: McFarland, 2017), 199.

3. K. Brown, *Penicillin Man: Alexander Fleming and the Antibiotic Revolution* (Stroud, UK: History Press, 2013), 25.

4. J. E. Lesch, *The First Miracle Drugs: How the Sulfa Drugs Transformed Medicine* (New York: Oxford University Press, 2007), 18–19, 44–50, 63, 159.

5. G. Domagk, "A Contribution to the Chemotherapy of Bacterial Infections," in Brock, *Milestones in Microbiology*, 195–198. First published 1935.

6. T. Hager, *The Demon under the Microscope: From Battlefield Hospitals to Nazi Labs, One Doctor's Heroic Search for the World's First Miracle Drug* (New York: Three Rivers Press, 2007), 126–132.

7. M. Kenny, "Chemotherapy in Obstetrics and Gynaecology," *BJOG* 52, no. 4 (1945): 372–388; Lesch, *First Miracle Drugs*, 60–63.

8. Lesch, *First Miracle Drugs*, 85–90; Domagk, "Chemotherapy of Bacterial Infections."

9. Lesch, *First Miracle Drugs*, 82.

10. Lesch, 84; A. Oliverio, "Daniel Bovet, 23 March 1907–8 April 1992," *Biographical Memoirs of the Fellows of the Royal Society* 39 (1994) 59–70.

11. Lesch, *First Miracle Drugs*, 105–106.

12. L. Colebrook and M. Kenny, "Treatment of Human Puerperal Infections, and of Experimental Infections in Mice, with Prontosil," *Lancet* 227, no. 5884 (1936): 1279–1281.

13. "Young Roosevelt Saved by New Drug," *New York Times*, December 17, 1936, 1; "Young Roosevelt Gets Tarpon," *New York Times*, January 21, 1937, 11.

14. S. Jayachandran, A. Lleras-Muney, and K. V. Smith, "Modern Medicine and the Twentieth Century Decline in Mortality: Evidence on the Impact of Sulfa Drugs," *American Economic Journal: Applied Economics* 2, no. 2 (2010): 118–146.

15. Lesch, *First Miracle Drugs*, 73, 101–102.

16. Lesch, 108–121; D. Jeffreys, *Hell's Cartel: IG Farben and the Making of Hitler's War Machine* (London: Bloomsbury, 2008), 374–375; *Trials of War Criminals Before the Nuernberg Military Tribunals under Control Council Law No. 10: Nuernberg, Oct. 1946–April 1949*, v. 7, 202–205, 247, v. 8, 1063 (Washington, DC: US Government Printing Office, 1952).

17. Medical Department United States Army, *Surgery*, vol. 2, ed. B. N. Carter and J. B. Coates (Washington, DC: Office of the Surgeon General, 1964).

CHAPTER 29

1. R. Hare, *The Birth of Penicillin and the Disarming of Microbes* (London: George Allen & Unwin, 1970), 57–58.

2. Allison, "Personal Recollections"; A. Fleming, "On a Remarkable Bacteriolytic Element Found in Tissues and Secretions," *Proceedings of the Royal Society B* 93 (1922): 306–317; J. H. Dowd, "A Doctor Has Discovered Antiseptic Properties in Tears," *Punch*, June 28, 1922, 528.

3. T. Williams, *Howard Florey: Penicillin and After* (Oxford: Oxford University Press, 1984), 67.

4. E. K. Lax, *The Mold in Dr. Florey's Coat: The Story of the Penicillin Miracle* (New York: Owl, 2005), 57; Williams, *Howard Florey*, 21, 36, 87.

5. D. Wilson, *Penicillin in Perspective* (London: Faber & Faber, 1976), 154; G. Macfarlane, *Alexander Fleming: The Man and the Myth* (London: Chatto & Windus, 1984), 281.

6. Lax, *Penicillin Miracle*, 82; Williams, *Howard Florey*, 91.

7. D. Masters, *Miracle Drug: The Inner History of Penicillin* (London: Eyre & Spottiswoode, 1946), 75–79.

8. R. G. MacFarlane, *Howard Florey: The Making of a Great Scientist* (Oxford: Oxford University Press, 1979), 312–316, 343; D. Cranston and E. Sidebottom, *Penicillin and the Legacy of Norman Heatley* (Oxford: Words by Design, 2016), 37–38; E. P. Abraham, "Ernst Boris Chain, 19 June 1906–12 August 1979," *Biographical Memoirs of Fellows of the Royal Society* 29 (1983): 42–91.

9. Masters, *Miracle Drug*, 95; E. Chain, H. W. Florey, A. D. Gardner, N. G. Heatley, M. A. Jennings, J. Orr-Ewing, and A. G. Sanders, "Penicillin as a Chemotherapeutic Agent," *Lancet* 236, no. 6104 (1940): 226–228.

10. Lax, *Penicillin Miracle*, 153.

11. Cranston and Sidebottom, *Legacy of Norman Heatley*, 42.

12. "Muriel Burge SRN RMN in interview with Dr. Max Blythe, 17 August 2000," The Royal College of Physicians and Oxford Brookes University Medical Sciences Video Archive MSVA 192, 9; Lax, *Penicillin Miracle*, 160.

13. G. L. Hobby, *Penicillin: Meeting the Challenge* (New Haven, CT: Yale University Press, 1985), 89.

14. Hare, *Birth of Penicillin*, 176–177.

15. Wilson, *Penicillin in Perspective*, 192–194.

16. Williams, *Howard Florey*, 134–136; E. P. Abraham, E. Chain, C. M. Fletcher, A. D. Gardner, N. G. Heatley, M. A. Jennings, and H. W. Florey, "Further Observations on Penicillin," *Lancet* 238, no. 6155 (1941): 177–189; Hobby, *Penicillin*, 72–75.

17. Hare, *Birth of Penicillin*, 179–180.

18. American Chemical Society, *Development of Deep-Tank Fermentation: Pfizer, Inc.* (Washington, DC: ACS, June 12, 2008).

19. Hobby, *Penicillin*, 189–190.

20. "Penicillin in the Field," *Lancet* 242, no. 6276 (1943): 737–738; "Paper Lauded for Help in Saving Life," *Milwaukee Sentinel*, October 17, 1943; M. Marshall, pers. comm.

21. Hobby, *Penicillin*, 155–156; "New Magic Bullet," *Time*, October 25, 1943, 38, 40.

22. Williams, *Howard Florey*, 148–149.

23. G. Shama, "Auntibiotics: The BBC, Penicillin, and the Second World War," *British Medical Journal* 337 (2008): 1464–1466; M. Burns and P. W. Dijck, "The Development of the Penicillin Production Process in Delft, the Netherlands, during World War II," *Advances in Applied Microbiology* 51 (2002): 185–200.

24. G. Shama and J. Reinarz, "Allied Intelligence Reports on Wartime German Penicillin Research and Production," *Historical Studies in the Physical and Biological Sciences* 32, no. 2 (2002): 347–367.

25. M. Wainwright, "Hitler's Penicillin," *Perspectives in Biology and Medicine* 47, no. 2 (2004): 189–198; Williams, *Howard Florey*, 144.

26. W. McDermott and D. E. Rogers, "Social Ramifications of Control of Microbial Disease," *Johns Hopkins Medical Journal* 151, no. 6 (1982): 302–312.

27. G. Bankoff, *The Conquest of Disease: The Story of Penicillin* (London: Macdonald, 1949), 175–176; B. Sokoloff, *The Miracle Drugs* (Chicago: Ziff-Davis, 1949), 254.

28. M. Barber, "Staphylococcal Infection Due to Penicillin-Resistant Strains," *British Medical Journal* 2, no. 4534 (1947): 863–865; D. Wheatley, L. P. Garrod, L. W. Batten, J. D. Nabarro, J. Fry, H. Joules, B. W. Lacey, and H. Cohen, "Discussion on the Use and Abuse of Antibiotics," *Proceedings of the Royal Society of Medicine* 48, no. 5 (1955): 355–364.

CHAPTER 30

1. W. Sheed, *In Love with Daylight: A Memoir of Recovery* (New York: Simon & Schuster, 1995), 26.

2. F. C. Robbins, *Reminiscences of a Virologist, in Polio*, ed. T. M. Daniel and F. C. Robbins (Rochester, NY: University of Rochester Press, 1999), 121–134.

3. D. M. Oshinsky, *Polio: An American Story* (Oxford: Oxford University Press, 2005), 55–58, 121–122.

4. S. L. Katz, C. M. Wilfert, and F. C. Robbins, "The Role of Tissue Culture in Vaccine Development," in *History of Vaccine Development*, ed. S. A. Plotkin (New York: Springer, 2011), 144–150; Robbins, *Reminiscences of a Virologist*, 125–126; Oshinsky, *Polio*, 123.

5. J. Kluger, *Splendid Solution: Jonas Salk and the Conquest of Polio* (New York: G. P. Putnam's, 2004), 109.

6. Robbins, *Reminiscences of a Virologist*, 126; T. M. Rivers and S. Benison, *Tom Rivers: Reflections on a Life in Medicine and Science: An Oral History Memoir* (Cambridge, MA: MIT Press, 1967), 446.

7. R. Carter, *Breakthrough: The Saga of Jonas Salk* (New York: Trident Press, 1966), 51–54, 61–63, 68–69.

8. Oshinsky, *Polio*, 95–96; Carter, *Breakthrough*, 81.

9. Carter, *Breakthrough*, 105–106, 114–115; Oshinsky, *Polio*, 125.

10. Carter, *Breakthrough*, 131.

11. L. K. Altman, "Dr. Dorothy Horstmann, 89; Made Strides in Polio Research," *New York Times*, January 21, 2001, 36.

12. Rivers and Benison, *Tom Rivers*, 407, 409.

13. A. Janus, *Mountain of Arabia* (Washington, DC: Smithsonian National Air and Space Museum, 2011); Oshinsky, *Polio*, 132.

14. Rivers and Benison, *Tom Rivers*, 246–247; Carter, *Breakthrough*, 123–124, 130.

15. Carter, *Breakthrough*, 137, 139–140; R. K. Vaughan, *Listen to the Music: The Life of Hilary Koprowski* (New York: Springer, 2012), 37; Rivers and Benison, *Tom Rivers*, 494–495.

16. Rivers and Benison, *Tom Rivers*, 497.

17. Oshinsky, *Polio*, 167, 171, 311n; A. L. Blakeslee, "Vaccine Ready for Big Test," *Cincinnati Enquirer*, January 27, 1953, 13; "Vaccine for Polio," *Time*, February 9, 1953, 43.

18. Carter, *Breakthrough*, 148–152, 156–62.

19. Carter, 231–232; H. M. Marks, "The 1954 Salk Poliomyelitis Vaccine Field Trial," *Clinical Trials: Journal of the Society for Clinical Trials* 8, no. 2 (2011): 224–234.

20. Carter, *Breakthrough*, 175; Marks, "Vaccine Field Trial."

21. Oshinsky, *Polio*, 175–176.

22. Carter, *Breakthrough*, 242, 264; W. L. Laurence, "Salk Polio Vaccine Proves Success," *New York Times*, April 13, 1955, 1; "3 U.S. Doctors Win Nobel Award," *New York Times*, October 23, 1954, 14.

23. G. Williams, *Virus Hunters* (New York: Knopf, 1971), 314.

24. "Fanfare Ushers Verdict on Tests," *New York Times*, April 13, 1955, 1; Laurence, "Salk Polio Vaccine Proves Success."

25. Williams, *Virus Hunters*, 315.

26. P. A. Offit, *The Cutter Incident: How America's First Polio Vaccine Led to the Growing Vaccine Crisis* (New Haven, CT: Yale University Press, 2007), 3, 85, 107; Oshinsky, *Polio*, 272.

27. W. M. Blair, "3 Scientists Urge Inoculation Halt," *New York Times*, June 23, 1955, 1; "O'Connor Scoffs at Vaccine Critic," *New York Times*, June 24, 1955, 1; Williams, *Virus Hunters*, 340.

28. Rivers and Benison, *Tom Rivers*, 542–545, 566–570; Oshinsky, *Polio*, 247, 250–253.

29. Offit, *Cutter Incident*, 125–127; D. A. Henderson, J. J. Witte, L. Morris, and A. D. Langmuir, "Paralytic Disease Associated with Oral Polio Vaccines," *JAMA* 190, no. 1 (1964): 41–48.

CHAPTER 31

1. World Health Organization, *The Global Eradication of Smallpox: Final Report of the Global Commission for the Certification of Smallpox Eradication* (Geneva: World Health Organization, 1980), 422.

2. L. A. Altman, "How Tiny Errors in Africa Led to a Global Triumph," *New York Times*, September 26, 2011, D5.

3. D. A. Henderson, *Smallpox: The Death of a Disease* (Amherst, NY: Prometheus, 2009), 69–75.

4. "US Will Help 18 Countries Fight Smallpox and Measles," *New York Times*, November 24, 1965, 13.

5. Henderson, *Smallpox*, 69–77, 85–87.

6. M. Dutta and W. Foege, "A Conversation between Dr. Mahendra Dutta & Dr. William Foege," *Global Health Chronicles*, July 9, 2008, https://globalhealthchronicles.org/items/show/3537.

7. A. D. Langmuir, "William Farr: Founder of Modern Concepts of Surveillance," *International Journal of Epidemiology* 5, no. 1 (1976): 13–18; World Health Organization, *Global Eradication of Smallpox*, 476.

8. W. H. Foege, *House on Fire: The Fight to Eradicate Smallpox* (Berkeley: University of California Press, 2012), 15–16, 56–59.

9. W. H. Foege, J. D. Millar, and D. A. Henderson, "Smallpox Eradication in West and Central Africa," *Bulletin of the World Health Organization* 52, no. 2 (1975): 209–222.

10. Foege, *House on Fire*, 54–58.

11. V. Harden and B. Foege, "Foege, William H," Global Health Chronicles, July 13, 2006, https://www.globalhealthchronicles.org/items/show/3516; W. H. Foege, "Smallpox Eradication in West and Central Africa Revisited," *Bulletin of the World Health Organization* 76, no. 3 (1998): 233–235.

12. World Health Organization, *Global Eradication of Smallpox*, 508–509, 526.

13. Henderson, *Smallpox*, 94–96, 118–127.

14. Henderson, 221, 223–224; J. B. Tucker, *Scourge: The Once and Future Threat of Smallpox* (New York: Atlantic Monthly Press, 2001), 114.

15. World Health Organization, *Global Eradication of Smallpox*, 438; Henderson, *Smallpox*, 86.

16. Henderson, *Smallpox*, 197; Dutta and Foege, "Conversation"; World Health Organization, *Global Eradication of Smallpox*, 513–516.

17. Henderson, 135, 165; Foege, *House on Fire*, 3.

18. World Health Organization, *Global Eradication of Smallpox*, 506

19. Henderson, *Smallpox*, 168, 177; World Health Organization, *Global Eradication of Smallpox*, 506.

20. Henderson, *Smallpox*, 178–182; S. Bhattacharya, *Expunging Variola: The Control and Eradication of Smallpox in India, 1947–1977* (New Delhi: Orient Longman, 2006), 192–195.

21. Foege, *House on Fire*, 3; Henderson, *Smallpox*, 182–183.

22. Tucker, *Scourge*, 115–116; Henderson, *Smallpox*, 236–239.

23. Tucker, *Scourge*, 117–118.

24. A. M. Nelson, "The Cost of Disease Eradication: Smallpox and Bovine Tuberculosis," *Annals of the New York Academy of Sciences* 894 (1999): 83–91; Tucker, 120–121, 132.

25. Henderson, *Smallpox*, 249.

26. Tucker, *Scourge*, 133; Henderson, 26–27.

27. "Eradication of Smallpox to be Announced Today," *New York Times*, May 8, 1980, A21.

EPILOGUE

1. L. Shaw-Taylor, "An Introduction to the History of Infectious Diseases, Epidemics and the Early Phases of the Long-Run Decline in Mortality," *Economic History Review* 73 (2020): E1–E19.

2. E. Smith-Greenaway, and J. Trinitapoli, "Maternal Cumulative Prevalence Measures of Child Mortality Show Heavy Burden in Sub-Saharan Africa," *Proceedings of the National Academy of Sciences* 117, no. 8 (2020): 4027–4033.

3. M. Peck, M. Gacic-Dobo, M. S. Diallo, Y. Nedelec, S. S. Sodha, and A. S. Wallace, "Global Routine Vaccination Coverage, 2018," *Morbidity and Mortality Weekly Report* 68 (2019): 937–942.

4. World Health Organization, *Progress on Drinking Water, Sanitation and Hygiene* (Geneva: WHO, 2017); G. Hutton and M. Varughese, *The Costs of Meeting the 2030 Sustainable Development Goal Targets on Drinking Water, Sanitation, and Hygiene* (Washington, DC: World Bank, 2016); World Health Organization, *Tuberculosis* (Geneva: WHO, 2020).

5. K. E. Jones, N. G. Patel, M. A. Levy, A. Storeygard, D. Balk, J. L. Gittleman, and P. Daszak, "Global Trends in Emerging Infectious Diseases," *Nature* 451, no. 7181 (2008): 990–993; J. Bedford, J. Farrar, C. Ihekweazu, G. Kang, M. Koopmans, and J. Nkengasong, "A New Twenty-First Century Science for Effective Epidemic Response," *Nature* 575 (2019): 130–136.

6. J. L. Geoghegan and E. C. Holmes, "Predicting Virus Emergence amid Evolutionary Noise," *Open Biology* 7, no. 10 (2017), https://doi.org/10.1098/rsob.170189.

7. J. R. Allan, O. Venter, S. Maxwell, B. Bertzky, K. Jones, Y. Shi, and J. E. M. Watson, "Recent Increases in Human Pressure and Forest Loss Threaten Many Natural World Heritage Sites," *Biological Conservation* 206 (2017): 47–55.

8. M. Hahn, R. Gangnon, C. Barcello, G. Asner, and J. Patz, "Influence of Deforestation, Logging, and Fire on Malaria in the Brazilian Amazon," *PLOS ONE* 9, no. 1 (2014), https://doi.org/10.1371/journal.pone.0085725; M. Pieper, A. Michalke, and T. Gaugler, "Calculation of External Climate Costs for Food Highlights Inadequate Pricing of Animal Products," *Nature Communications* 11, no. 6117 (2020), https://doi.org/10.1038/s41467-020-19474-6.

Index

Page numbers in italics refer to figures.

Elephantiasis, 205–207, 208, 214, 222
Emerson, Ralph Waldo, 162
Encephalitis, 222, 236
Enders, John, 272–274, 280–281, 283, 289–290
  tissue culture technique, 274, 276
Erythromycin, 270
Ethiopia, 296
Etiology, Concept, and Prophylaxis of Childbed Fever, The (Semmelweis), 95
"Etiology of Anthrax, Based on the Life Cycle of *Bacillus anthracis*, The" (Koch), 143–144
Europe, and the New World, 17–18. *See also* Smallpox; Syphilis

Fåhraeus, Robin, 15
Falloppio, Gabriel, 21–22
Fantine (*Les Misérables*), 69
Farr, William, 105–106, 110, 116–117, 118
Favus, 87
Ferdinand (king of Spain), 19
Fermentation, 123–125
Fewster, John, 56
Filariasis, 222
Filter-passing pathogens, 235. *See also* Virus and viruses
Finlay, Carlos, 208–209
First Congress of Italian Scientists, 100
First Miracle Drugs, The (Lesch), 250
Fischer, Emil, 202
Flagella, 207, 215
Fleming, Alexander, 249, 257–260
Flores, José, 66
Florey, Ethel, 264
Florey, Howard, 259–264, 265–266, 268
Flügge, Carl, 167–168
Foege, William, 292–294, 297
Fomites, 25, 26
Foot-and-mouth disease, 235
Foreign Correspondent (Hitchcock film), 264

Formalin, 277–278
Fosbroke, Thomas, 56
Fracastoro, Girolamo, 19, 25–26, 87
Francis, Thomas, Jr., 274, 282, 283–284
French Academy of Science, 115, 159
Frost, Wade Hampton, 110, 244
Further Observations on the Variolæ Vaccinæ (Jenner), 61

Galen, 12, 14, 31
Galileo Galilei, 32
Gandhi, Indira, 298
Gangrene, 132
Geison, Gerald L., 119–120, 125, 128, 146–147, 150, 153, 154, 181, 182
Gelatin, 158
General Board of Health (London), 78, 79, 104
General Register Office (London), 105, 106, 110, 112
George I (king of England), 44
Germinal rods, 218
Germ of an Idea, The (DeLacy), 33
Germs, fear of, 168
Germ theory, 84, 85, 87, 121, 135, 136, 138, 144, 172
Giardia, 12
Gillray, James, 64
Gloucestershire Medical Society, 54
Golgi, Camillo, 214, 217
Goniometer, 122
Gordon, Loney Clinton, 245–246
Grassi, Giovanni Battista, 219
Grassi's Law, 219–220
Grease (horsepox), 57
Great War, 223–225
  and war fevers, 227–228
Greenlees, James, 133
Grundy, Isobel, 45
Guaiacum wood, 22–23
Guilleman, Jeanne, 221–222
Gutenberg, Johannes, 20